DEPARTMENTAL CONTRIBUTORS

IN PSYCHIATRY

MARTHA M. BROWN, R.N., M.A.
Assistant Director, School of Nursing,
Washington University, St. Louis, Mo.

IN SURGERY

LILLIAN SHOLTIS BRUNNER, R.N., M.S.
Formerly Assistant Professor of Surgical Nursing,
Yale University School of Nursing,
New Haven, Conn.

IN OBSTETRICS

JAYNE F. DeCLUE, R.N., B.S., M. LITT.
Collegiate Instructor,
Boston Lying-in Hospital,
Boston, Mass.

IN MEDICINE

JANE TAYLOR TORRANCE, R.N., B.S., M.ED.
Visiting Lecturer in Nursing Education,
The University of Akron, Akron, Ohio;
Formerly Lecturer, Frances Payne Bolton School of Nursing,
Western Reserve University, Cleveland, Ohio

IN PEDIATRICS

GLADYS WILKINS, R.N., M.A.
Associate Professor of Pediatric Nursing,
University of Pittsburgh, School of Nursing,
Pittsburgh, Pa.

STUDY GUIDE
FOR
CLINICAL NURSING

A CO-ORDINATED SURVEY
INTEGRATED WITH ESSENTIALS
OF THE BASIC SCIENCES

Prepared Under the Direction of
EMILY C. CARDEW, R.N., M.S.
*Acting Director, University of Illinois
School of Nursing, Chicago*

Philadelphia   Montreal
J. B. LIPPINCOTT COMPANY

Distributed in Great Britain by
Pitman Medical Publishing Co., Limited
London

Library of Congress
Catalog Card Number
53–7644

PRINTED IN THE UNITED STATES OF AMERICA

PREFACE

This *Study Guide for Clinical Nursing* presents a method of organizing materials which will help students to synthesize and to apply the principles of the biologic, the physical and the social sciences in understanding and meeting the individual patient's needs.

The Guide is directed to three groups:

1. The *student* who during her period of clinical instruction will have the opportunity to develop skill in the use of resource materials in attempting to analyze and to solve nursing-care problems.
2. The *senior student* or graduate nurse attempting a systematic review, or orientation to the newer concepts of total nursing care, who will find the Guide a source for both purposes.
3. The *clinical instructor* who will find the content of assistance in:
   a. Organizing the clinical content around patients and their needs rather than in the traditional pattern of disease entities.
   b. Enriching the content of the course through the use of the suggested student projects, resources and references.
   c. Integrating the social and the health aspects of nursing.
   d. Stimulating the student to conduct independent inquiry and analysis.

In a "patient-centered approach," a real patient, known to the student, presents the ideal situation upon which to build the learning experiences. However, a patient is not always available when specific clinical course work is scheduled. Therefore, the patient studies here presented will assist the instructor to guide the student toward an understanding of the problems of patients.

When students are assigned to the care of patients similar to those being discussed in class, the patient problems frequently are solved *for* the student rather than *by* the student. The student must have her own experience in the analysis and the solution of nursing-care problems. The content affords the student an opportunity to recognize patient problems and to develop skill in planning individual nursing care. The opportunity to practice these skills must be provided. The presentation of patient studies with directed study projects and questions is used in this Guide as a means of providing good practice in problem-solving.

The patient studies around which the content is organized were selected not only in terms of incidence of the disease conditions but also because of the social, economic and emotional problems presented. Prevention and teaching have received emphasis throughout. Child growth, development and guidance are incorporated in both the obstetric and the pediatric sections.

Medical-surgical conditions more common to the child than to the adult have been incorporated into the pediatric section. Some communicable diseases have been considered in medical nursing; some, in pediatric

v

nursing. The instructor who wishes to use the patient studies in a clinical course organized around disease entities will find the index of assistance in the location of specific disease conditions.

Two new areas of content have been introduced. In the section on emergency, the student is introduced to problems of nursing care in civilian defense or in mass disaster.

"Summary" sections provide an opportunity for the student to develop skill in planning for the care of groups of patients and in the use of non-professional personnel.

The objective-type questions are included for 3 reasons: (1) to stimulate study, inquiry and use of resource materials, (2) to acquaint the student with this type of question and (3) to provide the student with an index of her own grasp of the material.

These questions were *not* designed for "achievement testing." Many items which could not be considered desirable in an achievement examination have been included because of the purposes of the Guide.

In questions where the responses are not purely factual, differences in the "correct" response may exist because of regional or institutional variations in practice. The authors believe that discussion or thought as to which item *is* correct, and *why*, will enhance the study method, and they have therefore included such items.

The study method recommended is the same for the beginning student as for the senior student, or graduate nurse, who wishes a comprehensive review. Each group must accept a systematic study method in order to achieve any real learning. The method recommended is an analysis of the situation, a thorough study of the suggested readings and an attempt to answer both the objective questions and those raised in the student projects.

A memorization of the responses to the objective questions will be of little or no value. First, because skill in the application of principles will *not* be acquired by this method. Such skill is necessary both for the practice of professional nursing and for the achievement of satisfactory scores on a well-constructed examination. Second, the student should realize that no objective questions available for review will be identical to questions in achievement or licensing examinations. If similarities exist, they are coincidental.

In summary, the *Study Guide for Clinical Nursing* is a student's working tool designed to aid in acquiring the knowledge and the skill basic to the provision of complete nursing care for the patient.

EMILY C. CARDEW

CONTENTS

PART ONE

Nursing Care of Adult Patients with Medical and Surgical Disorders

PART TWO

Nursing Care of Children

PART THREE

Nursing Care of the Psychiatric Patient

PART FOUR

Nursing Care of Mothers and the Newborn

Part One

Nursing Care of Adult Patients with Medical and Surgical Disorders

Section 1. Nursing Care of Patients with Disorders of the Respiratory Tract

STUDY SUGGESTIONS: Before beginning the study of this Section, the student will find it helpful to

A. Review
1. Anatomy and physiology: the respiratory tract.
2. Nursing arts: oxygen therapy, treatment for pediculosis.
3. Microbiology: *Acarus scabiei*, tubercle bacillus, pneumococcus.
4. Physics: pressure gases; suggested reference: Flitter, Hessel H.: An Introduction to Physics in Nursing, pp. 78-88, St. Louis, Mosby, 1948.

B. Study
1. In medical and surgical nursing texts: units on diseases of the respiratory system, scabies, syphilis.
2. In pharmacology texts: units on drugs affecting the respiratory tract, drugs affecting the skin, drugs used in the treatment of syphilis, drugs used in bacterial infection, sedative drugs, morphine sulfate.

C. Read the additional References listed before attempting to answer the questions relating to each patient study.

Background Review Questions

1. Match each of the following terms with the number of its correct definition:

    a._____cilia.
    b._____larynx.
    c._____nares.
    d._____alveoli.
    e._____pleura.
    f._____mediastinum.
    g._____diaphragm.

    (1) small air sacs at the end of a bronchiole.
    (2) aneurysm of the bronchi.
    (3) voice box.
    (4) wall dividing the chest.
    (5) floor of the thorax.
    (6) lining of the chest wall.
    (7) nostrils.
    (8) frontal sinus.

2. Match each of the following terms with the number of its correct definition:

    a._____dyspnea.
    b._____eupnea.
    c._____vital capacity.
    d._____hemoptysis.

    (1) amount of air expired by a normal expiration, after a normal inspiration.
    (2) amount of air which can be forcibly expired after a forcible inspiration.
    (3) normal air exchange.
    (4) difficulty in breathing.

3

    e.___ ___epistaxis.   (5) nose bleed.
    f._____anoxemia.   (6) listening for chest sounds.
    g._____auscultation.   (7) coughing up blood.
                              (8) incomplete oxygenation of blood.
                              (9) bloody emesis.

3. The lungs are constantly expanded even at the end of expiration due to

    a._____contraction of the diaphragm.
    b._____negative intrapleural pressure.
    c._____negative intrapulmonic pressure.
    d._____positive intrapulmonic pressure.

4. When an individual takes in air in inspiration, the air rushes into the lung air spaces because suddenly the pressure within the

    a._____alveoli is positive to atmosphere.
    b._____pleural space approaches atmospheric pressure.
    c._____alveoli of the lung is negative to atmospheric pressure.
    d._____pleural space becomes greater than atmospheric pressure.

5. The movement of carbon dioxide and oxygen into and out of the blood is due to the physical process of

    a._____diffusion.   c._____osmosis.
    b._____filtration.   d._____dialysis.

6. The chemoreceptors located in the carotid sinus and aortic arch are stimulated most powerfully by a (an)

    a._____excess of CO_2 in the blood.
    b._____excess of ketone bodies in the blood.
    c._____condition of anoxemia.
    d._____condition of acidosis.

7. Which one of the following stimulates respiration through its *direct* effect upon the respiratory center?

    a._____oxygen.   c._____increased H-ion concentra-
    b._____anoxemia.   tion of the blood.
                                     d._____carbon dioxide.

8. Expiration occurring during normal air exchange is due to the fact that efferent impulses from the

    a._____diaphragm inhibit the inspiratory center in the medulla.
    b._____cerebral cortex inhibit the inspiratory center in the medulla.
    c._____external intercostal muscles inhibit the inspiratory center in the medulla.
    d._____stretched alveoli inhibit the inspiratory center in the medulla.

9. Expiration during eupnea is easy and effortless because it results from the

    a._____stimulation of skeletal muscles lowering the thoracic cage.
    b._____stimulation of skeletal muscles decreasing the size of the thorax.

   c._____recoil of elastic tissue of the lungs and thorax.

   d._____relaxation of smooth muscle of the bronchioles.

10. Subjective symptoms of breathlessness will occur whenever the volume of air within the alveoli is less than normal, because the alveolar

   a._____air then becomes too overloaded with carbon dioxide.

   b._____air no longer has adequate quantities of oxygen to exchange with the blood.

   c._____blood vessels then become engorged with venous blood.

   d._____walls are not stretched sufficiently to inhibit the inspiratory desire.

11. If the right phrenic nerve is cut you would expect the

   a._____patient to be unable to breathe, since the diaphragm could no longer contract.

   b._____right lung partially to collapse because of right diaphragm paralysis.

   c._____afferent impulse going from the lung to the respiratory center to be stimulated.

   d._____left lung partially to collapse because of increased intrapleural pressure.

12. A pneumothorax partially (completely) collapses a lung because the

   a._____intrapulmonic pressure is now equal to that of atmospheric pressure.

   b._____intrapleural pressure now approaches or equals atmospheric pressure.

   c._____diaphragm can no longer contract on the affected side.

   d._____intrapulmonic pressure becomes negative to atmospheric pressure.

13. The tonsils and the adenoids are

   a._____useless in modern man.

   b._____lymphoid tissue protecting against infection.

   c._____one of the endocrine glands.

14. The function of the pleural space has significance for nursing because

   a._____this is where CO_2 and O_2 are exchanged.

   b._____this is a positive breathing area.

   c._____breathing is impaired if air enters the space.

Nursing Care of Patients with Disorders of the Nose and Throat

1. The primary infection in the common cold is

   a._____streptococcus.   c._____filtrable virus.
   b._____staphylococcus.   d._____mixed bacteria.

2. Avoidance of chilling and wet feet, etc., is important in the prevention of upper respiratory infections because such exposures

   a._____are direct causal factors of colds.
   b._____lower the general resistance.
   c._____irritate the mucous membrane of the upper respiratory tract.

3. The upper respiratory diseases responsible for from 40 to 50 per cent of all days lost from work and other activities are

   a._____tuberculosis.   c._____pneumonia.
   b._____"undifferentiated" upper d._____bronchiectasis.
      respiratory diseases.

4. The frequent use of nose drops in an oil base is contraindicated because oil

   a._____favors the growth of bacteria.
   b._____may be aspirated, causing lipoid pneumonia.
   c._____causes permanent changes in the mucous membrane.

5. Effective emergency treatment of severe nosebleed includes

   a._____having the victim blow his nose well; this usually is followed by a constriction of the small capillaries.
   b._____placing the victim in head-low (Trendelenburg) position because shock as well as hemorrhage must be combatted.
   c._____instructing the victim to remain in a sitting position, and inserting a pledget of cotton moistened with hydrogen peroxide and leaving it in the nostril for 10 to 15 minutes.
   d._____pressing the nostril on the bleeding side against the central partition of the nose for 4 or 5 minutes.
   e._____applying cloths over the nose that have been wrung out in cold water; it may also help to plug the nostril with a bit of cotton or gauze.

6. Most operations on the nose are done under local anesthesia, and the drug most commonly applied topically is cocaine. Toxic manifestations of this drug are

   a._____restlessness, garrulity, confusion, pulse and respiration increase, convulsive movements.

    b._____generalized blotching of the skin, dizziness, ringing in the ears, slowing of the pulse, faintness.
    c._____nervous excitability, insomnia, palpitation, dyspnea, tremors.
    d._____nausea, vomiting, burning of the mouth, the throat and the eyes, elevated blood pressure, a sense of constriction of the chest.

7. Because of the possible toxicity of cocaine, the nurse should check preoperative medication to note the presence of

    a._____atropine sulfate.   d._____caffeine sodium benzoate
    b._____morphine sulfate.   e._____scopolamine.
    c._____barbiturates.

8. A submucous resection is done to

    a._____repair a fracture of the nasal bones.
    b._____repair a deviated septum.
    c._____evacuate a peritonsillar abscess.
    d._____relieve a recurring septic sore throat.

9. Epidemics of septic sore throat usually are due to

    a._____contaminated water supply.
    b._____contaminated milk supply.
    c._____carriers without clinical symptoms.
    d._____sudden temperature changes.

10. The most likely time for hemorrhage after tonsillectomy is within the first 24 hours. The next most common time for postoperative hemorrhage is about the

    a._____third day.
    b._____end of the first week.
    c._____end of the second week.
    d._____end of the third week.

11. Hemorrhage may be detected in the fresh postoperative tonsillectomy patient by observing

    a._____a gradual decrease in the pulse rate.
    b._____infrequent swallowing.
    c._____an increasing pulse rate.
    d._____constant clearing of the throat.

12. Immediate treatment for hemorrhage in an adult following a tonsillectomy is to

    a._____place him in Trendelenburg position.
    b._____administer O_2 because respirations are impaired.
    c._____use a suction catheter to aspirate the blood.
    d._____place him in an upright sitting position.
    e._____have him use an ice-water gargle.
    f._____have emergency adrenalin ready for the surgeon.

13. The ideal position for an adult who has just had a tonsillectomy with cocaine anesthesia is

    a._____prone with the head turned to the side.
    b._____flat on the back with the head turned to the side.
    c._____Sims' lateral position.
    d._____Fowler's position.

Questions for Discussion and Student Projects

1. Discuss the economic effects of the common cold. If you were an industrial nurse, what program would you set up in your plant to attempt to prevent absenteeism from this cause?
2. Although everyone wishes to avoid the common cold, for which patients is such prevention of paramount importance?
3. Outline a lesson to present to high school freshmen on "the prevention of the common cold."
4. Discuss the use of the antihistaminic drugs for the prevention and treatment of the common cold. Include in your discussion their effectiveness as therapeutic agents, and their possible effects.
5. Make a nursing care plan for a patient with bronchiectasis, including assisting the patient with postural drainage, care of sputum, supportive treatment. What is the prognosis for a patient with well-established bronchiectasis? What forms of treatment are used?
6. Do tonsils or adenoids perform any useful function? Discuss.
7. What is the opinion of the medical men in your hospital or community with regard to the following:

    a. Tonsils and adenoids should (should not) be removed from all children before they are of school age. Why?
    b. T. and A. should (should not) be done in the late summer or early fall. Why?

8. Demonstrate the proper way of blowing one's nose. What are the dangers if this simple action is done incorrectly?
9. Are there any dangers involved in the promiscuous use of such nasal medications as nose drops and benzedrine inhalers? Discuss.
10. Discuss the problem of atrophic rhinitis from the following points of view:

    a. Why is it often a social problem and what can be done about it?
    b. The value of hormone therapy.

THE WHISPERER—PATIENT STUDY

Nine months ago, Mr. Smedley, a 60-year-old carpenter, was seen in the E.N.T. clinic. Mr. Smedley complained of a persistent hoarseness that had bothered him for the past 2 years. A laryngoscopy and roentgenograms showed an epidermoid cancer involving the whole left cord and most of the right cord of the larynx. Radiology was prescribed, but Mr. Smedley "refused" to finish therapy.

Mr. Smedley gave as his reasons for refusal the fact that he could not afford it, and that he would not think of accepting charity. His wife was ill and needed attention. Not only could he not afford the fees for treatment, but also time taken from work to come for treatment would result in a loss in pay. He decided to carry on without medical treatment as long as he could.

On December 6 he returned to the clinic because his hoarseness had progressed to a point where his voice was almost a whisper. He was emaciated and appeared ill. He admitted that he found it difficult to eat, and that smoking (he had always smoked excessively) was practically his only "comfort." He expectorated a thick prune-juice-colored sputum on occasion. Admission to the hospital was advised but he decided to wait until after Christmas.

Ironically, Mr. Smedley was admitted on Christmas Day in extreme distress. He had been unable to swallow food for a week, and had had progressive difficulty in breathing and pain over the larynx. His temperature was 102°, which was found to be due to an aspiration pneumonia.

Mr. Smedley was put to bed and penicillin 300,000 units b.i.d. was ordered. The second day he was taken to the O.R. and a tracheotomy was performed. Two days later a laryngoscopy was done in order that the surgeon might have a clear picture of what the next operation would entail.

On December 29 chest roentgenograms showed a clearing of the bronchopneumonia and orders were written for a laryngectomy on the thirtieth. These orders included

> Hykinone 2 mg.
> Ascorbic acid 200 mg.
> Luminal sodium gr. ii, h.s.
> Nembutal gr. iss @ 6:30 A.M.
> Morphine gr. ⅛ ⎫
> Atropine gr. ¹⁄₁₀₀ ⎭ when called

In the O.R. he was given pentothal sodium as the anesthetic. During surgery 100 cc. of blood and 1,500 cc. of 5 per cent glucose was given intravenously.

At the completion of the operation the surgeon wrote "prognosis poor, but will give or at least recommend x-ray therapy."

The postoperative orders included

> Demerol 75 mg. every 3 hours
> Resume pencillin and ascorbic acid
> Betabion 1 amp. daily
> O₂ at bedside, with nasal catheter
> 1,500 cc. of 10 per cent dextrose intravenously

On the first postoperative day a feeding catheter was inserted and 350 cc. of a prescribed high-caloric mixture was given every 2 hours for 8 hours. Unfortunately, 24 hours after "by mouth" feedings were begun Mr. Smedley developed an esophageal fistula which drained into the superior aspect of the tracheal stoma.

This had a marked effect on Mr. Smedley's mental state. He felt that he was regressing, and seemed to have lost confidence in the medical staff. He began to keep to himself and avoided the nurse as much as possible.

A few days later, a relative "slipped" an egg salad sandwich to him during visiting hours. The nurse noticed that he was able to eat it, and after that continued to eat without discomfort; the fistula was completely healed.

Mr. Smedley was discharged with instructions to return to E.N.T. clinic for follow-up and to x-ray for radiation therapy.

References

Greene, J. S.: Speech rehabilitation following laryngectomy, Am. J. Nursing 49:153, 1949.

Holmquist, E. W.: Nursing the adult tracheotomized patient, Am. J. Nursing 47:310, 1947.

Martin, H., and Ehrlich, H.: Nursing care following laryngectomy, Am. J. Nursing 49:149, 1949.

Questions Relating to the Patient Study

1. Carcinoma of the larynx is

   a._____more common in men.
   b._____more common in women.
   c._____more common in the age group 40 to 60.
   d._____more common in the age group 55 to 75.
   e._____more common than benign lesions of the larynx.
   f._____less common than benign lesions of the larynx.

2. Of all types of cancer in males, malignancy of the buccal cavity, pharynx and larynx ranks in incidence as follows:

   a._____most common.   d._____fourth most common.
   b._____second most common.   e._____fifth most common.
   c._____third most common.

3. The most common symptom of early laryngeal cancer is

   a._____shortness of breath.   d._____"tickle" sensation in throat.
   b._____hoarseness.   e._____excessive salivation.
   c._____offensive breath.

4. Luminal sodium is the same as

   a._____pentobarbital sodium.   d._____Pentothal Sodium.
   b._____Seconal.   e._____phenobarbital sodium.
   c._____Nembutal.   f._____Sodium Amytal.

5. Match the following:

   a.__3__vitamin B_1.   (1) Hykinone.
   b.__2__vitamin C.   (2) ascorbic acid.
   c._____vitamin D.   (3) Betabion.
   d._____vitamin G.
   e.__1__vitamin K.

f.___2___cevitamic acid.
g.___3___of value in correcting and
preventing anorexia.
h.___2___assists and promotes
wound healing.
i._____influences calcium and
phosphorus metabolism.
j.___1___maintains a normal prothrombin level in the
blood.
k._____aids in treating certain
lesions of the tongue, the
lips and the face.

6. It was noted by the nurse that the medication orders were not written consistently in either the metric or the apothecary system. Match the following:

a.___3___0.10 Gm.   (1) gr. $\frac{1}{150}$.
b.___4___0.008 Gm.   (2) gr. ii.
c.___1___0.0005 Gm.   (3) gr. 1½.
d.___6___0.2 Gm.   (4) gr. ⅛.
e.___2___0.13 Gm.   (5) gr. $\frac{1}{100}$.
f._____0.75 Gm.   (6) 200 mg.
g.___5___0.0006 Gm.   (7) 75 mg.
h.___7___0.075 Gm.   (8) 2 mg.
i._____0.002 Gm.

7. The nasal oxygen catheter should be passed a distance
a._____of 8 inches.
b._____of 10 inches.
c._____equal to the distance between the tip of the nose and the tip of the ear.
d._____equal to the distance between the tip of the nose and the supra-sternal notch.

8. Before inserting the nasal catheter the nurse should
a._____lubricate (heavily) with petroleum jelly.
b._____lubricate with a thin coating of water or oil.
c._____pinch off before inserting.
d._____allow O_2 to pass freely while inserting.

9. Steam inhalations were ordered to
a._____relax the surface tissues in the respiratory tract.
b._____contract the surface tissues in the respiratory tract.
c._____produce thinner secretions which may be expectorated more easily.
d._____reduce the evaporation of water from the mucous membrane.
e._____increase the oxygen content coming in contact with mucous membrane.

10. Since Mr. Smedley is a thin, bony and emaciated individual, it is necessary to give penicillin I.M. carefully in the following location:

    a._____outer aspect of the upper and outer quadrant of the buttock.
    b.__✓__inner aspect of the upper and outer quadrant of the buttock.
    c._____inner aspect of the lower and outer quadrant of the buttock.
    d._____outer aspect of the lower and outer quadrant of the buttock.
    e._____inner aspect of the upper and inner quadrant of the buttock.
    f._____outer aspect of the lower and inner quadrant of the buttock.

11. The reason for the extra caution recommended in giving intramuscular injections to Mr. Smedley is that there is less probability of

    a._____producing an abscess.
    b.__✓__injuring the sciatic nerve.
    c._____hitting the ischial tuberosity.
    d._____breaking the needle.
    e.__✓__entering a large blood vessel.

12. When an intravenous infusion is about to be started, a tourniquet is applied to the extremity between the desired site of injection and the main body. The reason for using a tourniquet is that

    a._____injected solution may then flow to the periphery of the extremity before returning to the heart.
    b.__✓__blood not being able to escape from the extremity pushes outward on the blood vessel and distends it.
    c._____the arterial system can be identified more easily, hence there is less danger of a major vessel becoming punctured.
    d._____the sensitive nerve system is pinched (desensitized), which allows for easy insertion of the needle with little discomfort.

13. The anesthetic of choice for Mr. Smedley was Pentothal Sodium.

    a. This anesthetic produces unconsciousness within

       (1)__✓__30 seconds.   (2)_____3 minutes.

    b. Duration of action is

       (1)_____long.   (2)__✓__brief.

    c. After-effects are

       (1)__✓__low incidence of nausea and vomiting.
       (2)_____moderate nausea and vomiting.

    d. Effects on respiration are

       (1)_____slight depressant of breathing.
       (2)__✓__powerful depressant of breathing.

14. Tracheotomy and laryngectomy tubes usually are made of sterling silver because

    a.__✓__it is least irritating to the tissues.
    b._____their parts are interchangeable.

  c._____it is more attractive than other metals.
  d._____it is less expensive than alloys.

15. To keep Mr. Smedley's airway patent, it is necessary to suction the trachea

  a._____at specified periodic intervals.
  b._____constantly.
  c._____whenever there is drainage in the tube or the trachea.
  d._____before every feeding.

16. In suctioning the tracheotomy, one should insert the catheter

  a._____only to the end of the tracheotomy tube.
  b._____about 3 inches.
  c._____about 5 inches.
  d._____as far as it will go easily.

17. During the first 3 postoperative days, the nurse should

  a._____change the outer tube daily.
  b._____insert the obturator when the inner tube is removed.
  c._____remove the inner tube for cleaning when necessary.
  d._____untie the tapes while removing the inner tube.

18. Morphine sulfate is contraindicated postoperatively for Mr. Smedley because

  a._____he may go to sleep and such relaxation will close off his airway.
  b._____opiates produce an irritating effect in a wound which is near the surface of the body.
  c._____it reduces the frequency of respirations, which in turn prevents the pooling of secretions.
  d._____it dulls the cough reflex; this mechanism is necessary to bring up secretions.

19. The best procedure for cleaning a tracheotomy or laryngectomy tube during the first few postoperative days is as follows:

Remove the inner cannula, and

  a._____immediately insert a functioning suction catheter into the outer cannula, clean the inner cannula with a fast-acting abrasive, rinse and boil the inner cannula, remove the suction catheter from the patient's outer cannula, reinsert the inner cannula.
  b._____submerge it into hydrogen peroxide, allowing the latter to bubble well as it dissolves the encrustations; immediately replace the inner cannula in the outer cannula.
  c._____clean it with soap and water using a brush or a gauze bandage threaded through a loop of wire, rinse well, boil for 10 minutes, suctioning the outer cannula before replacing the clean inner cannula.

20. In a partial laryngectomy, when a nurse is allowed to insert a nasal feeding catheter, she will observe that

a._____there is little difficulty or danger involved since the tube can be passed only into the esophagus.

b._____the progress of the tube may be into the trachea; this is known to have happened when, after instilling 2 drops of water, violent coughing is produced.

c._____the tube may proceed into the trachea or esophagus; however, since part of the larynx which closes off the air passageway still remains, there is no chance of fluid getting into the bronchi.

21. When the nurse gives Mr. Smedley his tube feedings, she should observe the following points:

a._____Serve the mixture as it comes from the icebox because it is more palatable.

b._____Heat the mixture to room temperature because it is more readily digested.

c._____Before attaching the funned to the catheter, aspirate the air from the tubing with a large syringe; pinch the end of the catheter until the feeding is in the funnel.

d._____To eliminate air from the catheter, tilt the funnel to a 30° angle and allow the mixture to flow in gradually; air will escape while the mixture enters the stomach.

e._____Precede and follow the mixture with water.

f._____Use no water with the mixture because the proportions are already fixed by the dietitian.

22. In a total laryngectomy, the following surgery has taken place:

a._____electrocoagulation of the invading carcinoma.

b._____removal of one vocal cord and adjacent cartilage.

c._____removal of the entire larynx and trachea.

d._____removal of the entire larynx and creation of a permanent tracheotomy.

e._____removal of the entire larynx, but the pharynx and trachea remain as previously.

23. Following a total laryngectomy, mouth care is

a._____unimportant because Mr. Smedley is no longer breathing through the nose or oropharynx.

b._____unimportant because Mr. Smedley is getting his feedings by means of a nasal feeding tube.

c._____important because of a tendency for the lips and mouth to become dry and cracked.

d._____important because of the presence of odors resulting from a certain inactivity of the mouth.

24. Radiation therapy not infrequently produces an x-ray burn of the tissues. Such a complication can be detected by early reporting of

a._____nausea and vomiting, fever, extreme malaise.

b._____chills, a drop in temperature, apprehension.

    c._____local pain, thirst, anoxia, an increased pulse rate.
    d._____inflammation of the area, hematemesis, dyspnea.

25. Because the inspiration of water is dangerous for an individual who has a tracheotomy or laryngectomy tube, the following activities are prohibited:

    a._____using a soap lather when shaving.
    b._____walking in the rain.
    c._____swimming.
    d._____taking a shower.

Questions for Discussion and Student Projects

1. What could have been done to persuade Mr. Smedley to have x-ray therapy, in the early stages of his illness, in view of his reasons for not following instructions? From the evidence of "cures" with early treatment of cancer of the larynx, what difference might have been made in his prognosis?
2. What do you suppose was in Mr. Smedley's mind, as he was rushed to the hospital on Christmas? If you were with him what could you say or do to help him?
3. List the equipment you would have at the bedside

    a. when Mr. Smedley is admitted.
    b. following the tracheotomy.
    c. following the laryngectomy.

4. List the fears a patient like Mr. Smedley undoubtedly has as he faces surgery. Indicate means of eliminating or lessening the effects of those fears.
5. Prepare a sample menu for an attractive and palatable semi-liquid diet for one day. Include several choices so that your patient may make a selection.
6. During the intravenous infusion of 10 per cent dextrose, suppose the needle comes out of the vein and fluid starts to run subcutaneously. If you do not observe this and stop the fluid, what will happen to the tissue cells in that area? Be explicit, explaining on the basis of the physiology of body fluids. Would the strength of the solution be a factor in this effect? Why?
7. Mr. Smedley was not able to write in English. Explain how you would establish an effective means of communication with him during the first few postoperative days.
8. Discuss the following complications from the point of view of (a) early symptoms, (b) causative factors, (c) preventive aspects, (d) treatment:

    (1) subcutaneous emphysema.   (2) esophageal fistula.

9. Outline in detail a teaching plan for Mr. Smedley to include

    a. clearing his laryngectomy tube of secretions.
    b. changing and cleaning the inner cannula.
    c. carrying on a conversation to the extent of his present ability.

10. Devise a simple method for setting up a suction system using equipment which is usually available in the home. Explain the principles of physics involved in your set-up.
11. Mr. Smedley has always enjoyed smoking. Will he be able to do so following his laryngectomy? Discuss.
12. What would you suggest for a man (a woman) who must wear a tracheotomy tube permanently which would make the tube less conspicuous?
13. What contribution has the National Hospital for Speech Disorders in New York City made in regard to the rehabilitation of the laryngectomized patient?
14. In 1859, Czermak devised the first mechanical larynx. It was a tube containing a reed which was connected to the laryngectomized patient's tracheal fistula and led to the mouth. All subsequent mechanical larynges have been modifications of this. List the advantages and disadvantages from the following points of view:

    a. voice sound.   b. contact with the fistula.   c. hygiene.

15. Speech rehabilitation following laryngectomy can be done by substituting esophageal for laryngeal function. Assume that you have a patient in need of such instruction. What local facilities are available to get your patient started in such a program? The actual teaching program may be a considerable distance from the community of the patient. How would this hurdle be overcome?
16. Inasmuch as Mr. Smedley has made a satisfactory recovery from his surgery, he should make a good candidate for esophageal speech rehabilitation. Discuss the merits of such a program, recognizing his financial situation, the illness of his wife and his guarded prognosis.
17. Assume that your patient has a temporary tracheotomy and goes through a process of decannulation.
    a. What is meant by decannulation?
    b. What is the procedure advocated in your hospital?
    c. What means can be improvised to bring about the same result?
    d. What part does the patient play in this?
18. Plan a program of possible activities in which Mr. Smedley may participate after he leaves the hospital. What additional information would you need to have before you can make a complete plan?

THE SICK VAGRANT
Background Review Questions

1. Scabies, a skin disorder produced by *Acarus scabiei*, is
    a._____noninfectious.   d._____an insect infestation.
    b._____contagious.   e._____a fungus infection.
    c._____an exanthema.

2. The characteristic lesion of scabies is
    a._____a scab.   d._____vesicles.
    b._____a burrow.   e._____desquamation.
    c._____a generalized rash.

3. The characteristic lesions are found most often

a._____in the hair.
b._____in the interdigital spaces.
c._____in the flexor surfaces of the wrists.
d._____in the soles of the feet.

e._____about the breast and axillae.
f._____in the genital regions.
g._____along the motor-nerve tracts.

4. The most outstanding symptom of scabies is

a._____excoriation.
b._____nocturnal itching.
c._____burning.

d._____maceration.
e._____urticaria.

5. Common secondary skin lesions of scabies include

a._____macules.
b._____papules.
c._____vesicles.

d._____fissures.
e._____pustules.

6. In long-neglected cases of scabies the following conditions may develop:

a._____carbuncle.
b._____eczema.
c._____ringworm.

d._____impetigo.
e._____psoriasis.

7. Treatment of scabies includes

a._____lancing the lesion.
b._____destruction of the parasite.
c._____destruction of the fungus.
d._____relief of itching.

e._____management of the cutaneous lesions.
f._____catharsis.

8. Complete the following table, summarizing your information on syphilis.

Stages	Symptoms	Diagnosis	Precautions Necessary to Prevent Infection	Treatment
Primary				
Secondary				
Tertiary				

THE SICK VAGRANT—PATIENT STUDY

Louis Adams was brought into the emergency ward by the police "paddy wagon." The driver stated that he had been called by the Salvation Army workers, who had discovered the patient collapsed on their doorstep.

The patient appeared to be about 35 years of age. He was incredibly dirty, and the acrid odor which surrounded him beggared description.

The nurse who prepared him for physical examination discovered evidence of body lice. His skin was encrusted with the scabs and tunnels of scabies.

Mr. Adams volunteered the information that he had dropped off a freight train the previous morning. He had not been feeling well. A cough had been bothering him, and he had a pain in his chest. It was cold, bleak and raining and he made his way to a nearby viaduct, hoping to find friends, a fire and, perhaps, a drink. He found no pals, was unable to start a fire, and by morning felt very sick and had a chill. He started for the Salvation Army Mission for some hot coffee.

Mr. Adams' temperature was 104°, pulse 120, respirations 30. His respirations were grunting and he had a constant racking nonproductive cough.

The patient was admitted to the male medical ward, with the diagnosis of lobar pneumonia, involving both lower lobes.

The following orders were written:

Complete rest.
Oxygen tent.
Force fluids to 4,000 cc.
Complete blood count.
Wassermann and Kahn.
Sputum for typing.
Penicillin 600,000 units daily.

Codein sulfate gr. ½ every 4 hours p.r.n. for pain and cough.
High-vitamin, high-caloric liquid to soft diet.
Special mouth care.
Isolation precautions.

In 48 hours Mr. Adams' temperature was normal. His blood test showed a 4 + Kahn. A lumbar puncture, with colloidal gold test, was negative. Penicillin therapy was continued for 10 days with daily doses of 600,000 units in oil and beeswax.

After the third day, treatment for scabies and energetic "clean-up" measures were taken.

Mr. Adams was reticent about his past but did mention that he had been in World War II and was dishonorably discharged for stealing.

He was discharged after 2 weeks with clean clothing, a referral for employment, and instructions for continuation of treatment. Although appreciative of his treatment, clean clothes and counselling, one had the feeling that he would soon take again to the open road.

References

Anderson, Donald C.: Penicillin, Am. J. Nursing 45:18, 1945.
Barach, Alvan L.: Physiologic Therapy in Respiratory Diseases, Philadelphia, Lippincott, 1948.

Buch, Frances S.: Venereal Disease Control Manual for Nurses, Division of Venereal Diseases, U.S. Public Health Service, 1948.

Curtis, Arthur C., et al.: Penicillin treatment for syphilis, J.A.M.A. **145**:1223, 1951.

Elliott, M., and Merrill, F. E.: Social Disorganization, Chapter 2, New York, Harper, 1942.

Faddis, Margene O.: Penicillin, Am. J. Nursing **47**:31, 1947.

Fox, E. C., and Shields, T. L.: Résumé of skin diseases most commonly seen in general practice, J.A.M.A. **140**:763, 1949.

Gist, Noel, and Halbert, L. A.: Urban Society, 3d ed., Chapter 9, New York, Crowell, 1948.

Gould, William George: Prostitution, promiscuity, venereal disease, Public Health Nursing **38**:173, 1946.

Johnson, Artell E.: Penicillin aerosol therapy, Am. J. Nursing **46**:834, 1946.

Kaiser, Albert D.: Treatment of pediculus capitis in school children with DDT powder, Am. J. Pub. Health **36**:1133, 1946.

Means, J. H.: The patient with pneumonia, Am. J. Nursing **38**:1299, 1938.

Mercer, E.: Nursing care in lobar pneumonia, Am. J. Nursing **37**:1211, 1937.

Molner, Joseph G.: Treatment of pediculosis capitis, Am. J. Pub. Health **35**:1302, 1945.

Mower, Ernest: Disorganization, Personal and Social, Chapter 4, Philadelphia, Lippincott, 1942.

Pickens, M. Elizabeth: The nurse in a changing VD program, Pub. Health Nursing **39**:253, 1947.

Slepyan, A. H.: A rapid treatment for scabies, J.A.M.A. **124**:1127, 1944.

Additional References on "Vagrancy"

Anderson, Nels: The Hobo, Chicago, University of Chicago Press, 1923.

Gilmore, Harlan W.: The Beggar, Chapel Hill, University of North Carolina Press, 1940.

Park, Robert E.: The Mind of the Hobo, Chapter 9, "The City," by Park, Burgess, and McKenzie, Chicago, University of Chicago Press, 1925.

Reckless, Walter C.: Why women become hoboes, American Mercury **31**:175, 1934.

Reitman, Ben L.: Sister of the Road, New York, Macaulay, 1937.

Sutherland, E. H., and Locke, Harvey J.: Twenty Thousand Homeless Men, Philadelphia, Lippincott, 1936.

Questions Relating to the Patient Study

1. Sputum specimen for typing should be secured
   a.____before therapy is instigated.
   b.____at a time convenient to the patient.
   c.____after 3 doses of penicillin.
   d.____before breakfast.

2. The drug selected for chemotherapy will depend primarily upon the
   a.____degree of illness.
   b.____causal organism.
   c.____temperature cycle.

3. If Mr. Adams is a typical case of pneumococcus pneumonia the nurse would expect the sputum to be

    a._____clear, thin, white.
    b._____rusty, tenacious.
    c._____thin, coffee-colored.

4. Mr. Adams' cyanosis is due probably to

    a._____cardiac involvement.
    b._____decreased circulation.
    c._____low oxygenation of blood in the lungs.
    d._____anemia.
    e._____malnutrition.

5. The optimum position for Mr. Adams will be

    a._____semi-Fowler's.
    b._____high Fowler's.
    c._____lying on the unaffected side.
    d._____lying on the affected side.
    e._____determined by the comfort of the patient.

6. During the first evening the physician left an order for morphine, gr. ¼ p.r.n. The nurse would

    a._____withhold it if the patient has difficulty in expectorating.
    b._____give it only for severe pain.
    c._____give it for evidence of increased moisture in the lungs.
    d._____give it for extreme restlessness.

7. The nursing care of primary concern for Mr. Adams will be

    a._____energetic treatment of pediculosis.
    b._____energetic treatment of scabies.
    c._____energetic treatment of syphilis.
    d._____rest and relaxation.
    e._____hyperventilation and stir-up exercises.

8. Penicillin should be stored

    a._____in a locked area of the medicine closet.
    b._____in a warm, moist place.
    c._____under refrigeration.

9. The nurse will be sure that Mr. Adams' cubicle is damp-dusted every day because

    a._____this is good hospital routine.
    b._____pneumococci survive in dust.
    c._____the scabs of scabies produce an infectious dust.

10. Treatment for scabies and body lice was postponed until the third day because

    a._____the drugs used in this treatment would conflict with those used for pneumonia.
    b._____the energetic type of treatment would be too disturbing for the patient.
    c._____nursing service could not be expected to care for an acutely ill patient and also treat scabies and pediculosis.

d.____of oversight; this treatment should have been instigated immediately.

11. Sulfur ointment would be effective in the treatment of

a.____body lice.   c.____tertiary syphilis.
b.__✓__scabies.

12. Sulfur ointment was ordered applied to Mr. Adams' skin. This treatment should be carried out

a.__✓__twice daily.   c.____on alternate days.
b.____4 times daily.   d.__✓__once daily.

Questions for Discussion and Student Projects

1. Discuss the transmission of pneumonia. How can you explain the incidence of the disease in individuals who have had no contact with a patient ill with pneumonia?

2. Discuss the reasons for vagrancy. What may be done to assist these men? Do you think the "exposure" to clean environment, good food, comfort, etc., will change Mr. Adams' way of life?

3. Prepare a total nursing care plan for Mr. Adams including (a) care of oxygen tent, (b) adaptations of nursing care while the patient is in the tent, (c) isolation precautions, (d) supportive care, (e) prevention of complications.

4. Several days before discharge the physician told Mr. Adams that he had syphilis and advised continued treatment. How would you answer Mr. Adams if he asked you why he should continue treatment when he has no symptoms?

5. Discuss the legal measures taken for the control and prevention of syphilis.

6. Write to your state department of public health for educational materials on the prevention of syphilis.

7. Discuss the incidence and prevalence of syphilis. In what area of the United States is the highest incidence? Among what groups? What factors might account for these differences?

8. Inasmuch as antibiotics and chemotherapy are so effective in combatting venereal disease, why should promiscuity be discouraged and how can this be best accomplished? What is the incidence of re-infection with these diseases? What can be done about this?

9. Discuss the nursing measures necessary to correct pediculosis of the scalp, of the body. For what reasons, other than for Mr. Adams' comfort, would energetic measures be taken to correct these conditions? Can any complications result? Do body lice transmit disease?

10. Sulfonamides sometimes are used in the treatment of pneumonia. Discuss the relative advantages and disadvantages of the treatment by chemotherapy and antibiotics under the following headings:

    a. effectiveness against causal organisms.   d. excretion.
    b. development of resistance.   f. cost.
    c. toxic effects.

THE MOTHER WITH A COUGH
Background Review Questions

1. Pulmonary tuberculosis

   a. The tubercle bacillus belongs to a group of organisms which are

      (1)＿＿＿＿acid-fast.
      (2)＿＿＿＿motile.
      (3)＿＿＿＿gram-positive.
      (4)＿＿＿＿gram-negative.
      (5)＿＿＿＿non-spore-forming.

   b. The characteristic lesion of tuberculosis is the

      (1)＿＿＿＿node.
      (2)＿＿＿＿tubercle.
      (3)＿＿＿＿cavity.
      (4)＿＿＿＿caseation.
      (5)＿＿＿＿ulcer.

   c. The tuberculin test consists of

      (1)＿＿＿＿cutaneous application of tubercle bacilli extract.
      (2)＿＿＿＿injection of purified protein derivative of tubercle bacilli.
      (3)＿＿＿＿injection of attenuated tubercle bacilli.
      (4)＿＿＿＿injection of killed tubercle bacilli.
      (5)＿＿＿＿injection of vaccine of tubercle bacilli.

   d. The tuberculin test is useful to determine

      (1)＿＿＿＿the presence of organism in the blood.
      (2)＿＿＿＿the presence of organism in the tissues.
      (3)＿＿＿＿allergy to the organism.
      (4)＿＿＿＿the strain of the organism.
      (5)＿＿＿＿the degree of infection present.

   e. The development of tuberculosis in an individual depends on

      (1)＿＿＿＿age.
      (2)＿＿＿＿degree of exposure.
      (3)＿＿＿＿obesity.
      (4)＿＿＿＿duration of exposure.
      (5)＿＿＿＿malnutrition.
      (6)＿＿＿＿type of occupation.
      (7)＿＿＿＿overwork.
      (8)＿＿＿＿resistance.
      (9)＿＿＿＿body build.
      (10)＿＿＿＿heredity.

   f. Prevention of tuberculosis depends on

      (1)＿＿＿＿hospitalization of infected cases.
      (2)＿＿＿＿systematic rest periods for workers.

      (3)_____mass x-ray examinations.
      (4)_____universal use of vaccination.
      (5)_____segregation of persons with positive sputa.

  g. Complications of tuberculosis are

      (1)_____pleurisy.
      (2)_____pneumonia.
      (3)_____spontaneous pneumothorax.
      (4)_____hemorrhage.
      (5)_____brain abscess.

2. Proper feeding is important in treatment:

  a. Over-all diet rules are

      (1)_____Caloric intake should be sufficient only to maintain body weight at normal or slightly above normal.
      (2)_____Caloric intake should be above normal for body maintenance because of very high basal metabolism.
      (3)_____Protein intake should be liberal.
      (4)_____Carbohydrates should be restricted because they increase respiratory volume.
      (5)_____Fats should be restricted because they increase respiratory volume.

  b. A vitamin-rich diet is necessary because

      (1)_____a tuberculosis patient requires a higher daily intake of vitamin C than the normal person.
      (2)_____Vitamin D is essential in absorbing and retaining calcium from milk.
      (3)_____Vitamin B is important in rebuilding tissues.
      (4)_____Vitamin K produces prothrombin which helps prevent hemoptysis.
      (5)_____Vitamin A is essential to maintaining protein-carbohydrate balance.

  c. The tuberculous patient's appetite varies because

      (1)_____of the toxic products of the disease.
      (2)_____his body needs increase as he is more active.
      (3)_____he becomes bored with the constant diet of milk and proteins.
      (4)_____he frequently suffers from indigestion.
      (5)_____frequent nourishment destroys his appetite for meals.

  d. Characteristics of a diet for a bed patient with tuberculosis are

      (1)_____large amounts of laxative vegetables and fruits.
      (2)_____ample fluids, especially milk.
      (3)_____a high-caloric diet.
      (4)_____limited use of animal fats, including cream and butter.
      (5)_____small servings, carefully arranged.

3. Public health measures for control include

    (1)_____eradication of tuberculosis in cattle.
    (2)_____pasteurization of all milk supplies.
    (3)_____universal vaccination.
    (4)_____inspection of meat.
    (5)_____chest roentgenogram of all food handlers.
    (6)_____sanitation of water supplies.
    (7)_____routine examination of industrial employees.
    (8)_____spraying the community with DDT to destroy insects.
    (9)_____active immunization.
    (10)_____isolation of children with fever.

4. Pulmonary tuberculosis is characterized by

    (1)_____an elevation of temperature in the morning.
    (2)_____an elevation of temperature in the afternoon.
    (3)_____coughing and expectoration.
    (4)_____a loss of weight and strength.
    (5)_____an abnormal weight gain with loss of strength.

THE MOTHER WITH A COUGH—PATIENT STUDY

Mrs. Allen, a 25-year-old housewife, stopped one morning at a mobile unit which was parked in the neighborhood shopping center. Her two children, 6 months and 3 years old, were with her. Mrs. Allen had a photofluorograph taken of her chest and felt happy that she had spared a few minutes for the picture. She had been worried recently about a persistent cough that produced blood-tinged sputum.

A few days later, Mrs. Allen received a card requesting her to call at the Tuberculosis Clinic for another roentgenogram. Mrs. Allen was quite worried; the nurse at the clinic told her that the doctor needed a larger roentgenogram for a more complete examination.

In a few days, a nurse from the Tuberculosis Clinic called at her home and talked with her about the chest roentgenogram. The nurse stated that some damage was evident in the roentgenogram and that it was important for her to have a complete physical examination immediately. The "cigarette cough," fatigue, loss of weight, indigestion and irritability which had been apparent since the birth of her last child were due probably to changes in her chest. The nurse made an appointment for the mother to have a physical examination at the clinic the next evening when her husband could accompany her.

The physical examination confirmed the suspected diagnosis of acute pulmonary tuberculosis, moderately advanced.

Within 2 weeks, satisfactory arrangements had been made: the grandmother would care for the children in her own home, the husband would board with relatives and the mother would go to the sanatorium.

During the first night at the sanatorium, Mrs. Allen had a hemoptysis of approximately 1 ounce of bright red blood. Nearby ambulatory patients urged her not to move, and called a nurse.

During the next few weeks, Mrs. Allen was kept on bed rest, high-caloric diet with supplementary vitamins, and streptomycin therapy.

References

Bloom, Sophia: Some economic and social problems of the tuberculosis patient and his family, U.S. Public Health Report 448–455, April 1948.

Bosworth, H. W.: The care and education of the tuberculosis patient, Am. J. Nursing 46:764, 1946.

Boynton, Tood, Meyers: The control of tuberculosis in nursing students, Am. J. Nursing 51:496, 1951.

Coleman, J. V., et al.: Psychiatric contributions to the care of the tuberculosis patient, J.A.M.A. 135:699, 1947.

Hilleboe, Herman E.: Rehabilitating the tuberculous, (ed.), U.S. Public Health Report 969–971, July 4, 1947.

Horbein, Ruth, and Patterson, Winifred: Tuberculosis—a social and emotional problem, Am. J. Nursing 47:376, 1947.

Rosenthal, Sol Roy, et al.: B.C.G. vaccination in all age groups, J.A.M.A. 136:73, 1948.

Smith, Austin: Streptomycin in treatment of tuberculosis, J.A.M.A. 138:584, 1948.

Weber, Francis J.: The modern pattern of tuberculosis control, U.S. Public Health Report 1591–1592, November 7, 1947.

Wilson, Charles C.: Educating the older tuberculosis patient and his family, Public Health Nurse 40:363, 1948.

Questions Relating to the Patient Study

1. The following clinical methods were employed to aid in verifying Mrs. Allen's diagnosis and in selecting the proper treatment:

   a._____serum iodide test.
   b._____sedimentation rate.
   c._____microscopic examination of the sputum.
   d._____electrocardiogram.
   e._____roentgen therapy.
   f._____complete blood count.
   g._____urinalysis.

2. The most important single measure in protection of the worker against contracting tuberculosis from patients is

   a._____well-informed and co-operative patients.
   b._____strict isolation technic for all cases of tuberculosis.
   c._____immunization programs.
   d._____optimum health habits and condition of the worker.
   e._____frequent sputum tests and chest roentgenograms of the worker.

3. Toxic manifestations of streptomycin which the nurse should report immediately are

   a._____decreased auditory acuity.
   b._____increased auditory acuity.
   c._____vertigo.

d._____thickening of the tongue.
e.__✓__skin rashes.

4. The usual daily dosage of streptomycin is

a._____gr. $\frac{1}{150}$–gr. $\frac{1}{200}$.   d.__✓__1–4 Gm.
b._____50 mg.–100 mg.   e._____0.5 cc.–1.0 cc.
c._____300,000–600,000 units.

5. P.A.S. (para-aminosalicylic acid) is given to

a._____hasten the effectiveness of streptomycin.
b.__✓__delay the development of resistance to streptomycin.
c._____prevent brain damage.
d._____destroy tubercle bacilli.

6. Mrs. Allen's dietary treatment would be characterized by

a._____high-caloric feeding until the disease is arrested.
b.__✓__normal well-balanced intake of nutrients.
c._____high fat for efficient use of protein.
d.__✓__slightly increased amounts of protein.
e._____many iron-containing foods.
f.__✓__increased amounts of vitamins A, C and K.

7. Mrs. Allen should not smoke because smoking

a._____increases her RBC.
b._____reverses her tuberculin reaction.
c._____makes the x-ray picture cloudy.
d.__✓__decreases her appetite.
e.__✓__irritates the mucous membrane of the lung.

8. Mrs. Allen may have received her exposure to tuberculosis from

a._____contamination from food.
b._____contamination from milk.
c._____contamination from well water.
d._____cough spray from a passing stranger.
e.__✓__long exposure to a person with undiagnosed tuberculosis.

9. Tuberculosis is most common during the following ages:

a._____under 10 years.
b.__✓__between 15 and 25 years.
c._____between 25 and 45 years.
d._____between 30 and 50 years.
e._____between 45 and 60 years.

10. Linen used in the care of Mrs. Allen may be disinfected by

a._____soaking in chloride of lime.
b._____soaking in alcohol.
c._____washing in boiling water.
d.__✓__washing in hot soapy water with detergents.
e._____exposing to·sunlight before washing.

Questions for Discussion and Student Projects

A. Related to Patient Study
1. Describe specifically the program which should be carried out adequately to protect Mrs. Allen's family.
2. Describe how you would help Mrs. Allen accept the necessity of sanatorium care. What are the important reasons why sanatorium care is recommended?
3. Outline a teaching plan for Mrs. Allen, to be carried out
   a. during her first few weeks in the sanatorium.
   b. preparatory to going home.
   What would you need to know about Mrs. Allen, her home and her family to carry out a teaching program?
4. List the steps you should take, in the order in which they should be taken, when patients notify you that Mrs. Allen is having a hemorrhage.
5. What worries might Mrs. Allen have? How would you know if she were worried? What might be done to relieve these worries?

B. Related to Tuberculosis in General

1. What environmental factors may predispose to tuberculosis? How can these be corrected?
2. How do racial and nationality groups compare in susceptibility to tuberculosis? Name some factors accounting for these differences?
3. Compare the morbidity and mortality rates of tuberculosis since 1900. What factors are responsible for these changes?
4. What is being done in your community to prevent tuberculosis? What agencies are responsible for a preventive program?
5. What is meant by rehabilitation of tuberculosis patients? When does this begin? What agencies in your community are responsible for this program?
6. What are the costs to society for tuberculosis in this country?
7. What are the facilities for the care of the tuberculosis patient in your community? In your state? Are these facilities adequate for all patients needing care?
8. What is the recommended nurse-patient ratio for the care of sanatorium patients? How does this compare to the recommended ratio for patients in general hospitals?
9. Locate references on use of new antituberculosis drugs. What effect may this research have on need for additional facilities?

THE MOTHER WITH A COUGH—PATIENT STUDY—(*Continued*)

After several weeks in the sanatorium, Mrs. Allen suffered from pleurisy with effusion which persisted for several months. Left pneumothorax was unsuccessful and a pneumoperitoneum was done.

Later a phrenic emphraxis was done. When cavitation was noted, she was placed on streptomycin therapy and a thoracoplasty was recommended.

References

Ellison, Bess M.: Nursing care in collapse therapy, Am. J. Nursing 50:473, 1950.

Fortune, Gwendolyn: Positive pressure therapy, Am. J. Nursing 47:108, 1947.

Keill, Kenneth: The emotions in tuberculosis, Am. J. Nursing 47:601, 1947.

Lacy, Marion, and Hitchcock, M. O.: Retained secretions following thoracic surgery, Am. J. Nursing 51:607, 1951.

Lincoln, Louise: Thoracoplasty—nursing care, Am. J. Nursing 44:1022, 1944.

Lindnuff, Florence S.: Physical therapy and chest surgery, Physiotherapy Rev. 27:94, 1947.

Lloyd, M. S.: Chest surgery demands skilled nursing care, Trained Nurse and Hosp. Rev. 112:344, 1944.

Oatway, W. H.: Aseptic technic in the care of tuberculous patients, Am. J. Nursing 50:164, 1950.

Smith, B. G.: Spontaneous pneumothorax, Am. J. Nursing 43:553, 1943.

Questions Relating to the Patient Study

1. The surgeon decided to collapse Mrs. Allen's left upper lobe by performing a 2-stage thoracoplasty. The reason for performing the operation in two stages is to

   a._____achieve better collapse.
   b._____prevent undue deformity.
   c._____decrease the trauma to the circulatory and respiratory systems.
   d._____facilitate the technical aspects for the surgeon.

2. A rongeur is a surgical instrument used in a thoracoplasty. Its chief function is to

   a._____act as a rib separator.   c._____peel off periosteum.
   b._____cut the rib.   d._____nibble off sharp edges of
                                             the rib.

3. In observing Mrs. Allen as she recovers from a general anesthetic, the nurse must be certain that Mrs. Allen's head is

   a._____low and erect.
   b._____elevated to the semi-Fowler position and erect.
   c._____low and turned to the side.
   d._____elevated to the semi-Fowler position and turned to the side.

4. For a short while, Mrs. Allen was placed in an oxygen tent following her second-stage thoracoplasty. Chief precautions which must be observed by the nurse are:

   a._____Have the electric bell cord within the tent so that the patient can ring for the nurse.

     b._____Do not allow anyone to smoke in the room where oxygen is flowing.

     c._____Keep the temperature in the tent low since the oxygen is more pure at a lower temperature.

     d._____Lubricate all valves on the regulator with oil while the tent is in use.

     e._____Undo the bottom of the tent when caring for Mrs. Allen because oxygen is less likely to escape this way.

5. Postoperatively, Mrs. Allen should be encouraged to

     a._____cough, turn on the operated side.
     b._____refrain from coughing, turn on the operated side.
     c._____cough, turn on the unoperated side.
     d._____refrain from coughing, turn on the unoperated side.
     e._____have cough medicine as often as necessary to prevent coughing.

6. Following thoracoplasty, Mrs. Allen

     a._____is cured permanently.
     b._____is cured temporarily.
     c._____may be required to alter her manner of life.
     d._____may resume active normal living without limitations.

7. Sand bags or pillows are used for added pressure on the operative side because

     a._____they make the patient more comfortable.
     b._____support is needed inasmuch as several ribs were removed.
     c._____atelectasis can be prevented this way.
     d._____collapse of the lung can be maintained more effectively.

8. Unless the advice indicated in question 5 is followed, the result may be

     a._____mucus plugs causing airlessness of the lobe or entire lung.
     b._____rupture of small blood vessels in the alveoli.
     c._____the formation of small pockets of pus in the bronchi.
     d._____deposits of fluid at the base of the lobes.

9. The condition described in question 8 is known as

     a._____hemoptysis.   c._____atelectasis.
     b._____emphysema.   d._____pneumonitis.

10. The arm on the affected side should have

     a._____passive and active movement.
     b._____passive movement only.
     c._____immobilization measures.

Questions for Discussion and Student Projects

1. Of what significance to the physician is a laminogram (sectionogram or planogram) in Mrs. Allen's case? How would you prepare Mrs. Allen and care for her during this diagnostic aid?
2. Compare the principles of medical and surgical aseptic technic. What does Mrs. Allen need to know of either or both of these procedures?
3. The attempted pneumothorax was unsuccessful due to the presence of adhesions. What treatment is often resorted to when this is the case? Describe the nursing responsibilities before, during and after this procedure.
4. If the thoracoplasty is done in one, two or three stages, will there be appreciable differences in the pre- and postoperative care? Why?
5. What kinds of fluids will Mrs. Allen receive postoperatively? Why?
6. How would you plan to insure proper body elimination during the time that activity is so limited?

Nursing Care of Patients with Other Disorders of the Lungs and the Bronchi

1. Foreign bodies of vegetable origin in the bronchi

    a._____produce temporary irritation.
    b._____are absorbed rapidly.
    c._____produce symptoms of acute bronchitis.
    d._____are of little or no clinical significance.

2. Foreign bodies in the bronchi usually are

    a._____removed by incision of the chest wall.
    b._____removed by bronchoscopy.
    c._____ignored unless early symptoms are alarming.
    d._____ignored as they seldom cause difficulty.

3. Bronchiectasis is a chronic disease characterized by

    a._____stricture of the bronchial tubes.
    b._____dilatation of the bronchial tubes.
    c._____pulmonary edema.
    d._____dry, nonproductive cough.

4. The most characteristic symptom of bronchiectasis is

    a._____slow pulse.
    b._____pain in the chest.
    c._____intermittent fever.
    d._____profuse sputum.
    e._____hectic flush.

5. X-ray examination to determine bronchiectasis includes

    a._____Priodax.   c._____Lipiodal.
    b._____Bromosulphalein.   d._____Diodrast.

6. Bronchograms are essential to the diagnosis of

    a._____lung abscess.   d._____bronchiectasis.
    b._____tuberculosis.   e._____empyema.
    c._____carcinoma.

7. The most frequent symptom of lung cancer is

    a._____bloody sputum.   d._____persistent cough.
    b._____chest pain.   e._____frequent chest colds.
    c._____dyspnea.

8. The chief diagnostic aid in detecting carcinoma of the lung is

    a._____bronchogram.   d._____x-ray therapy.
    b._____roentgenogram.   e._____radium therapy.
    c._____exploratory thoracotomy.   f._____bronchogenic biopsy.

9. The most satisfactory treatment for carcinoma of the lung is

    a._____pneumonectomy.   d._____x-ray therapy.
    b._____pneumothorax.   e._____radium therapy.
    c._____pneumonotomy.

10. Conservative treatment of lung abscess includes

    a._____intratracheal aspiration.
    b._____ketogenic diet.
    c._____pneumothorax.
    d._____thoracentesis with penicillin instillation.
    e._____bronchoscopy with penicillin instillation.

11. The position for the patient having postural drainage for a lung abscess in the upper right lobe is

    a._____lying on the right side.
    b._____the Trendelenburg position, lying on the left side.
    c._____with the head and chest lower than the rest of the body.
    d._____sitting up, turned to the left side.

12. The chief action of terpin hydrate elixir is to

    a._____depress the annoying cough reflex.
    b._____increase or liquefy mucus and facilitate its removal from the trachea, bronchi or lungs.
    c._____assist in producing a cough so that mucus can be removed more easily.
    d._____thicken secretions, thereby shrinking their volume.

13. Codeine is often used with an expectorant because it

    a._____is effective in the reduction of cough.
    b._____makes coughing less painful.

    c._____has a systemic sedating effect.

    d._____counteracts the toxic effects of terpin hydrate.

14. Treatment for fractured ribs is to

    a._____surgically remove fractured segments.

    b._____splint the chest wall with adhesive strapping.

    c._____perform an immediate thoracentesis.

    d._____get the patient to bed for he needs rest most.

15. At the scene of an accident, a victim is found to have a hissing wound of the chest. Which of the following would you do?

    a._____Let the wound alone for it proves that the patient is still able to breathe.

    b._____Place any available cloth loosely over the wound so that air being sucked into the chest is at least filtered clean.

    c._____Place some covering, such as a folded handkerchief, directly over the wound and bind snugly to prevent the air leak.

    d._____Look for other injuries because one of them may be more serious than this one.

Section 2. Nursing Care of Patients with Disorders of the Cardiovascular System and the Blood*

STUDY SUGGESTIONS: Before beginning the study of this Section, the student will find it helpful to

A. Review

1. Anatomy and physiology: the heart and circulatory system, physiology of blood formation and clotting.
2. Nursing arts: oxygen therapy, preparation for surgery, surgical aseptic technic.
3. Physics: pressure in liquids; suggested reference: Flitter, Hessel H.: Introduction to Physics in Nursing, pp. 77–78, St. Louis, Mosby, 1948.

B. Study

1. In medical nursing texts: units on cardiovascular disease, diseases of the blood and blood-forming organs.
2. In surgical nursing texts: surgery for diseases of the circulatory system, amputation, infection and healing.
3. In pharmacology texts: drugs affecting the circulation, the blood and blood-forming organs, narcotics and sedatives, drugs affecting the urinary system, diuretics.
4. In nutrition texts: diet therapy in heart disease, diet therapy in the anemias.
5. See also section on nursing in neurologic conditions, cerebrovascular accident for material on arteriosclerosis.

C. Read the additional References listed before attempting to answer the questions relating to each patient study.

THE MAN WHO COULDN'T BREATHE

Background Review Questions

1. When the ventricles of the normal heart become temporarily overfilled with blood, the muscle fibers

   a._____relax, resulting in a decreased cardiac output.
   b._____stretch, bringing about a more forceful contraction.
   c._____stretch, resulting in a weakened contraction.
   d._____prevent the normal flow of blood through the coronary arteries.

2. When there is a temporary increase in venous return to the normal heart, the pressure within the auricles and vena cavas tends to rise, stretching those parts and irritating a reflex

---

* Cardiovascular diseases and blood dyscrasias are also considered in the pediatric section.

33

    a._____fall in arterial blood pressure.
    b._____ventricular fibrillation.
    c._____decrease in the heart rate.
    d._____increase in the heart rate.

3. Any factor which brings about a temporary inhibition in the normal conveyance of impulses from the atrioventricular node through the bundle of His will result in

    a._____the auricles beating at a slower rate than the ventricles.
    b._____the ventricles beating at a slower rate than the auricles.
    c._____ventricular fibrillation.
    d._____tachycardia.

4. The higher the diastolic arterial blood pressure, the

    a._____greater the resistance offered to the blood ejected by the ventricle during the systole.
    b._____easier it is for the ventricles to open the semilunar valves.
    c._____greater the load placed upon the auricles during systole.
    d._____lower the resistance offered to the auricles in opening the atrioventricular valves.

5. The second heart sound is due to

    a._____closure of the semilunar valves.
    b._____closure of the atrioventricular valves.
    c._____contraction of the ventricles as they enter systole.
    d._____contraction of the auricles as they enter systole.

6. The time interval between first and second heart sounds denotes

    a._____auricular systole.
    b._____ventricular systole.
    c._____ventricular diastole.
    d._____auricular diastole.

7. In taking blood pressure in man, the systolic value is determined by the height of the column of mercury when the pressure within the

    a._____cuff exceeds the maximum pressure within the brachial artery.
    b._____brachial artery slightly exceeds that within the cuff.
    c._____brachial artery is slightly lower than that within the cuff.

8. In which of the following instances would you expect an individual to exhibit bradycardia?

    a._____following an injection of adrenalin.
    b._____overstimulation of the left vagus.
    c._____increased return of venous blood to the left atrium.
    d._____overstimulation of the sympathetic nerves to the heart.

9. The principal factor involved in closing the bicuspid valves is a rise in pressure within the

    a._____right auricle above that in the right ventricle.
    b._____right ventricle above that in the right auricle.

c.____left ventricle above that in the left auricle.
d.____left auricle above that in the left ventricle.

10. If a patient has aortic insufficiency (the aortic valve cannot close completely), there will be regurgitation of blood back into the

   a.____right ventricle during diastole.
   b.____right ventricle during systole.
   c.____left ventricle during systole.
   d.____left ventricle during diastole.

11. A patient suffering from right heart failure (decompensation) probably would show symptoms of edema of the

   a.____lungs, due to an increased venous filtration pressure.
   b.____ankles, due to an increased venous filtration pressure.
   c.____face and abdomen, due to a fall in plasma osmotic pressure.
   d.____entire body, due to a fall in plasma osmotic pressure.

12. With intense muscular exercise all except one of the following physiologic changes would take place. Which one would not occur? A marked increase in

   a.____diastolic blood pressure.   c.____systolic blood pressure.
   b.____pulse pressure.   d.____heart rate.

13. Pulse pressure indicates the

   a.____amount of blood which can flow through a capillary per unit of time.
   b.____amount of blood ejected from the left ventricle per unit of time.
   c.____pressure at which blood spurts through the brachial artery from beneath the cuff.
   d.____pressure at which the blood flow in the brachial artery becomes continuous beneath the cuff.

14. Rapid filling of the ventricles occurs while

   a.____the auricles are in systole.
   b.____the ventricles are in systole.
   c.____both auricles and ventricles are in systole.
   d.____both auricles and ventricles are in diastole.

15. In the normal individual the heart rate is controlled by the

   a.____atrioventricular node.   c.____auricles.
   b.____bundle of His.   d.____sino-atrial node.

16. Which one of the following blood pressure values is within normal limits for a young adult?

   a.____120/30.   c.____120/110.
   b.____110/72.   d.____150/100.

17. Which of the following is a normal value for pulse pressure?

   a.____80 mm. Hg.   c.____4 mm. Hg.
   b.____120 mm. Hg.   d.____40 mm. Hg.

18. A large overdose of atropine will have marked inhibitory effects on the parasympathetic nerve endings to the heart. The nurse reasonably could expect a

    a._____marked decrease in the heart rate.
    b._____marked increase in the heart rate.
    c._____marked increase in the pulse pressure.
    d._____partial heart block.

19. A rise in the blood pressure in the carotid sinus initiates a normal reflex

    a._____increasing the heart rate.
    b._____slowing the heart rate.
    c._____constricting the splanchnic arterioles.
    d._____dilating the splanchnic arterioles.

20. Arterial blood pressure could fall to zero in which one of the following circumstances?

    a._____overstimulation of the sympathetic nerves to the smooth muscle in the walls of the splanchnic arterioles.
    b._____sudden, complete dilatation of the splanchnic arterioles.
    c._____complete dilatation of the arterioles in the brain.
    d._____complete constriction of the arterioles in the skeletal muscles.

21. Diastolic arterial blood pressure is used as an index of the

    a._____constant maximum pressure being exerted against the arterial walls.
    b._____volume of blood being forced out of the ventricles with each systole.
    c._____constant minimum pressure being exerted against the arterial walls.
    d._____volume of blood being forced out of the ventricles with each diastole.

22. If you had a patient with a clinical diagnosis of heart block, you should expect the patient's radial pulse to be

    a._____slower in rate than normal and probably irregular in rhythm.
    b._____faster in rate than normal and probably irregular in rhythm.
    c._____regular in rhythm and more rapid in rate than normal.
    d._____regular in rhythm and slower in rate than normal.

23. The hormone thyroxin influences the action of the heart by

    a._____depressing the sino-atrial node.
    b._____stimulating the atrioventricular node.
    c._____directly depressing the myocardium.
    d._____directly stimulating the myocardium.

24. The most important physiologic effect of the hormone adrenalin on the action of the heart is to bring about a (an)

    a._____increased heart rate.
    b._____increased force of ventricular contraction.
    c._____increased force of auricular contraction.
    d._____decreased heart rate.

25. If the parasympathetic nerve control of the heart is stimulated the result is

    a._____slowing of the heart beat.
    b._____acceleration of the heart beat.
    c._____fibrillation of the ventricles.
    d._____a rise in diastolic blood pressure.

26. If a drug inhibiting the vagus is given you should expect

    a._____an increased heart rate.
    b._____a decreased heart rate.
    c._____a more forceful contraction of the heart.
    d._____a rise in blood pressure.

27. When you take a patient's pulse, you are actually observing the results of

    a._____the pumping action of the heart.
    b._____contraction of the right ventricle.
    c._____contraction of the left ventricle.
    d._____the discharging of impulses by the sino-atrial node.

THE MAN WHO COULDN'T BREATHE—PATIENT STUDY

Mr. Keith, a 67-year-old retired policeman, was brought to the emergency room by a neighbor following a heart attack at home. He was in great distress with orthopnea, dyspnea, pallor, some cyanosis and tremendous edema of his trunk and extremities. The chaplain was called; he administered the last rites of the Roman Catholic church.

Mr. Keith was well known to the Medical Service through numerous hospitalizations and clinic visits. He was admitted to the Medical Ward immediately and the following diagnosis was written:

1. Hypertensive cardiovascular disease with failure (cardiac failure at rest).
2. Anasarca.
3. Hydrothorax bilateral.
4. Bronchopneumonia.

His admission orders included:

Bed rest.
Soft, low-sodium diet.
Limit fluids to 1,500 cc. per day.
Apical-radial pulse b.i.d.
Morphine gr. ¼ p.r.n.
Digitalis gr. ½ t.i.d.
Ammonium chloride 4 Gm. b.i.d. today and tomorrow.

Thoracentesis this evening.
Paracentesis tomorrow.
Mercurin suppository 0.5 Gm. q. 3 day.
Blood specimen for n.p.n.

The fever subsided after a few days and chest sounds indicated that patches of possible bronchopneumonia had disappeared. The patient had lost 16.5 kilograms of weight. Minimal pitting edema of the thighs was still apparent. Following thoracentesis the patient had relief from the respiratory distress.

He continued to be somewhat orthopneic and dyspneic; the arteriosclerotic heart disease had not been cured. However, his condition was improved sufficiently to permit discharge after 3 weeks. His wife will care for him at home. She is trying, through the Social Service Department, to have his pension increased in order to assist with the added expense of hospitalization and necessary home care.

References

Covalt, Nila K.: Early exercise for the convalescent patient, Am. J. Nursing 47:544, 1947.

Crenshaw, Virginia: Teaching patients, Am. J. Nursing 50:666, 1950.

Crowley, Evelyn M.: Convalescent care in heart disease, Am. J. Nursing 44:1124, 1944.

Dale, Lucy S.: Diversional activities for patients, Am. J. Nursing 47:384, 1947.

Elman, Robert: Fluid balance from the nurses' point of view, Am. J. Nursing 47:222, 1947.

Harrison, Tinsley R.: The abuse of rest as a therapeutic measure for patients with cardiovascular disease, J.A.M.A. 125:1175, 1944.

Hollander, Lester: Care of the skin in older people, Am. J. Nursing 47:219, 1947.

Jones, Meredith: The basic 7 dietary pattern, Am. J. Nursing 50:224, 1950.

Manwell, Elizabeth Moore: Three basic needs, Am. J. Nursing 40:403, 1940.

Metropolitan Life Insurance Company: Encouraging trends in heart disease, Statistical Bulletin, Vol. 27, No. 8, 1946.

Nagle, R. A.: Patients' spiritual needs, Am. J. Nursing 50:65, 1950.

Questions Relating to the Patient Study

1. The optimum choice of a room for Mr. Keith would be a (an)

   a._____corner unit of a 4-bed ward.
   b._____2-bed room with a similar patient.
   c._____single room near the bath.
   d._____single room near the nurses' station.
   e._____8-bed convalescent ward.

2. An apical-radial pulse is ordered to determine

   a._____pulse deficit.
   b._____digitalis toxicity.
   c._____bigeminal pulse rate.
   d._____pulse tension.

3. Pulse deficit is

    a._____a description of a weak fluttery pulse.
    b._____a description of the pulse in heart block.
    c._____the difference between the rate of the apical and the radial pulse.
    d._____the difference between the resting pulse and the pulse after exercise.

4. Digitalis usually is administered in

    a._____large dosages until optimum concentration in the body has been obtained.
    b._____small dosages until tolerance has been developed.

5. The average maintenance dosage of digitalis for an adult is

    a._____1.0 Gm. per day.   d._____0.05 Gm. per day.
    b._____0.1 Gm. per day.   e._____0.005 Gm. per day.
    c._____0.01 Gm. per day.

6. The most common symptoms of digitalis toxicity are

    a._____marked slowing of the pulse rate.
    b._____marked increase of the pulse rate.
    c._____anoxemia.
    d._____anasarca.
    e._____nausea and vomiting.
    f._____constipation.

7. When symptoms of digitalis toxicity occur the nurse should

    a._____give the drug and report to the doctor.
    b._____omit the drug and report to the doctor.
    c._____omit one dose of the drug and resume.
    d._____cancel the order for the drug.

8. The pulmonary congestion indicated by Mr. Keith's pulmonary edema is caused by failure of the

    a._____left ventricle.   d._____mitral valve.
    b._____right ventricle.   e._____semilunar valve.
    c._____tricuspid valve.

9. Simple exercises, such as pushing the feet against the footboard, should be started

    a._____on the day of admission.
    b._____after dyspnea ceases.
    c._____after the temperature becomes normal.
    d._____several days after admission.
    e._____the day before getting out of bed.

10. The best guide in determining the effect of activity on Mr. Keith is the

    a._____degree of cyanosis.
    b._____amount of dyspnea.

c._____comfort of the patient.
d._____pulse rate.
e._____temperature reaction.

11. Careful back care for Mr. Keith is

    a._____contraindicated because of need for rest.
    b._____of less importance than for most patients, since edema "pads"
    the coccygeal region.
    c.___✓___of more importance than for most patients, since edematous
    tissue readily breaks down.

12. The position most likely to keep dyspnea at a minimum while caring
for Mr. Keith's back is with the patient

    a._____lying on either side with the bed flat.
    b._____lying prone with the head of the bed elevated at a 45° angle.
    c._____lying on the right side with the pillow under the head.
    d.___✓___sitting up, resting the arms and head over the bed table.

13. Mr. Keith's weight loss probably was due to the

    a._____debilitating effects of disease.
    b._____complete loss of appetite.
    c.___✓___loss of fluid from the tissues.

14. For Mr. Keith the action of digitalis primarily desired is

    a._____slowing of the pulse rate.
    b._____acceleration of the pulse rate.
    c.___✓___increased strength of contraction of the heart muscle.
    d._____sedative action on the heart muscle providing "rest" to the
    heart.

15. The desired action of ammonium chloride is to

    a.___✓___increase the action of Mercurin.
    b._____decrease the toxicity of Mercurin.
    c._____alkalize the urine.
    d._____increase the appetite.

16. The desired action of the mercurin suppository is

    a.___✓___diuretic, because of its irritant action on the tubules.
    b._____diuretic, because of its stimulation of the circulation.
    c._____antiseptic to the lower bowel.
    d._____mild catharsis, through mild irritation of the lower bowel.

17. Ammonium chloride usually is administered in

    a._____solution, orally.
    b.___✓___enteric-coated pills, orally.
    c._____solution, intravenously.
    d._____solution, intramuscularly.
    e._____petrolatum, rectally.

18. From your knowledge of the action of ammonium chloride, and from a careful interpretation of the physician's orders, you would administer the ordered drugs as follows:

    a.____first day, Mercurin and ammonium chloride; second and third days, ammonium chloride; fourth day, Mercurin.
    b.____first and second days, ammonium chloride; third day, Mercurin.
    c.____first day, Mercurin and ammonium chloride; second day, ammonium chloride; third day, Mercurin.

19. The stock bottle of ammonium chloride is labeled "grains xxx." In order to administer 4 Gm. you should give

    a.____½ tablet.   c.____2 tablets.
    b.____1 tablet.   d.____4 tablets.

20. In order to interpret Mr. Keith's weight loss the nurse should understand that 1 kilogram equals approximately

    a.____½ pound.   d.____4 pounds.
    b.____1 pound.   e.____5 pounds.
    c.____2 pounds.

Questions for Discussion and Student Projects

1. Describe the nurse's responsibility in preparing for and during the administration of the sacrament of last rites (extreme unction).
2. Discuss various preparations of digitalis. How do you account for the wide range of dosages between the preparations? What is meant by a "biologic assay" of digitalis?
3. Describe the method of taking and recording the apical-radial pulse.
4. Plan a distribution of fluids to provide for Mr. Keith's needs and comfort during the 24-hour period.
5. What is meant by heart block? What are the symptoms? Treatment?
6. Outline the nursing responsibilities in carrying out

    a. paracentesis.
    b. thoracentesis, including

       (1) equipment (indicate which articles should be sterile).
       (2) preparation of patient (mental and physical).
       (3) position of patient.
       (4) precautions.
       (5) care after procedure.

7. Mr. Keith was much concerned about a definite increase in the amount of urine voided. How would you explain this to him?
8. When Mr. Keith told Mrs. Keith he had lost considerable weight, she expressed concern and felt that his dislike of the low-sodium diet was a factor. What should you tell her?
9. Discuss the differences in the effect of right and left heart failure. Why are these conditions seldom seen separately?

10. Outline the teaching plan you would give to Mrs. Keith before the patient goes home. What portions of this teaching should Mr. Keith also receive?
11. Plan a week's diet for Mr. Keith considering the "seven basic foods," the family's income, food habits and facilities, and the necessity of high-protein, low-sodium content. What information in addition to a suggested diet would Mrs. Keith need before assuming the responsibility for preparing his food?
12. What are the measures for the prevention of heart disease? What would you instruct a person to do who thought he had heart disease?
13. How does heart disease compare with other illnesses in regard to mortality rate? Incapacitation? Crippling?
14. What is the program of the American Heart Association? How is it financed?

THE MAN WITH THE HEART ATTACK—PATIENT STUDY

Mr. Clark, a 49-year-old American, was brought to the emergency room with excruciating chest pain, dyspnea, cyanosis and symptoms of shock. He had collapsed at the football stadium and was seen by the ambulance intern, who rushed him to the hospital. Mr. Clark indicated that the pain extended from his chest into his left shoulder and arm. He was given morphine immediately and admitted to a single room. His orders were:

Absolute bed rest.	Routine laboratory tests of blood
Liquid diet.	and urine.
Morphine sulfate gr. ¼ p.r.n.	Sedimentation rate.
Papaverine gr. 1½ b.i.d.	Electrocardiogram.
Dicumarol 100 mg. daily.	Chest roentgenogram.
	Place on dangerously ill list.

Mrs. Clark was called; she came to the hospital at once. She stated that Mr. Clark was a foreman for the Western Union Telegraph Co. and had gone to supervise Western Union arrangements at the stadium for the football game. She appeared to be intelligent, attractive and well dressed, and very much concerned about her husband. She indicated that he had been healthy until 3 years before when he had an attack which the doctor said was angina. He was advised to limit his activities. His wife had noticed he was a little short of breath when climbing stairs and occasionally was nauseated. His work required little physical effort but involved much emotional and nervous strain.

On the basis of the history, physical examination, laboratory findings and electrocardiogram, a diagnosis was made of hypertensive and arteriosclerotic heart disease with coronary occlusion.

Mr. Clark improved gradually and after 18 days was delighted to be able to feed himself. On the nineteenth day he developed thrombophlebitis of his left arm and again was placed at complete rest. The arm was elevated on a pillow and ice packs were applied continuously for several days. This condition improved in a comparatively short time.

Mr. Clark was a naturally sociable person and was lonely in a single room. Later, when he was feeling better, he was moved to a 3-bed ward where he seemed happier.

He was discharged to his home after 4 weeks, his condition much improved. He was advised to continue bed rest for a period of several weeks and then gradually to increase his activity.

References

Brown, A. F.: Coronary occlusion—nursing care, Am. J. Nursing **42**:248, 1942.
Stallman, Dorothy Prange: Nursing care in cardiac catheterization, Am. J. Nursing **49**:215, 1949.
Webster, R. J.: Educating the cardiac patient, Trained Nurse and Hosp. Rev. **120**:257, 1948.
Wright, I. S., et al.: Anticoagulant therapy of coronary thrombosis with myocardial infarction, J.A.M.A. **138**:1074, 1948.

Questions Relating to the Patient Study

1. Mr. Clark's sudden severe attack of coronary occlusion was

   a._____atypical of this condition, which usually develops progressively.

   b._____typical of this condition, which usually has sudden, severe onset.

   c._____more typical of acute cardiac failure than of coronary occlusion.

2. Immediately following Mr. Clark's acute attack the following symptoms would be expected:

   a._____an increase in blood pressure.

   b._____a fall in blood pressure.

   c._____temperature elevated.

   d._____temperature subnormal.

3. Several hours following Mr. Clark's acute attack the following changes would be expected:

   a._____an increase in blood pressure.

   b._____a fall in blood pressure.

   c._____temperature slightly elevated.

   d._____temperature slightly subnormal.

   e._____an increase in white blood cells.

   f._____an increase in red blood cells.

4. The optimum position for Mr. Clark would be

   a._____flat in bed.

   b._____semi-Fowler's position.

   c._____high Fowler's position.

   d._____Trendelenburg position.

5. Mr. Clark should be encouraged to

    a._____move about freely, hyperventilate, do stir-up exercises frequently.

    b._____assume responsibility for much of his own bathing, feeding, etc.

    c.✓_____remain as immobile as possible, permitting the nurses to do everything for him.

6. Routine personal hygiene (bathing, change of linen, etc.) for Mr. Clark should be

    a._____omitted if the patient is resting.

    b._____rigidly carried out, regardless of the patient's protests.

    c.✓_____of less importance than complete rest of the patient.

    d._____of greater importance for patients with this condition than for most patients.

7. During the first few days Mr. Clark's morphine order would be used

    a.✓_____liberally to provide rest.

    b._____sparingly to prevent addiction.

    c._____only during the night.

    d._____only for excruciating pain.

    e._____only in case of symptoms of a second attack.

8. While placing Mr. Clark in an oxygen tent, the nurse should

    a._____warn him that oxygen is combustible.

    b.✓_____remove cigarettes and matches.

    c._____place a signal cord outside the tent.

    d._____protect exposed skin with oil.

9. A substance which may ignite spontaneously in contact with oxygen under high pressure is

    a._____safety matches.

    b.✓_____oil.

    c._____talcum.

    d._____helium.

10. In observing the oxygen tank to determine the adequacy of the supply, the nurse should know that 100 pounds of oxygen will last approximately

    a._____15 minutes.

    b.✓_____1 hour.

    c._____2 hours.

    d._____6 hours.

11. Dicumarol was given to Mr. Clark to

    a._____delay the destruction of red blood cells.

    b.✓_____delay the clotting time of the blood.

    c._____hasten the clotting time of the blood.

    d._____retard the coronary circulation.

    e._____improve the coronary circulation.

12. The following symptoms would indicate untoward action of Dicumarol:
    a.____bleeding from the mouth, ears or rectum, or blood in the urine.
    b.____increased salivation, profuse diaphoresis, restlessness.
    c.____decreased salivation, dry hot skin, stupor.
    d.____increased dyspnea, cardiac pain, slow weak pulse.

13. During the time Dicumarol is being administered it is important to provide for
    a.____prothrombin determinations twice daily.
    b.____sedimentation rates daily.
    c.____strict measurement of intake and output.
    d.____regular electrocardiogram readings.

14. The effect of Dicumarol is
    a.____rapid, and persists for several days.
    b.____rapid, and effective for a brief period.
    c.____delayed, and persists for several days.
    d.____delayed, and effective for a brief period.

15. In the event the nurse observes symptoms of untoward reaction of Dicumarol she should prepare to administer
    a.____morphine sulfate.
    b.____oxygen therapy.
    c.____vitamin K.
    d.____stimulants.

16. Papaverine, which was ordered for Mr. Clark, is a
    a.____habit-forming alkaloid of opium.
    b.____non-habit-forming alkaloid of opium.
    c.____habit-forming barbiturate.
    d.____non-habit-forming barbiturate.

17. The primary action of papaverine desired for Mr. Clark is
    a.____relaxation of involuntary muscles of the gastro-intestinal tract.
    b.____to relieve pain and apprehension.
    c.____increased collateral circulation in vascular beds.
    d.____absorption of blood clots.

18. When recovery from attack is complete, Mr. Clark probably will be advised to
    a.____seek employment which will involve more physical exercise.
    b.____seek employment which will involve less emotional tension.
    c.____remain in the same employment, as it involves relatively little activity.

Questions for Discussion and Student Projects

1. List the nursing responsibilities in the use of the oxygen tent, including precautions, maintenance of oxygen concentration, and temperature of the tent. What adaptations are desirable when bathing and feeding the patient?

2. What is meant by absolute bed rest? List the usual activities of a patient on bed rest which would not be desirable for a cardiac patient on absolute bed rest.
3. List the instructions the nurse should give family and friends in regard to visiting this patient. How can she elicit their co-operation?
4. Mr. Clark seemed to dislike being fed by the nurse. How can the nurse make this procedure more acceptable to the patient?
5. Outline the instructions you should give Mr. Clark and his wife before his discharge. What would you need to know about his living arrangements to help them plan his activities?
6. Should Mr. Clark return to the same position? If not, what type of employment do you believe would be more desirable? What agencies or groups would be helpful in securing different employment?

Nursing Care of Patients with Other Cardiovascular Diseases

Background Review Questions

1. The cause of essential hypertension is

    a._____chronic nephritis.
    b._____hemolytic infections.
    c._____frequent upper respiratory infections.
    d._____unknown.

2. Essential hypertension

    a._____is definitely hereditary.
    b._____shows a tendency to run in families.
    c._____is more frequent in men than in women.
    d._____shows no difference in incidence between the sexes.
    e._____usually develops before the age of 40.
    f._____usually develops after the age of 40.

3. Malignant essential hypertension is

    a._____hypertension associated with carcinoma.
    b._____hypertension resulting from carcinoma of the blood vessels.
    c._____rapidly progressing hypertension.
    d._____chronic subclinical.

4. Cardiac rhythm indicates the

    a._____force of the heart beat.   c._____sequence of the heart beat.
    b._____rate of the heart beat.

5. Arrhythmia refers to a

    a._____rapid pulse.   d._____irregular pulse.
    b._____normal pulse.   e._____weak pulse.
    c._____slow pulse.

6. Sinus arrhythmia describes the

    a._____pathology of the endocardium.
    b._____pathology of the coronary artery.
    c._____heart rate varying with respiration.
    d._____decreased reflex sensitivity of the pacemaker.
    e._____increased reflex sensitivity of the pacemaker.

7. Paroxysmal tachycardia describes the

    a._____pathology of the auricles.
    b._____pathology of the ventricles.
    c._____sudden onset of rapid, regular rhythm.
    d._____sudden onset of slow, irregular rhythm.
    e._____heart rate fluctuating with respirations.

8. Paroxysms of thoracic pain relieved by nitrites and with no apparent discomfort between attacks probably are caused by

    a._____acute indigestion.   d._____angina pectoris.
    b._____pulmonary infarct.   e._____pleuritic pain.
    c._____coronary occlusion.

9. Bacterial endocarditis develops most frequently

    a._____in patients with damaged heart valves.
    b._____in patients with emotional disorders.
    c._____in any patients, following bacterial infections.
    d._____in patients with congenital heart defects.

10. A patient with acute bacterial endocarditis is receiving penicillin every 3 hours. The night nurse should

    a._____administer the drug promptly even though the patient is asleep.
    b._____withhold the drug when the patient is asleep.
    c._____withhold one dose of the drug, to allow at least 6 hours of sleep.

11. Cardiac catheterization describes

    a._____tapping the heart for a blood sample.
    b._____tapping the heart for pericardial fluid.
    c._____tapping the heart for excess fluids.
    d._____tapping the kidney of a cardiac patient.
    e._____removing urine from a cardiac patient.

Questions for Discussion and Student Projects

1. Distinguish between auricular and ventricular paroxysmal tachycardia, considering the cause, treatment and implications for prognosis.
2. Distinguish between auricular fibrillation and auricular flutter, considering the physiology, etiology, symptoms and diagnosis, treatment and prognosis.
3. Which of the cardiac arrhythmias are essentially of little clinical importance? Which are of considerable clinical significance? How would you advise a friend who described to you an arrhythmia which is a "normal" phenomena?

4. What type of heart disease has shown a percentage increase since 1910? How would the age of the population affect these figures?
5. Discuss the relationship to heart disease of (a) bacterial infections, (b) syphilis, (c) nutritional deficiencies, (d) thyroid function.

THE MAIL CARRIER WITH NUMB FEET

Background Review Questions

1. The term used to mean thickening and hardening of the blood vessel walls is

    a.＿＿hyperplasia.   c.＿＿ischemia.
    b.＿＿arteriosclerosis.   d.＿＿infarct.

2. Atherosclerosis is a disease which occurs within

    a.＿＿the aorta and its large branches.
    b.＿＿the arterioles.
    c.＿＿any of the arteries of the body.
    d.＿＿the large veins.

3. Atherosclerosis is most dangerous when it attacks the

    a.＿＿coronary arteries.   c.＿＿iliac arteries.
    b.＿＿aorta.   d.＿＿renal arteries.

4. At the present time, it appears that one of the predisposing factors involved in the development of atherosclerosis is faulty metabolism of

    a.＿＿carbohydrates.   c.＿＿calcium.
    b.＿＿proteins.   d.＿＿fat.

5. Differentiate between the following two conditions:

    a. thrombophlebitis.
    b. phlebothrombosis.

    (1)＿＿slight temperature elevation (1–2°F.).
    (2)＿＿minimal or no signs of leg pain or tenderness.
    (3)＿＿edema and pain in the extremity.
    (4)＿＿redness and swelling along the course of the vein.
    (5)＿＿evidence of an embolus.
    (6)＿＿pain in the calf.

6. A blood clot which is moving about freely in the circulatory system is called a (an)

    a.＿＿thrombus.   d.＿＿phlebothrombosis.
    b.＿＿phlebus.   e.＿＿thrombophlebus.
    c.＿＿embolus.

7. Thrombophlebitis is a disease of

    a.＿＿veins, characterized by an inflammation of the vessel wall with clotting of the blood.
    b.＿＿veins, characterized by dilatation, stagnation of the blood and ultimately ulceration of adjacent tissue.

c.____arteries, characterized by acute inflammation of the vessel wall with the formation of thrombi.

d.____arteries, characterized by the formation of calcified plaques.

8. Hemorrhoids (or piles) is a disease process due to

   a.____the formation of blood clots within the hemorrhoidal arteries.
   b.____an obstruction to venous outflow from the hemorrhoidal veins.
   c.____a marked dilatation of the superficial veins of the leg, accompanied by stagnation of blood.
   d.____an acute inflammation of the deep veins predisposing to the formation of thrombi.

9. If one of the blood clots forming on a plaque in the intima of the aorta should break, it might easily become lodged within which of the following vessels?

   a.____portal vein.   d.____femoral vein.
   b.____splenic artery.   e.____renal artery.
   c.____pulmonary artery.   f.____pulmonary vein.

10. A thrombus formed in the femoral vein of a bed-ridden postoperative patient may become dislodged when he gets up and moves about. The thrombus would most likely lodge next within the

   a.____coronary artery.   c.____portal vein.
   b.____renal artery.   d.____pulmonary artery.

11. Thrombi are most likely to develop in the veins of bed-ridden postoperative patients because

   a.____postoperative patients characteristically show a rise in the plasma prothrombin level.
   b.____they are more prone to infection resulting in inflammation of the blood vessel.
   c.____inactivity of the skeletal muscle leads to slowing of the venous blood flow.
   d.____poor nutrition in postoperative patients leads to formation of calcium plaques on the vessel wall.

12. Preventive measures against venous complications in the lower extremities which the nurse can carry out in the postoperative care of surgical patients are as follows:

   a.____Resort to passive exercises for the lower extremities until the patient is able to move them about himself, then remind him to exercise every 3 or 4 hours.
   b.____Move the lower extremities as little as possible until the physician allows the patient to get out of bed.
   c.____Be on the alert for any complaints of tenderness or pain in the lower extremities; massage these parts well.
   d.____Flex the lower part of the bed so that pressure is exerted on the space back of the knees; the legs will then be dependent, which is desirable.

13. Dicumarol, administered as a drug, acts within the body to

    a._____prevent the formation of thrombi.
    b._____prevent the formation of emboli.
    c._____dissolve thrombi formed within the blood vessels.
    d._____prevent retraction of the clot.

14. The physiologic action of Dicumarol is to

    a._____inhibit the formation of thrombin.
    b._____depress the production of prothrombin.
    c._____inhibit the formation of thromboplastin.
    d._____depress the production of fibrinogen.

15. A drug which is used as an emergency anticoagulant is

    a._____sodium citrate.   d._____thromboplastin.
    b._____heparin.   e._____vitamin K.
    c._____Dicumarol.

16. During an operation, blood pressure is taken because

    a._____vital tissue fluid cannot form when it is too low.
    b._____oxygen and nutrient cannot diffuse out of blood to the cells
          when it is too low.
    c._____blood cannot flow when arterial pressure is less than capillary
          pressure.

THE MAIL CARRIER WITH NUMB FEET—PATIENT STUDY

Two years ago, John Black appeared in the clinic complaining of numbness in both feet.

Mr. Black was a Negro, but with Caucasian features. He had completed high school before enlisting in World War I. He has been divorced twice, but his present marriage seems more successful. He and his third wife have 3 teen-age children.

Until recently, Mr. Black had been a mail carrier. He states that occasionally, during Christmas rush periods, he found it necessary to drink whisky several times a day to get a lift and to complete his rounds in the cold weather.

Three weeks prior to his clinic visit Mr. Black noticed symptoms of coldness, numbness and burning of his feet while marching in a Memorial Day parade. At night he has had cramps in his toes. He could walk only 2 blocks without pain.

Mr. Black claims that he drinks very seldom now, and that, although he had smoked regularly, he had given it up.

Physical examination revealed absence of dorsalis pedis and popliteal sensations. A diagnosis of Buerger's disease was made. He was admitted to the hospital and Buerger's exercises instigated. In about a week feeble lower leg pulsations were felt.

During his hospitalization Mr. Black showed a tendency to be nervous, dependent and often undependable. The physician had directed him not to smoke but there was frequent evidence that he disregarded these instructions.

A bilateral sympathectomy was done. He responded very well and was discharged with the following instructions:

> Discontinue tobacco completely.
> Keep off the feet as much as possible.
> Continue with Buerger's exercises.
> Report to the clinic regularly.

His clinic reports showed that he was able to increase his exercise tolerance satisfactorily. Subjectively, he had benefited considerably by the sympathectomy.

References

Palumbo, L. T.: Some recent advances in surgery of the autonomic system, Am. J. Nursing 52:700, 1952.

Smithwick, R. H., and Kinsey, Dera: Surgical treatment of hypertension, Am. J. Nursing 47:153, 1947.

Spinney, J. M.: Buerger's disease, Am. J. Nursing 49:119, 1949.

Questions Relating to the Patient Study

1. Buerger's disease is

   a. the same as

      (1)_____arteriosclerosis of the lower extremities.
      (2)_____atherosclerosis of the lower extremities.
      (3)_____thrombo-angiitis obliterans.

   b. found most commonly in

      (1)_____young (25–45 years) Jewish males.
      (2)_____older (45–60 years) Negro males.
      (3)_____men (25–60 years) of the Polish race.

   c. characterized by

      (1)_____blanching of the skin of a lower extremity, burning pain precipitated by exposure to cold, relief of pain when heat is applied.
      (2)_____persistent coldness of a lower extremity, color changes dependent on the position of the extremity (cyanosis, pallor, rubor), susceptibility to ulcers from minor injuries.
      (3)_____edema, mottled cyanosis, warmth of the extremity, systemic manifestations of anorexia, malaise, fever and leukocytosis.

2. Mr. Black's condition was aggravated by

   a._____tobacco.
   b._____alcohol.
   c._____immobilization.
   d._____exposure to cold.
   e._____exposure to heat.

3. Methods of administering passive postural exercises to allow the intermittent filling and emptying of capillaries, venules and arterioles are

a._____an oscillating bed.　　　d._____a Stryker frame.
b._____an alternating pressure　e._____electric suction and a pressure boot.
　　mattress.
c._____an Unna paste boot.

4. A sympathectomy results in the following:

a._____Smooth muscle tone is decreased, therefore there is greater peripheral resistance to blood flow through smaller vessels.
b._____Because smooth muscle tone is decreased, there is less peripheral resistance to blood flow through smaller vessels.
c._____The magnitude of reflex responses (such as occur after pain, cold or emotional stimuli) is modified.
d._____There is an increase in the activity of the adrenals.

5. The temperature of the contrast baths should be

Cold	*Warm*
a._____40°–50°.	a._____100°–105°.
b._____32°–40°.	b._____ 80°– 90°.
c._____32°–40°.	c._____100°–105°.
d._____32°–40°.	d._____120°–130°.
e._____40°–50°.	e._____120°–130°.

6. Following a sympathectomy, one can expect the patient to show the following reaction until he readjusts to his "new circulation":

a._____headache, a sense of fullness in the head, a throbbing sensation in the ears.
b._____pain in the hands and the feet, heartburn, nystagmus followed by diplopia.
c._____dryness of the mouth, a tingling sensation of the hands and the lower extremities, abdominal distention.
d._____syncope, palpitation, light-headedness, an unsteady feeling.

7. The unpleasant reaction referred to in the preceding question may be alleviated as follows:

a._____Have the patient roll to the unoperated side before he slowly rises to the sitting position.
b._____Administer a sedative about 20 minutes before getting the patient out of bed.
c._____Apply ace bandages (or rubber hose) and a tight abdominal binder before the patient gets out of bed.
d._____Instruct the patient to perform Buerger's exercises before he attempts to get out of bed.

8. Instructions to Mr. Black on the care of the feet should include

a._____to maintain cleanliness, to use a soap which contains naphtha or borax.

b._____after washing the feet, to dry briskly (especially between the toes) with a turkish towel.

c._____to prevent drying and cracking of the skin, to use a mild astringent such as alcohol.

d._____to help prevent irritation, to place lamb's wool between the toes.

e._____to aid in the absorption of perspiration, to wear warm woolen socks in the summer.

9. If Mr. Black discovered an ingrown toenail he should

a._____swab the toe gently with iodine tincture.

b._____cut the nail straight across.

c._____soak his foot in epsom salt solution.

d._____visit a chiropodist.

e._____come to the vascular O.P.D. where he is known.

10. If contrast baths had been ordered for Mr. Black, he should have been instructed to

a._____place his foot in a cold bath for 1 minute, then in a warm bath for 1 minute, continuing this procedure for 15 minutes.

b._____place one foot in cold water, the other in warm water; reverse in 15 minutes.

c._____bathe his feet in warm water in the morning, and in cold water in the evening.

THE MAIL CARRIER WHO LOST HIS LEGS

Background Review Questions

1. Inflammatory reaction of tissue varies from the simplest to the most violent, depending upon many factors. When a foreign substance enters the body, remains localized, and is of low irritation, the method of disposal is usually as follows:

a._____Phagocytosis takes place by local macrophages with the destruction of the foreign body or its incorporation in scar formed from proliferated macrophages.

b._____Phagocytosis takes place by local macrophages plus microphages (polymorphs).

c._____Phagocytosis takes place by reticulo-endothelial macrophages scattered throughout the body and destroyed with the formation of antibodies, fever and leukocytosis.

2. Examples of exogenous foreign substances which may enter the body are

a._____fibrin.   d._____silica dust.
b._____infarcts.   e._____cholesterol esters.
c._____bacteria.   f._____catgut and sutures.

3. Consider the events that follow the introduction of a sufficient number of staphylococci into the tissues. Check the series of activities which

take place *in the order* of progression. Number only those spaces which are correct and pertinent, beginning with 1, 2, 3, etc.

a. ___1___ transient vasoconstriction followed by marked dilatation.
b. _____ transient vasodilatation followed by marked constriction.
c. ___2___ the phenomena of (a) or (b) take place first in the arterioles, then in the venules and last in the capillaries.
d. _____ the phenomena of (a) or (b) take place first in the capillaries, then in the venules and last in the arterioles.
e. ___3___ hyperemia takes place in the entire affected area.
f. ___3___ there is an increased exudation of plasma fluid and proteins from capillaries to intercellular space, with swelling.
g. ___4___ there is a retardation of blood flow.
h. ___5___ leukocytes wander to the walls of the vessels, squeeze through and begin to move forward toward the focus of infection.
i. ___6___ complete cessation of blood flow occurs.
j. _____ status quo in tissues is regained following ingestion of foreign body by leukocytes.
k. ___7___ blood in the injured vessels coagulates (thrombosis).
l. ___8___ the area of tissue involved becomes highly toxic and necrosis follows.
m. ___9___ dead cells gradually disintegrate and the leukocytes set free their powerful proteolytic enzymes.
n. _____ dead cells gradually disintegrate and are dissolved by the ingestive action of the fibroblasts.
o. __10__ because of increasing osmotic pressure which develops, fluid is drawn toward the dissolving area.
p. __11__ a mass of fluid containing dead and living cells develops to form pus and the area is called an abscess.
q. __12__ lymphocytes, plasma cells and macrophages remove the débris.
r. __12__ granulation tissue fills the cavity.
s. __13__ new-formed tissue is converted into a contracted fibrous scar.

4. An abscess is incised and drained most effectively when

a. _____ the inflammation is noted; allowing it to progress untreated causes unnecessary spread of infection.
b. _____ it is, so called, "cold"; such an abscess is localized and limited tissue damage results.
c. _____ it is localized; this is evidence that the abscess is encapsulated and drainage of it will prevent its spread to uninvolved tissue.
d. _____ it is diffuse; the advantages of a more extensive blood supply mean the more rapid dissolution of the foreign substance.

5. The removal of necrotic tissue by careful dissection with a surgical scissors and forceps is called

a. _____ sloughing.   c. _____ saucerization.
b. _____ débridement.   d. _____ sequestrectomy.

6. Débridement is the technic of

a._____cleansing a wound by a styptic agent such as a silver nitrate stick.

b._____removing bone fragments with the aid of a rongeur.

c._____mechanically cleaning a contaminated wound by irrigation.

d._____removing devitalized tissue from wounds.

7. *Pyocyaneus* wound infection is a serious surgical problem because it

a._____spreads rapidly.

b._____is pathogenic.

c._____is often extremely resistant to eradication.

d._____is anaerobic.

e._____has a selective affinity for nerve tissue.

8. Acceptable methods for treating acute inflammation are to

a._____remove or destroy the cause by excision, drainage or drug action.

b._____concentrate the toxins for easier evacuation by limiting fluid intake.

c._____support circulation to the part by keeping it active (passive if not active exercise is acceptable).

d._____increase carbohydrate and vitamin intake to meet greater combative energy requirements.

9. The repair of an open wound, an ulcer or a cavity takes place by the formation of granulation tissue. Steps in this process are described as

a._____new blood capillaries form by budding from previously existing capillaries; these buds become canalized, grow in length and anastomose with other new capillaries.

b._____new blood capillaries form from flagellated extensions of arterioles and venules; these extensions form an intricate network because of the increasing pressure of blood, the extensions are forced open.

c._____fibroblasts and other connective-tissue cells now also multiply between the newly formed capillaries.

d._____intercellular fluid seeps in between the newly formed capillaries to produce mass.

10. Repair of tissue or closure of a wound can be handicapped seriously by

a._____hypovitaminoses A, B and D.

b._____hypovitaminoses C and K.

c._____hyperproteinemia.

d._____tight suturing of wounds.

e._____regulated diabetes mellitus.

11. Wound healing by "third intention" refers to a wound in which

a._____primary healing takes place without delay and without infection.

b._____healing is inhibited or retarded because of poor approximation or because infection develops.

c.———healing is by secondary suture; this takes place after a wound is left open for some purpose (such as after infection with delayed healing).

THE MAIL CARRIER WHO LOST HIS LEGS—PATIENT STUDY—(*Continued*)

One and one-half years following the bilateral sympathectomy, Mr. Black was again in difficulties. He had stubbed his third left toe, and, in spite of epsom salt soaks, the wound discharged a small amount of pus. At the same time, his right leg up to the midcalf was swollen, red and tender.

Mr. Black was admitted to the vascular ward. The toe was dressed, but it continued to throb and to ooze pus, and the infection spread to the adjacent toes. The nail of the third toe was removed, and finally it was necessary to amputate the toe.

Mr. Black stated that he had been fine since his sympathectomy. He had considered himself "cured" of his former difficulties. He admitted to smoking about 6 cigarettes daily and to having several drinks each evening.

One week following the toe amputation, Mr. Black showed signs of confusion. He got out of bed at night, wandered about, begged for and got cigarettes and disturbed other patients. His confusion was thought to be due to sedation, to infection, to cerebral Buerger's disease or to a combination of these factors.

As his left leg continued to show progressive infection, a left mid-thigh amputation was performed. He reacted well to this surgery. After 4 days his mental symptoms had almost completely disappeared.

Meanwhile, the right toes had become completely gangrenous. Débridement, local and general medications, even radical cleaning of the bone with a rongeur helped little. *Pyocyaneus* infection created an additional problem.

When a right posterior tibial nerve crush failed, it was decided to pack his limb in ice, and to do a mid-calf amputation.

Again, Mr. Black responded well to surgery. The stumps healed satisfactorily. Mr. Black made a fine adjustment and with the help of his wife has developed an optimistic philosophy of life. He is enthusiastically promising to show the fellows that he will be walking on his "new legs" by Christmas.

References

Glover, J. R.: The major amputations, Am. J. Nursing 50:544, 1950.

Knocke and Knocke: Orthopaedic Nursing, pp. 460–478, "Crutch Walking," Philadelphia, Davis, 1951.

Moshoff, M. E., and Sloan, J.: Nursing care for the amputee, Am. J. Nursing 50:550, 1950.

Questions Relating to the Patient Study

1. Débridement of the wound refers to

   a.———cauterization of gangrenous tissue.

   b.———packing of the wound with medicated gauze.

c.____removal of necrotic tissue by dissection.
d.____amputation of a toe or a finger.

2. Mr. Black's limb was packed in ice in order to

   a.____reduce pain.
   b.____reduce toxemia.
   c.____increase the amount of blood available to other
   parts of the body.
   d.____accelerate healing.
   e.____prevent shock.

3. The most satisfactory method of packing the limb in ice is to

   a.____apply a tourniquet distal to the incision site, place a rubber sheet under the limb, pack ice completely around the limb and send the patient to the O.R. in his bed.
   b.____place ice bags around the area where the tourniquet is to be applied, elevate the leg for 5 minutes prior to tourniquet application, apply the tourniquet, place the limb on a rubber sheet and pack in ice which has been well salted.
   c.____chill the area where the tourniquet is to be applied with ice bags, elevate the leg for 10 minutes prior to tourniquet application, then pack the limb in ice, being sure that the temperature does not reach the freezing point.

4. The following measures will assist in maintaining comfort during the ice pack:

   a.____Apply ice quickly, chill the rest of the body with ice bags and give iced beverages.
   b.____Keep the trunk warm, place a blanket on the other leg and drain off water.
   c.____Apply ice quickly, drain off water and apply an ice cap to the head.

5. Postoperatively, the stump should be elevated for

   a.____4 to 12 hours.
   b.____24 to 48 hours.
   c.____1 week.
   d.____entire hospitalization.

6. Emergency equipment which should be at the bedside is

   a.____a sterile suture tray.
   b.____a tourniquet.
   c.____a transfusion set.
   d.____an aspiration needle and syringe.

7. Contractures in the amputated limb can be prevented best by

   a.____gentle massaging of the stump.
   b.____placing the stump in the position of least pain.
   c.____insisting that the stump go through the normal range of motion at least once every 4 hours.
   d.____splinting the joint nearest the stump site so that no flexion takes place.

8. A stump sock is worn to

    a._____prevent infection. d._____take the place of a dressing
    b._____prevent friction. over the incision.
    c._____prevent perspiration. e._____absorb moisture.

9. A posterior plaster splint was applied to the below-the-knee stump for the first week postoperatively. The purpose of such a splint is to

    a._____prevent hemorrhage and tension on the wound.
    b._____develop a permanent straight contracture of the knee joint.
    c._____prevent involuntary flexion of the knee.
    d._____allow for easy turning from one side to the other.

10. Bed exercises which will help to strengthen those muscles which are used in crutch walking are

    a._____grasping an over-bed trapeze in moving about in bed to strengthen the biceps.
    b._____push-up exercises done in the sitting position with the arms straight and the hands planted in the bed to develop the triceps.
    c._____stretching the arms over the head while lying flat in bed to strengthen the tissues under the arm for weight bearing.
    d._____flexion and extension of the foot of the good leg to keep those muscles active and to prevent foot drop.

11. Hip-flexion contractures can occur very easily in an amputee. Ways of preventing this deformity are to

    a._____have the patient lie on his abdomen for short periods during the day.
    b._____allow the patient to be up in a wheel chair for short periods and then have him return to bed to assume a semi-Fowler or Fowler's position.
    c._____let the patient lie flat on his back on a pillow so placed that it extends from his shoulders to a point even with his hip joint.

12. A satisfactory method for measuring crutches while the patient is still in bed is as follows: Having him lie flat on his back with his heel against a footboard,

    a._____measurement is taken from the anterior fold of the axilla straight down to the footboard (without shoes).
    b._____with his shoes on, measurement is taken from the anterior fold of the axilla straight down to the footboard.
    c._____without his shoes on, measurement is made from the axilla to a point about 4 inches out from the side of the foot.
    d._____measurement is taken from the anterior axillary fold down to the foot minus 2 inches.

13. Muscles in which greater strength than usual will be needed for crutch walking are

    a._____those of the hand, wrist and forearm.
    b._____the flexors of the upper arm.

  c._____the extensors of the upper arm.
  d._____the quadriceps femoris on the side of amputation.
  e._____the spinal-extensor muscles.

14. The normal crutch stance is to place the crutches

  a._____adjacent to the middle outer side of each foot.
  b._____about 4 inches out to the side and 4 inches to the back of each
    foot.
  c._____about 4 inches out to the side and 4 inches in advance of each
    foot.
  d._____about 10 inches out from the middle outer aspect of each foot.

15. The purpose(s) of resilient padding on the axillary bar of the crutch
  is (are) to

  a._____allow the patient to have a temporary support which is used
    when he tends to slump from being tired (for the beginner).
  b._____provide a comfortable support since he bears most of his body
    weight at this point when he "swings through" the crutches.
  c._____prevent the likelihood of the crutch slipping out of the be-
    ginner's axilla.
  d._____absorb axillary secretions since there is a greater than normal
    tendency to perspire.

16. The bulk of the patient's weight in conventional crutch walking is
  borne by the

  a._____axilla.   c._____forearm.
  b._____upper arm.   d._____palm of the hand.

17. Crutch paralysis may develop

  a._____when a patient reaches the point of fatigue.
  b._____from pressure exerted on the superficial radial nerve.
  c._____from poor circulation in the axilla.
  d._____from pressure exerted on the brachial plexus.
  e._____from weakness of the deltoid due to repeated intramuscular
    injections.

18. Match the following crutch-walking gaits with the correct definition:

  a._____2-point gait   (1) when assistance in bearing
                                  weight on both lower extremi-
                                  ties is needed.
  b._____3-point gait   (2) those who can bear weight on
                                  only one extremity and can
                                  lift the weight of the body on
                                  crutches.
  c._____4-point gait   (3) those who are allowed partial
                                  or assisted weight bearing on
                                  one leg and full weight bear-
                                  ing on the other.

d._____swing-to and swing-
        through gait

(4) those who can bear weight on
    both extremities and can lift
    the weight of the body on
    crutches.

e._____rocking-chair gait

(5) when it is physically impossi-
    ble to perform other gaits.

Questions for Discussion and Student Projects

1. Mr. Black's history for the past 10 years shows the results of disregard
   of precautions on the progression of Buerger's disease. What have you
   learned from this patient study which you can use in assisting other
   patients in avoiding the complications Mr. Black experienced?
2. In your hospital, what type of skin preparation is used prior to an
   amputation of an extremity? Why is there more concern for a good
   skin preparation in cases involving surgery of the bone than in other
   types of operations? Is this difference justified?
3. What is meant by normal range of motion? With the physical therapist, plan a program of exercises which would help Mr. Black develop
   normal range of motion in his mid-thigh and mid-calf stumps.
4. Demonstrate an acceptable way of bandaging a mid-thigh stump.
   What are the purposes of applying a snug, well-fitting stump bandage?
5. "Phantom limb pain" can be a serious problem which may lead to
   morphine or other drug addiction, acute alcoholic debauchery or suicide. What is it? How can it be prevented? How can it be treated effectively? How can the nurse help her patient with such a problem?
6. Since it takes from 6 to 8 weeks for the construction of an artificial
   limb, a patient will be at home for the greater part of this period. Plan
   a detailed daily regimen for him to follow which will prepare him for
   his prosthetic. (Check with the physical therapist.) In the plan include the following:

   a. exercises.
   b. bandaging stump.
   c. use of crutches.

   d. inspection and care of the
      stump.

7. When a patient such as Mr. Black has an amputation of both legs,
   how are crutches measured? What are the steps he will have to follow
   to use them effectively?
8. What are the advantages of the suction socket leg prosthesis over the
   other types of leg prostheses? What precautions must be taken by the
   wearer?
9. What is a guillotine amputation? When is it used? What nursing
   problems are involved in this type of amputation which are different
   from other types?
10. Assume that your patient has an ulcer of the foot. The surgeon plans
    to do a mid-thigh amputation. List the reasons which you can present
    to your patient in justifying what appears to be radical and unneces-
    sary surgery.

11. If a patient with diabetes mellitus has a mid-thigh amputation, for what complications would you be on the alert in addition to those of any other amputee?

12. A postoperative traumatic amputee may appear to be unusually cheerful and optimistic during the first 24 to 48 hours. Often this is followed by a "quiet period" or a time when he seems withdrawn. Is this natural? How do you account for it? What sequelae might you expect? What can you do about it?

THE DAY WORKER WITH VARICOSE VEINS—PATIENT STUDY

Mrs. Czerny is a rather obese, Hungarian woman in her late forties. She comes to the O.P.D. for treatment of a leg ulcer, which she states "broke open" about a year ago. She says that she has had varicose veins for years, and that, since the ulcer appeared, she has been bandaging the area with a clean beige nylon stocking. She felt this was helpful, because when she made the bandage tight, the drainage was less.

Mrs. Czerny's personal problems are very real. Her husband is a chronic alcoholic, who is unemployed. She has 5 small children, whom she supports by doing housework for hire 3 or 4 days a week. Recently she has not been able to work as many days as she finds necessary.

Her reaction to the physician's instructions to stay off her feet as much as possible is a hopeless "How can I, until the children are old enough to help?"

References

Ochsner, Kay, DeCamp, Hutton, and Balla: Newer concepts of blood coagulation with particular reference to postoperative thrombosis, Ann. Surg. **131**:652, 1950.
Stalker, L. K.: Varicose veins and their treatment, Am. J. Nursing **42**:638, 1942.
Williams, Dorothy E.: The care of the feet, Am. J. Nursing **41**:650, 1941.

Questions Relating to the Patient Study

1. A varicosity is

   a.____a saccular outpouching of a weakened vessel wall.
   b.____an inflammatory process which usually is localized to veins of the leg.
   c.____dilatation of veins resulting from valvular deficiency.
   d.____an ulceration in a thrombophlebitic process.
   e.____an arteriovenous outpouching usually found in peripheral circulation.

2. Varicose veins develop as a result of

   a.____sitting too much; this prevents muscular tissue from developing and supporting superficial veins of the leg.
   b.____congenital weakness of the veins.

    c._____increased intra-abdominal pressure as in pregnancy or pelvic tumor.

    d._____a poor functioning system of the deep veins; the superficial vessels have twice as much work to do.

3. Symptoms of varicose veins of the lower extremity are

    a._____easy fatigue of the leg; cramps in the leg at night; enlarged and tortuous superficial veins.

    b._____a throbbing sensation over the vessel; a saccular out-pouching of the vessel wall.

    c._____burning of the soles of the feet when standing in one position for a while; intermittent claudication.

    d._____venous stasis with secondary edema; lowered resistance to infection and trauma.

4. Conservative measures which assist Mrs. Czerny are to

    a._____wear circular garters which are able to hold the stockings snugly to the leg.

    b._____when sitting, rest the involved leg by crossing it over the good leg.

    c._____elevate the legs on a pillow as she relaxes several times a day.

    d._____immerse the legs in a warm (110°F.) saline bath for 20 minutes 3 times a day.

5. A sclerosing drug used for the injection of varicose veins

    a._____dissolves clots and prevents pooling of stagnant blood.

    b._____is a type of local anesthetic which relieves tensions of the veins.

    c._____strengthens the intima and aids in overcoming the tendency to relax.

    d._____produces a chemical thrombosis which closes the vein.

6. Since Mrs. Czerny must earn her livelihood by physical work, she feels she must be on her feet. Suggest ways in which she may "save her legs" in

    a. preparing meals.   d. cleaning a room.
    b. washing clothes.   e. marketing.
    c. ironing.   f. caring for a vegetable garden.

7. Mrs. Czerny cannot afford such items as sterile gauze and adhesive. Outline step-by-step directions which she can use in dressing her ulcer, which will make use of improvised dressings and means of sterilization and yet maintain aseptic technic.

Nursing Care of Patients with Other Disorders of the Circulatory System

1. Match the following:

   a. Raynaud's disease   (1)_____affects the arteries.
   b. Buerger's disease   (2)_____affects the veins.
   c. arteriosclerosis   (3)_____affects the lymphatics.
   d. elephantiasis   (4)_____affects the arteries and
   e. thrombophlebitis   the veins.

2. Elephantiasis (lymphedema) is a condition in which there is

   a._____an occlusion of the lymphatic vessels.
   b._____an acute inflammation of the lymph nodes.
   c._____a gradual enlargement of the lymph nodes.
   d._____a malignant disease invading the lymphatic system.

3. Surgery is usually the last resort in elephantiasis. The usual procedure is to

   a._____amputate the extremity.
   b._____ligate the superficial venous and lymphatic vessels.
   c._____carefully dissect and resect the involved sections of the lymphatic system.
   d._____remove the thickened fibrosed subcutaneous fat and much of the excess skin.

4. The chief postoperative instructions to a patient who has had surgery (Kondoléon) for elephantiasis is to

   a._____take precautions to avoid injury and infection.
   b._____move to a warm, dry climate.
   c._____give up the idea of ever bearing weight on the involved limb.
   d._____secure a satisfactory prosthesis.

5. Homan's sign is

   a._____the downward flexion of the great toe when the sole of the foot is stroked forcibly in a prescribed fashion.
   b._____the presence of a definite line of demarkation in an extremity between an area having sensation and one in which there is no feeling.
   c._____the puffing outward of a superficial vein; it is usually tortuous and bluish in color.
   d._____pain in the calf of the leg, aggravated when the foot is dorsiflexed.

6. The significance to the nurse of Homan's sign is that it should prompt her to report it to the surgeon immediately because it may suggest

a.———Buerger's disease; any massage or movement may instigate the rapid development of the process of necrosis.

b.———an aneurysm which is an outpouching of a weakened vessel; if it is untreated and in a place where there is great pressure it may rupture.

c.———a phlebothrombosis; massage may dislodge a blood clot which may endanger the life of the patient.

7. Protamine sulfate, Priscoline and epsilan phosphate are recent drugs which have been used for various vascular problems. Discuss their uses, merits and future potentialities.

8. Compare the two anticoagulants, heparin sodium and Dicumarol, under the following headings:

a. Cost.
b. Rapidity of action.
c. Duration of action.
d. Precautionary measures.
e. Mode of action (physiologic).

9. Frostbite and "immersion foot" are two conditions which have received considerable medical attention during the Korean conflict. How are they treated?

10. How would you give emergency treatment to an individual who has a frozen ear? What is the physiologic basis for your treatment?

THE GRIEVING MOTHER

Background Review Questions

1. Of the following substances, the one *not* normally present in the blood or other body fluids is

a.———fibrinogen.
b.———prothrombin.
c.———thromboplastin.
d.———ionized calcium.

2. Vitamin K is essential for the

a.———retraction of the clot which helps seal off ruptured blood vessels.
b.———production of bile salts by the liver.
c.———formation of thrombin from prothrombin.
d.———formation of prothrombin by the liver.

3. The *chief* source of thromboplastin is derived from

a.———fragmented leukocytes.
b.———fragmented platelets.
c.———injured tissue cells.
d.———specialized liver cells.

4. The normal action of thrombin is to bring about the

a.———conversion of fibrinogen to fibrin.
b.———release of thromboplastin.
c.———formation and maturation of platelets.
d.———production of prothrombin.

5. Thromboplastin is essential for

a.———the conversion of fibinogen to fibrin.
b.———the conversion of prothrombin to thrombin.

   c._____clot retraction.

   d._____platelet formation.

6. Substances such as sodium and potassium oxalate act as anticoagulants. They inhibit the clotting mechanism by

   a._____depressing the formation of prothrombin.

   b._____inhibiting the formation of fibrin.

   c._____inhibiting the formation of thrombin.

   d._____combining with and removing calcium ions from the blood.

7. The intrinsic factor essential for the formation of the anti-anemia principle is

   a._____found in many of the foods in the average diet.

   b._____formed by the cells of the reticulo-endothelial system.

   c._____produced by the cells lining the stomach.

   d._____absorbed in the stomach in the presence of hydrochloric acid.

8. Which one of the following best describes the fate of the iron derived from fragmented and worn-out erythrocytes?

   a._____It is deposited in bilirubin and excreted as bile.

   b._____It is stored in the liver and if present in excessive amounts leads to jaundice.

   c._____It is returned to the red bone marrow to be used again.

   d._____It is attracted to normoblasts where it is present in large amounts.

9. The anti-anemia principle is essential for

   a._____removal of damaged red blood cells from the blood.

   b._____maturation of the erythrocytes.

   c._____formation of the intrinsic factor.

   d._____absorption of iron from the digestive tract.

10. The anti-anemia principle normally is stored in the

   a._____duodenum.   c._____red bone marrow.

   b._____reticulo-endothelial sys-   d._____liver.
        tem.

11. In the normal adult, erythrocytes are produced by cells of the

   a._____spleen.   c._____red bone marrow.

   b._____lymph nodes.   d._____liver.

12. In the normal adult, granular leukocytes are produced by cells of the

   a._____reticulo-endothelial sys-   c._____liver.
        tem.   d._____red bone marrow.

   b._____lymph nodes.

13. Pernicious anemia is known also as

   a._____Addison's.   c._____Castle.

   b._____Minot.   d._____sickle-cell.

14. Pernicious anemia is classified on the basis of cell indices as

   a._____microcytic hypochromic.   d._____macrocytic.
   b._____normocytic hypochromic.   e._____aplastic.
   c._____microcytic normochromic.

15. Pernicious anemia is thought to be caused by a (an)

   a._____lack of intrinsic factor in the gastric juices.
   b._____loss of blood from hemorrhage.
   c._____iron-deficient diet.
   d._____malignancy of the blood-forming organs.

16. In order to establish a diagnosis of pernicious anemia it is necessary to

   a._____place the patient on therapy several weeks to determine empiric results.
   b._____complete the blood picture before therapy, before the picture has been obscured.

17. Extracts made from liver are given as therapy to patients with pernicious anemia because the liver

   a._____is the source of the extrinsic factor.
   b._____stores the anti-anemia principle.
   c._____is the source of the intrinsic factor.
   d._____produces prothrombin.

18. Erythrocytes will not develop to the mature state without the stimulus given the hemopoietic tissue by

   a._____vitamin K.   c._____the intrinsic factor.
   b._____the extrinsic factor.   d._____the anti-anemia principle.

19. Blood platelets are important in the clotting of the blood because they are a source of

   a._____ionized calcium.   c._____thromboplastin.
   b._____prothrombin.   d._____fibrinogen.

20. The anticoagulant heparin acts rapidly after its entrance into the body because it

   a._____precipitates ionized calcium.
   b._____prevents the liver from forming prothrombin.
   c._____prevents the conversion of prothrombin to thrombin.
   d._____prevents the conversion of thrombin to fibrin.

21. If a laboratory report on a blood study is returned stating that "band cells" are present, you should know that this means

   a._____immature neutrophils.   c._____immature monocytes.
   b._____immature erythrocytes.   d._____fragmented erythrocytes.

22. The normal individual living for several weeks at a high altitude will develop a (an)

    a._____anemia, because a lowered oxygen concentration of blood de-
presses the red bone marrow.

    b._____anemia, because an increase in oxygen concentration of the
blood depresses the hemopoietic tissue.

    c._____polycythemia, because a lowered oxygen concentration of the
blood stimulates the red bone marrow.

    d._____polycythemia, because an increased oxygen concentration of
the blood stimulates the hemopoietic tissue.

23. The site of production of polymorphonuclear leukocytes is the

    a._____pulp of the spleen.   c._____nodules of the lymph nodes.
    b._____sinusoids of the liver.   d._____red bone marrow.

24. If a biopsy is to be done on an adult, the purpose of which is to examine
a living sample of erythrocyte-producing tissue, which one of the following structures most likely would be used?

    a._____liver.   c._____spleen.
    b._____lymph node.   d._____sternum.

25. Write in the following blanks the values which would make a normal
differential white count:

    a. neutrophils_____
    b. eosinophils_____
    c. basophils_____
    d. monocytes_____
    e. lymphocytes_____
    f. band cells_____

26. Write in the following blanks the normal values for the following blood
constituents:

    a. erythrocytes _4-4.5 r/c mn_
    b. leukocytes _5-9000 c/mm_
    c. hemoglobin _11-13 GM /1000_
    d. acetone_____
    e. bilirubin_____
    f. glucose _80-123 mg/1000_

27. Place the number of the phrase in the right-hand column which defines the following terms in the space provided:

    a._7_leukopenia.   (1) tumor of the lymphatic system.
    b._9_leukocyte.   (2) reduction of lymphocytes.
    c._11_leukoma.   (3) increased white blood cells.
    d._7_leukoplakia.   (4) malformed and oversized red blood
    e._3_leukocytosis.   cells.
    f._14_lymphocytosis.   (5) abnormally large red blood cells.
    g._2_lymphocytopenia. (6) poikilocytes in the blood.
    h._10_lymphocyte.   (7) white patches in the mouth.

i. _6_ poikilocytosis.
j. _4_ poikilocyte.
k. _8_ anisocytosis.
l. _13_ anisochromia.
m. _5_ macrocytes.
n. _16_ erythrocyte.

(8) inequality in size of the red blood cells.
(9) white blood cells.
(10) variety of white blood cells.
(11) opacity of the cornea.
(12) abnormally shaped blood platelets.
(13) variation in color of the red blood cells.
(14) excess lymphocytes.
(15) excess lymphoblasts.
(16) red blood cells.
(17) reduced white blood cells.

THE GRIEVING MOTHER—PATIENT STUDY

Mrs. Archer, a 55-year-old housewife, was admitted to the medical ward on a stretcher. She was very pale, and so weak that she was scarcely able to move her extremities.

Mrs. Archer had been comparatively healthy until about 6 months ago. At that time her only son was killed in a motor accident, and since then Mrs. Archer has grieved constantly. She has avoided seeing her friends, has neglected her personal appearance and has eaten indifferently. She sought medical advice only recently, upon the insistence of her husband, when she complained of numbness of her fingers.

The physician sent her to the hospital for diagnosis, with the impression of anemia.

Following physical examination, extensive blood work and a gastric analysis, the diagnosis of pernicious anemia was made.

The following orders were written:

Bed rest.
High-caloric, high-vitamin, soft diet.
Liver extract, 1 unit daily.
Dilute hydrochloric acid 4 cc. t.i.d.
Vitamin B_{12} 1 microgram daily i.m.
Special mouth care t.i.d.

Mrs. Archer was quite querulous and difficult for several weeks. However, as her blood picture changed in response to therapy, she also seemed to have a completely new outlook on life. She became less irritable and nervous, enjoyed visitors and demonstrated a mild interest in her trays.

After 4 weeks she had responded well to treatment and was discharged with instructions to return to the clinic in 1 week.

References

Blank, Mildred: Nursing care in Hodgkin's disease, Am. J. Nursing 48:563, 1948.

Fouts, Paul J.: Neurological conditions in pernicious anemia, Am. J. Nursing 49:523, 1949.

Hall, B. E., et al.: Vitamin B_{12} and coordination exercises for combined degeneration of the spinal cord in pernicious anemia, J.A.M.A. **141**:257, 1949.

Heinle, Robert W.: An evaluation of folic acid: a critical appraisal of the effectiveness of this vitamin in the treatment of macrocytic anemias, Am. J. Nursing **48**:381, 1948.

Mitchell, Helen S.: How vitamins function, Am. J. Nursing **51**:96, 1951.

Spies, Tod D.: Effect of folic acid on persons with macrocytic anemia in relapse, J.A.M.A. **130**:474, 1946.

————et al.: Tentative appraisal of vitamin B₁₂ as a therapeutic agent, J.A.M.A. **139**:521, 1949.

West, Randolph, and Reisner, Edward H., Jr.: Treatment of pernicious anemia with crystalline vitamin B₁₂, Am. J. Med. **5**:643, 1949.

Questions Relating to the Patient Study

1. If Mrs. Archer presents the usual clinical picture of pernicious anemia, the following findings would be expected:

   a. Physical examination and history:

   (1) Mouth:
   (a) normal color.
   (b) smooth red tongue, soreness.
   (c) white patches.
   (2) Skin:
   (a) faint yellow tinge.
   (b) cyanosis.
   (c) waxy pallor.
   (3) G.I. tract:
   (a) nausea, diarrhea, anorexia.
   (b) occult blood, constipation, anorexia.
   (4) Neurologic:
   (a) numbness, tingling, paresthesia.
   (b) tremor, twitching, nervousness.
   (5) Mental:
   (a) lassitude, confusion, depression.
   (b) exhilaration, restlessness, excitability.

   b. Laboratory examination:

   (1) Blood picture:
   (a) reduced red count, low color index, macrocytes.
   (b) reduced red count, high color index, macrocytes.
   (c) reduced red count, high color index, large number reticulocytes.
   (2) Gastric analysis:
   (a) fasting
   (1) HCl acid 0
   (2) HCl acid+
   (b) post-histamine
   (1) HCl acid 0
   (2) HCl acid+

2. Mrs. Archer's depression probably is

    a.＿＿＿due entirely to her son's death.
    b.＿＿＿common in patients with pernicious anemia.
    c.＿＿＿indicative of neurotic tendencies, aggravated by her son's death.

3. To prepare Mrs. Archer for the gastric analysis the nurse should

    a.＿＿＿omit breakfast.
    b.＿＿＿give a fat-free breakfast.
    c.＿＿＿give the regular breakfast.

4. The purpose of the gastric analysis is to

    a.＿＿＿determine the motility of   c.＿＿＿examine for bleeding.
         the G.I. tract.   d.＿＿＿determine free and total
    b.＿＿＿examine the gastric mu-   hydrochloric acid.
         cosa.

5. Drugs used during a gastric analysis are

    a.＿＿＿7% alcohol per tube.
    b.＿＿＿histamine phosphate subcutaneously.
    c.＿＿＿barium sulfate orally.
    d.＿＿＿tetraiodophenolphthalein sodium intravenously.

6. If Mrs. Archer presents the usual symptoms, you would expect her to find the following types of foods unpalatable:

    a.＿＿＿bland.   e.＿＿＿soft.
    b.＿＿＿acid.   f.＿＿＿chewy.
    c.＿＿＿hot.   g.＿＿＿spicy.
    d.＿＿＿cool.

7. The nurse should anticipate that Mrs. Archer will be

    a.＿＿＿sensitive to cold, requiring the use of flannel gowns, blankets, etc.
    b.＿＿＿sensitive to heat, requiring cotton gowns, fans, icebags, etc.

8. The most satisfactory type of mouth care for Mrs. Archer would be

    a.＿＿＿vigorous massage of the gums with a stiff toothbrush.
    b.＿＿＿use of a highly astringent mouthwash.
    c.＿＿＿gentle cleansing with cotton swabs.
    d.＿＿＿usual care with brush and dentifrice.

9. The purpose of dilute HCl acid for Mrs. Archer is to

    a.＿＿＿supply an intrinsic factor which is lacking.
    b.＿＿＿supply an extrinsic factor which is lacking.
    c.＿＿＿facilitate the absorption of vitamins from the G.I. tract.
    d.＿＿＿alleviate gastric symptoms.

10. To administer dilute HCl acid to Mrs. Archer the nurse should

    a._____dilute with ½ glass of water.
    b._____dilute with 1 ounce of water.
    c._____add no water since the drug is already diluted.

11. A drinking tube is used with dilute HCl acid in order to

    a._____make the drug more palatable.
    b._____prevent staining of the teeth.
    c._____prevent erosions of the mouth.

12. Mr. Archer has expressed concern about his wife's depression. The nurse can best reassure him by

    a._____advising him to help his wife forget their son.
    b._____telling him that depression is common in this condition and probably will disappear with medical treatment.
    c._____advising him to seek psychiatric help.

13. When Mrs. Archer leaves the hospital she should understand that

    a._____she will need treatment for several weeks.
    b._____she will need treatment for the rest of her life.
    c._____she must be aware of symptoms of recurrence and seek treatment at that time.
    d._____if she eats an adequate diet she will have no further difficulties.

14. Symptoms which would indicate progressive neurologic deterioration would include

    a._____incontinence.   c._____loss of memory.
    b._____excitement.   d._____paralysis.

Questions for Discussion and Student Projects

1. Mrs. Archer has been in the hospital for a period, has responded well to therapy, and is now ready to be discharged. What are the important points in regard to treatment that the nurse should have taught her while she was hospitalized?
2. How would you convince Mrs. Archer on discharge that she should return to the clinic for treatment?
3. Discuss the use of preparations of liver extracts and vitamin B_{12} for Mrs. Archer. How are they administered? What are the evidences of sensitivity?
4. Estimate the approximate weekly cost of the maintenance dose of the necessary drugs for Mrs. Archer.
5. Plan a week's diet, specifying the types of food Mrs. Archer should have. Discuss the relationship of diet to this disease condition.
6. Prepare a hematologic chart of a patient receiving treatment for pernicious anemia in your hospital, showing the blood picture on admission and daily changes. Compare these findings with the normal blood picture. Trace the changes in the patient's emotional and physical responses. Do you see any relationship between these responses and the blood picture?

Nursing Care of Patients with Other Diseases of the Blood

Questions for Discussion and Student Projects

1. Discuss the prevention of anemia of iron deficiency.
2. Discuss the management of a patient with lymphoma and with leukemia. What types of disorders are included in these categories? What encouragement may be offered to the patient and his family? What provisions may be made for chronic care? What community facilities and resources are available for these patients?
3. Discuss the nurse's responsibility for the care of a patient suffering from purpura, hemophilia and prothrombin deficiency.
4. What symptoms would lead you to believe a patient was experiencing untoward effects from x-ray or radium therapy?
5. Discuss the use of radioactive isotopes in the treatment of neoplastic disease. What are the therapeutic and toxic effects? When do they appear and what is their significance and value of treatment? Discuss the results of experimental studies of nitrogen mustard and folic acid antagonists. Review clinical use, dosage, therapeutic complications and importance of treatments.

Section 3. Nursing Care of Patients with Disorders of the Digestive System*

STUDY SUGGESTIONS: Before beginning the study of this Section, the student will find it helpful to

A. Review
1. Anatomy and physiology: the autonomic nervous system, the digestive system.
2. Nursing arts: colonic irrigation, enemata, gastric suction, intravenous infusion.
3. Microbiology: *Bacillus shiga, Endameba histolytica,* virus.
4. Physics: subatmospheric pressure, suction; suggested reference: Flitter, Hessel H.: Introduction to Physics in Nursing, pp. 89–94, St. Louis, Mosby, 1948.

B. Study
1. In medical nursing texts: units on diseases of the alimentary and biliary tracts, nonbacterial infections of the intestine.
2. In nutrition texts: diet therapy for constipation, cholecystitis, diarrhea, peptic ulcer, ulcerative colitis.
3. In surgical nursing texts: surgery of the alimentary tract.

C. Read the additional References listed before attempting to answer the questions relating to each patient study.

THE WOMAN WITH THE SORE TONGUE

Background Review Questions

1. Digestion is initiated in the mouth in the following manner. Saliva containing

   a._____ptyalin begins the digestion of starches.
   b._____pepsin begins the digestion of sugars.
   c._____pepsin begins the digestion of proteins.
   d._____ptyalin begins the digestion of sugars.

2. The only substances absorbed from the stomach are

   a._____alcohol and small amounts of glucose.
   b._____proteases and peptones.
   c._____fatty acids and glycerol.
   d._____amino acids.

3. Which one of the following has an inhibitory action on both gastric motility and secretion of gastric juice?

   a._____stimulation of the vagus nerve.
   b._____starchy foods.

* Conditions of the gastrointestinal tract peculiar to children are considered in the pediatric section.

   c._____foods rich in fat content.

   d._____meats and other foods high in protein content.

4. The most potent single factor involved in stimulating the pancreas to secrete pancreatic juice is

   a._____the hormone cholecystokinin liberated by the cells of the duodenum upon arrival of fats within the duodenum.

   b._____stimulation of the sympathetic outflow to the abdominal viscera.

   c._____the hormone secretin liberated by the cells of the duodenum upon stimulation of the acid chyme.

   d._____the arrival of bile within the duodenum, initiating a reflex stimulating the pancreas.

5. The cardiac sphincter normally is opened only by

   a._____liquids.

   b._____waves of peristalsis.

   c._____stimulation reaching it via the splanchnic nerves.

   d._____pressure of food in the esophagus.

6. An over-stimulation of the vagal branches to the stomach would result in

   a._____increased gastric motility and hypersecretion of gastric juice.

   b._____decreased gastric motility and hypersecretion of gastric juice.

   c._____hyposecretion of gastric juice and increased gastric motility.

   d._____decreased motility and hyposecretion of gastric juice.

7. Which of the following chemicals acts to stimulate secretion of gastric juice?

   a._____Alcohol and histamine.   c._____Glucose and fatty acids.

   b._____Alcohol and glucose.   d._____Fatty acids and histamine.

8. The functions of the stomach are described most accurately by:

   a._____The stomach changes food into chyme, hydrolyzes some fat into fatty acids and glycerol, converts glucose to glycogen.

   b._____The stomach changes food into chyme, converts glucose to glycogen, absorbs iron and rejects any excess amount.

   c._____The stomach hydrolyzes some fat into fatty acids, secretes pepsin, changes food into chyme.

   d._____The stomach converts glucose to glycogen, absorbs iron and rejects any excess amount, secretes gastric protease.

9. The acid factor seems to account for the incidence of peptic ulcer in the

   a._____greater curvature of the stomach.

   b._____lesser curvature of the stomach.

   c._____proximal duodenum.

   d._____distal duodenum.

   e._____magenstrasse.

10. Factors leading to hyperacidity in the stomach are

   a._____overactivity of the vagus.
   b._____an unstimulated vagus.
   c._____an overly active individual.
   d._____failure to neutralize excessive acid by duodenal regurgitation.

11. That the acid factor is strongly associated with peptic ulcer is suggested by the

   a._____absence of peptic ulcer in people with hyperchlorhydria.
   b._____peptic ulcer of the jejunum adjacent to the stoma of an unsuccessful gastro-enterostomy, with high gastric acidity.
   c._____high incidence of ulcer along the anterior wall of the distal duodenum.
   d._____cure of peptic ulcer by antiacid treatment.

12. Alcohol has a pronounced local action upon gastric mucosa,

   a._____stimulating it to secrete gastric juice.
   b._____inhibiting the production of gastric juice.
   c._____stimulating gastric motility.
   d._____inhibiting gastric motility.

13. Cancer of the stomach and pernicious anemia characteristically are accompanied by

   a._____hyperchlorhydria.
   b._____achlorhydria.
   c._____a lowered prothrombin level of the blood.
   d._____a lack of absorption of vitamin K.

14. Ulcer patients usually secrete

   a._____gastric juice rich in mucin and low in acid content.
   b._____scanty amounts of gastric juice of low acidity.
   c._____excessive quantities of gastric juice of relatively high acidity.
   d._____gastric juice of very low acidity.

15. Symptoms of hunger are due to

   a._____depletion of the body's reserve food supply because of starvation.
   b._____powerful peristaltic waves passing over the empty stomach.
   c._____the thought and odor of food an individual has learned to like especially well.
   d._____peristaltic waves passing over the empty small intestine.

16. One cause of vomiting is a lowering of the threshold of excitability of the vomiting center in the medulla so that stimuli entering the medulla which normally would have no stimulating effect upon the cells may result in exciting them. One important cause of this lowered threshold is

   a._____an increased carbon dioxide supply to the medulla.
   b._____a decreased oxygen supply to the medulla.

c.____an excessive secretion of the hormone adrenalin
d.____eating food contaminated by toxic substances.

17. When vomiting becomes excessive, the result may be

a.____hypochloremia.
b.____lowering of the blood non-protein nitrogen.
c.____alkalemia.
d.____acidosis.
e.____ketosis.
f.____azotemia.

18. When protein has been lost from the body or there has been an insufficient intake of protein, edema occurs. This is due to changes of pressure. Development of an edema is indicated by

a.____hydrostatic pressure at the arterial end of a capillary is 35 mm. of mercury; protein osmotic pressure is 22 mm. of mercury; blood pressure at the venous side of a capillary is 22 mm. of mercury.
b.____hydrostatic pressure at the arterial end of a capillary is 35 mm. of mercury; blood pressure at the venous end of a capillary is 15 mm. of mercury; protein osmotic pressure is 12 mm. of mercury.
c.____hydrostatic pressure at the arterial end of a capillary is 22 mm. of mercury; protein osmotic pressure is 35 mm. of mercury; hydrostatic pressure at the venous end of a capillary is 12 mm. of mercury.

19. Interstitial fluid contains large amounts of

a.____sodium.   d.____magnesium.
b.____bicarbonate.   e.____chlorides.
c.____protein.   f.____phosphorus.

20. Wound healing is favored by

a.____alkalosis.   b.____acidosis.

21. The amount of salt in 1,000 cc. of normal saline is 9.0 Gm. The average patient requires

a.____1–2 Gm. of salt daily.   d.____6–8 Gm. of salt daily.
b.____2–4 Gm. of salt daily.   e.____8–10 Gm. of salt daily.
c.____5–6 Gm. of salt daily.

22. The amount of fluid secreted by the gastro-intestinal tract in 24 hours is approximately

c.____3,000–4,000 cc.
a.____1,000–2,000 cc.   d.____4,000–6,000 cc.
b.____2,000–3,000 cc.   e.____7,000–8,000 cc.

23. The basic elements of proteins are

a.____hydrogen.	f.____potassium.
b.____oxygen.	g.____phosphorus.
c.____carbon.	h.____nitrogen.
d.____magnesium.	i.____sodium.
e.____sulfur.	

24. "Complete" proteins may be obtained from

a.____cereals.	d.____nuts.
b.____legumes.	e.____cheese.
c.____fowl.	f.____fruit.

25. In a surgical patient, hypoproteinemia results in

a.____impaired prothrombin formation, weakened blood capillaries, delayed wound healing.

b.____atrophy of epithelial tissues, infections of mouth and salivary glands, gastro-intestinal infection.

c.____anorexia, vomiting, deficient absorption of tissues, serious liver damage.

d.____peripheral edema, visceral edema, inhibition of gastro-intestinal motility, interference with wound healing.

THE WOMAN WITH THE SORE TONGUE—PATIENT STUDY

Miss Flosser, a 51-year-old retired office worker, was admitted to the hospital complaining of difficulty in swallowing and a lump on her tongue.

Until her present illness, she has been living with two elderly aunts in the aunts' home. She has two married brothers and a sister who is in a convent. She seldom has visitors, but quickly rationalizes by saying, "Well, you know, they're busy with their families." Miss Flosser is concerned about her post-hospital care, knowing that her aunts will not be able to help her.

Four months prior to her admission, Miss Flosser discovered a sore on the right side of her tongue. Later, at the same site, an ulceration appeared; this was painful.

One month ago, she noted pain over the anterior part of the right ear and also beneath the right jaw. It was sharp and radiated to the right temporal region. She could not take anything but fluids. A weight loss of 15 pounds was noted.

When a biopsy confirmed the diagnosis of epidermoid carcinoma, Miss Flosser had radiation treatment. This was followed by full mouth dental extraction. While waiting for the sockets to heal, her tongue increased in size so that she had difficulty in closing her mouth, eating, drinking and talking. A palliative hemi-glossectomy was done. However, it failed to relieve her of much discomfort. Because of continued difficulty with eating and an added problem of dyspnea, tracheotomy as well as gastrostomy was done. Miss Flosser was "willing to face anything for relief." She tolerated the surgery well and showed some improvement. Her case is one of terminal carcinoma, and she has only a few months to live.

References

Clarke, Carl D.: Facial and body prosthesis, Am. J. Nursing 48:82, 1948.
Flood, Josephine A.: Nursing in cancer of the mouth, Am. J. Nursing 43:536, 1943.
Miller, Charles J.: Cancer of the mouth, Am. J. Nursing 43:531, 1943.

Questions Relating to the Patient Study

1. Individuals with cancer of the tongue usually give a history of

   a._____drinking hot coffee.   c._____sucking sourball candy.
   b._____possessing a jagged tooth.   d._____chewing tobacco.

2. Radiation therapy for oral cancer may produce the following symptoms in Miss Flosser:

   a._____excessive watery saliva.   d._____serous exudate.
   b._____lack of saliva ("cotton   e._____difficult swallowing.
   mouth").   f._____leukoplakia.
   c._____ropy, sticky saliva.

3. Skin which is irritated from x-ray treatment should be cared for by

   a._____washing with soap and water frequently.
   b._____the application of dry sterile dressing fastened with adhesive.
   c._____cleansing every 4 or 6 hours with cotton dipped in mineral oil.
   d._____doing nothing, for the condition may become worse.

4. Following oral surgery, Miss Flosser must be watched carefully for signs of respiratory distress. This is manifested by

   a._____audible congestion of the upper trachea.
   b._____mild cyanosis.
   c._____excessive drooling.
   d._____edematous tongue.

5. Following mouth surgery, a patient occasionally returns from the O.R. with the tongue sutured to the lip (one stitch). This may mean that

   a._____the surgeon has forgotten to remove the stitch.
   b._____edema of the tongue is expected.
   c._____there is danger of obstruction to the airway.
   d._____this will inhibit tumor growth.

6. Following a hemi-glossectomy, Miss Flosser

   a._____will not be able to talk.
   b._____will have no speech handicap.
   c._____will lisp.
   d._____may stutter.
   e._____will have some impairment which may be overcome easily.

7. The most satisfactory mouth irrigation for Miss Flosser is

   a.____sodium bicarbonate (1T to 1 quart of water), temp. 115°F., irrigating can 2 feet above the mouth.
   b.____normal saline solution, temp. 125°F., irrigating can 18 inches above the mouth.
   c.____equal parts of hydrogen peroxide and water, temp. 105°F., irrigating can 1 foot above the mouth.
   d.____KMnO₄ 1:10,000, temp. 120°F., irrigating can 3 feet above the mouth.

8. To help Miss Flosser most successfully with her problem of constant salivation, the nurse should

   a.____administer atropine sulfate to dry secretions.
   b.____insert cotton dental rolls in the mouth to absorb secretions.
   c.____insert a gauze wick in the corner of the mouth to drain secretions into a basin.
   d.____encourage her to swallow excess secretions to prevent undue fluid loss.

9. Indications that a nasal feeding catheter is being passed correctly are

   a.____a wheezing sound, the tube is seen in the throat on the side of insertion, bubbles appear when the catheter end is submerged in water.
   b.____no wheezing sound, the tube is seen in the throat on the side of insertion, bubbles do not appear when the catheter is submerged in water.

10. When Miss Flosser has her gastrostomy feeding, water should be

    a.____always given before, but never after, the feeding.
    b.____never given before, but always after, the feeding.
    c.____always given before and after a feeding.
    d.____never given.

11. When giving a liquid feeding to Miss Flosser via her gastrostomy tube, it is best to

    a.____use a syringe; a steady force on the plunger will hasten the procedure.
    b.____instill about 10 cc. at a time so that the reception of the liquid is not shocking to the stomach.
    c.____allow the fluid to flow by gravity; this should take about 15 to 20 minutes.

12. Since the normal phenomenon of swallowing does not precede the entrance of food into the stomach (in gastrostomy) the following discomforts may be noted occasionally:

    a.____feeling of fullness.   d.____regurgitation.
    b.____hiccough.   e.____nausea.
    c.____belch.

Questions for Discussion and Student Projects

1. From your knowledge of Miss Flosser, would you think it wise to tell her she has cancer? Support your views.
2. What is the significance of the pain Miss Flosser experienced near her right ear and jaw?
3. What symptoms would you expect to note as the malignancy spreads? In what possible ways does such a lesion metastasize?
4. Assuming that Miss Flosser is your patient, how would you arrange for posthospital care in your community?
5. Since Miss Flosser will now be on liquid foods, what help can you give her to prevent diarrhea? (This is a common problem with older people who are on liquids exclusively.)
6. A soft, bland diet usually is recommended for a patient with a gastric difficulty. When an individual has had trauma or surgery of the mouth, the same diet is prescribed. List the foods which the latter patient may have but which are restricted for the patient with gastric difficulty.
7. Obtain the formula for gastrostomy feeding which your physician and/or dietition recommend. From the ingredients of the formula, ascertain the amount of the following in a 24-hour quantity of formula:

   a.____calories.
   b.____protein.
   c.____fat.
   d.____calcium.
   e.____iron.

   f.____vitamin A.
   g.____thiamine.
   h.____riboflavin.
   i.____niacin.
   j.____ascorbic acid.

   Do these amounts meet the needs of an adult? Discuss.
8. Secure the prices of various food blenders and liquefiers. Describe the advantages and disadvantages of each type which would be helpful to Miss Flosser.
9. "The older person is inclined to think that any unusual sore in the mouth is a canker sore and that it will clear up within a few days."* What are the dangers of such a belief? What can be done to provide better information?

Nursing Care of Patients with Other Mouth Disorders

1. Ludwig's angina is an infection of the

   a.____heart.
   b.____gums.
   c.____lips.
   d.____tongue.

   e.____larynx.
   f.____roof of the mouth.
   g.____floor of the mouth.

* Newton, Kathleen: Geriatric Nursing, p. 161, St. Louis, Mosby, 1950.

2. Ludwig's angina is an infection characterized by the classical symptoms of

    a._____earache, toothache, face ache, weight loss.

    b._____hard, boardlike swelling in the sublingual region, edematous tongue, dyspnea, general toxicity.

    c._____swelling, soreness and bleeding gums, hemorrhage under the mucous membranes of the palate.

    d._____redness and tenderness of the gums, a coated and slightly swollen tongue, salivation.

3. Another name for Ludwig's angina is

    a._____Vincent's angina.   d._____pyorrhea.

    b._____stomatitis.   e._____canker sores.

    c._____thrush.   f._____cellulitis.

4. The use of vitamin A preoperatively is important in potential mouth surgical patients in order to prevent

    a._____keratinization.   c._____abnormal calcification of

    b._____hypovitaminosis.   bone.

                                            d._____anorexia.

5. Surgical "mumps" is

    a._____a swelling of lymph glands which happens to occur when a patient has had major surgery.

    b._____an infection of the parotid gland brought about by inactivity and subsequent invasion by mouth micro-organisms.

    c._____a condition which can be compared to Hodgkin's disease, although not malignant.

    d._____an infection of the sublingual gland owing to the presence of pathogenic organisms in the blood stream.

6. Treatment recommended to prevent surgical "mumps" is

    a._____chewing gum or sucking hard candy.

    b._____no food or fluids by mouth.

    c._____sucking penicillin lozenges.

    d._____rinsing the mouth with equal parts of glycerin and water q. 3 hours.

7. The most satisfactory way of caring for a sutured incision of the lip is to

    a._____apply a dry sterile dressing, holding it in place with adhesive.

    b._____swab with compound benzoin tincture and apply a dressing and adhesive.

    c._____swab with compound benzoin tincture, allow it to dry; do not apply dressing.

8. Lip wounds heal easily because of

    a._____great opportunity for contact with air.

    b._____the inherent qualities of epithelial tissue.

    c._____acceleration of the process from moistening by the tongue.

    d._____adequacy of blood supply.

9. Proper treatment of incision of a lip includes

    a._____a medicated dressing to inhibit possible infection.

    b._____a dry, sterile dressing to keep the wound clean.

    c._____no dressing since it might harbor organisms.

10. The highest incidence of lip cancer occurs in

    a._____young females.   c._____young males.

    b._____elderly females.   d._____elderly males.

11. Factors which seem to have clinical significance in the etiology of cancer of the lip are

    a._____thumb sucking.   d._____long exposure to sunlight.

    b._____pipe smoking.   e._____indelible lipstick.

    c._____tobacco chewing.

12. External mouth and chin dressings can be kept in place and removed easily by using

    a._____Montgomery adhesive straps.

    b._____Barton dressing, using 2-inch gauze bandage.

    c._____sterile cotton mask.

    d._____elastic bandage, 3-inch width.

Questions for Discussion and Student Projects

1. Of what value is a dentifrice which is "ammoniated" and which also contains "chlorophyll"?
2. What is the effect of fluorine on the prevention of dental caries? How can it be administered effectively? How can a community supply this chemical to its citizens? How expensive is it? Are there any untoward effects?
3. Investigate the provisions in your community for dental care of

    a. pregnant women in the prenatal clinic.

    b. preschool children.

    c. adults.

    d. hospitalized adults.

    Are these provisions adequate? If not, how could more adequate care be provided?
4. If a patient is to have procaine anesthesia for the first time, a small wheal should be raised on one arm by injecting 2 or 3 drops of 2 per cent procaine, to determine any reaction. Why is this test done? What reaction would indicate that such an anesthesia is safe? What reaction would contraindicate this anesthesia?
5. Outline a method for minimizing the inevitable psychologic trauma which results when an individual has a disfiguring condition of the face. Include

Preparation of family.   Possibilities of plastic surgery.

Availability of prosthetics, cosmetics, etc. Control of odors.

THE TRUCK DRIVER WITH INDIGESTION—PATIENT STUDY

A 22-year-old Italian, Mr. Pasha, was admitted for diagnosis. He stated that he had had persistent, gnawing pains in the gastric region for "as long as I can remember. Oh, ever since I was 18." These pains were relieved by a patent ("stomach") medicine and he thought nothing of them until a friend told him that it might be cancer. Therefore he came to the clinic.

Mr. Pasha is a truck driver and works for a cross-country moving company. He was born in Italy and moved here with his family when he was 12 years old.

Mr. Pasha is a devout Roman Catholic. His wife, a very attractive girl, is of no particular religious faith. "That doesn't bother me, except I don't know what we'll do if we have kids." He seems extremely proud of his wife, but "I have to watch her—she's so darned pretty—and I'm away a lot."

His life is very irregular, as he is on the road so much. This he enjoys as "I can't bear just sitting around." When questioned about his habits, he states that he snatches a bite at hot-dog stands, catches naps in the truck, and smokes constantly when driving. He seldom drinks "hard" liquor but likes wine with his meals. His wife has learned to do Italian cooking like his mother.

The patient was placed on bed rest, had a routine physical examination, G.I. x-ray series and gastric analysis. Following the examinations he was put on milk and cream every 2 hours when awake, phenobarbital gr. ¼ t.i.d. and gr. 1½ h.s.

Mr. Pasha, although co-operative, complained about the "strictness" of his treatment as "I'm not that sick." After 10 days of the milk and cream diet, the physician left the following order:

> Gradually increase diet to modified Sippy regimen.
> Belladonna tincture 10 minims t.i.d.
> Allow up and about.

References

Beck, Sr. M. Berenice: The Nurse, Handmaid of the Divine Physician, Philadelphia, Lippincott, 1945.

Bertram, Harold F.: Nonoperative treatment of perforated duodenal ulcer, Ann. Surg. 132:1075, 1950.

Co Tui, et al.: The hyperalimentation treatment of peptic ulcer with amino acids and dextrimaltose, Gastroenterology 5:5, 1945.

Dragstedt and Woodward: Appraisal of vagotomy for peptic ulcer after seven years, J.A.M.A. 145:795, 1951.

Merrill, I., and O'Neal, M.: Nursing care of peptic ulcer, Am. J. Nursing 46:520, 1946.

Mittelmann, Wolf, and Scharf: Emotions and gastroduodenal function: Experimental studies on patients with gastritis, duodenitis, and peptic ulcer, Psychosomatic Med. 4:5, 1942.

Portis, Sidney A.: The clinical significance of emotional disturbances affecting the stomach, duodenum, and biliary tract, Psych. Med. VI:71, 1944.

Questions Relating to the Patient Study

1. In order to prepare Mr. Pasha for a G.I. series the nurse should

   a.____force fluids during the night, giving nothing by mouth after 6 A.M.
   b.____force fluids until the patient is called to x-ray.
   c.____give nothing by mouth after midnight.
   d.____give the usual fluids and foods before x-ray.

2. During the G.I. series the patient is given

   a.____intravenous dye.   c.____histamine phosphate sub-
   b.____barium sulfate by mouth.   cutaneously.
                                     d.____glucose intravenously.

3. Unless preventive measures are taken, Mr. Pasha may, as a result of the G.I. series, have

   a.____nausea and vomiting.   c.____urticaria.
   b.____constipation.   d.____diarrhea.

4. Mr. Pasha's gastric analysis would be expected to show

   a.____free acid in gastric juice.
   b.____absence of free acid in gastric juice.

5. The primary purpose of phenobarbital for Mr. Pasha is to

   a.____prevent pain.   c.____decrease tension.
   b.____decrease peristalsis.   d.____improve his appetite.

6. The action of belladonna tincture is

   a.____parasympathetic blocking. c.____sympathetic stimulation.
   b.____parasympathetic stimula- d.____sympathetic blocking.
   tion.

7. The action of belladonna tincture desired for Mr. Pasha is

   a.____decrease of secretions.   d.____mild catharsis.
   b.____increase of secretions.   e.____sedation.
   c.____relaxation of the muscles
   of the G.I. tract.

8. Symptoms of toxicity of belladonna include

   a.____dryness of the throat and flesh, dilated pupils, rapid pulse, excitement.
   b.____dryness of the throat, pallor, constricted pupils, slow pulse, depression.
   c.____weak rapid pulse, cold clammy skin, depression, depressed respirations.
   d.____weak slow pulse, flushed skin, nausea, dilated pupils.

9. The dosage of 10 minims of belladonna tincture is equal to

   a.____1.5 cc.   c.____0.6 cc.   e.____0.15 cc.
   b.____1 cc.   d.____0.06 cc.

10. There are certain objectives of dietary treatment for peptic ulcer. Match the objectives listed in column I with the dietary descriptions listed in column II.

              I   II

a._____Omission of chemically irritating foods.
    (1) Low-residue diet.

b._____Neutralization of gastric HCl.
    (2) Bland diet.
    (3) Frequent small feedings.

c._____Prevention of distention of the stomach.
    (4) High CHO diet.
    (5) Use of meat extractives.

d._____Reduction of stomach motility.
    (6) High fat intake.
    (7) Alkaline-ash diet.

e._____Omission of mechanically irritating foods.
    (8) High-protein diet.

f._____Inhibition of HCl secretion.

g._____Promotion of healing of ulcerated area.

11. Of the following accessories found on a hospital tray, one should remove from Mr. Pasha's tray the

a._____salt shaker.
    d._____butter (1 pat).

b._____pepper shaker.
    e._____bread (1 slice).

c._____sugar bowl.
    f._____cream pitcher.

12. Check the following dietary practices which apply to the treatment of Mr. Pasha:

a._____To omit non-essential foods high in calories.

b._____To serve foods at frequent intervals.

c._____To serve foods which combine quickly with the free HCl acid.

d._____To limit the intake of concentrated sources of sugars.

e._____To serve all the essential food in quantities to meet the minimum requirements of all nutrients.

f._____To serve small amounts at any one time.

g._____To serve foods which total in calories more than the patient's requirements.

h._____To avoid serving foods which will have mechanical, chemical or psychic stimulation.

13. The chief advantage of Amphojel over other antacids is that it

a._____tastes better.
    c._____is less apt to cause alkalosis.

b._____is less expensive.
    d._____does not have to be taken so frequently.

14. Complications which can occur following a spreading chronic peptic ulcer are

a._____cicatrization with stenosis of the pylorus.

b._____perigastric adhesions.

    c._____perforation with local or general peritonitis.
    d._____erosion of vessels with hematemesis and melena.

15. Milk and cream are given as frequently as every 2 hours in order to

    a._____assure adequate caloric intake.
    b._____assure adequate fluid intake.
    c._____keep the gastric juice neutralized.
    d._____provide protein for tissue repair.

16. Foods which would be added to the diet during the first few days of the modified Sippy regimen would include

    a._____whole-wheat cereals, meat soups, ginger ale.
    b._____eggs, cottage cheese, custard.
    c._____toast, coffee, ginger ale.
    d._____small quantities of meat, cooked vegetables and fruit.

17. In order to promote digestion, Mr. Pasha should be taught to

    a._____exercise after meals.   c._____rest after meals.
    b._____exercise before meals.   d._____take a daily enema or cathartic.

18. During the early stages of his hospitalization the resident wrote the following note on Mr. Pasha's chart: "Symptoms may be of functional origin." The best interpretation of this statement is that the patient is

    a._____deliberately faking symptoms to secure attention.
    b._____imagining his symptoms.
    c._____experiencing a physiologic reaction to emotional stress.
    d._____experiencing pain from an organic lesion.

19. Although the etiology of peptic ulcer is not understood clearly, recent investigation indicates that ulcers tend to develop

    a._____after physical trauma.
    b._____after bacterial infection of the G.I. tract.
    c._____during periods of emotional stress.
    d._____from irritation from highly seasoned foods.

20. The most dangerous complication of peptic ulcer is

    a._____secondary anemia.   d._____perforation.
    b._____pernicious anemia.   e._____pyloric obstruction.
    c._____hemorrhage.

21. Patients with ulcer frequently fear cancer. Records show that

    a._____40 per cent of duodenal ulcers become cancerous.
    b._____gastric ulcers of the greater curvature usually are cancerous.
    c._____duodenal ulcers never become cancerous.
    d._____gastric ulcers of the lesser curvature occasionally become cancerous.
    e._____untreated ulcers, regardless of site, are potentially cancerous.

22. Overstimulation of the vagus nerve, as may occur in some instances of emotional tension, results in the

   a._____production of large quantities of gastric juice of low acidity.
   b._____production of relatively small quantities of gastric juice of low acidity.
   c._____production of abnormally large quantities of gastric juice of high acidity.
   d._____inhibition of gastric juice.

Questions for Discussion and Student Projects

1. What phases of Mr. Pasha's type of employment are undesirable for this type of patient? Are there any desirable aspects? If you believe a change of employment is desirable, discuss the type of employment he might secure. Where can he receive assistance in seeking a new job?
2. What factors in Mr. Pasha's personal life might aggravate his condition? Discuss the relationship of tenets of the Roman Catholic church to his family life. Where might he secure help in resolving some of his worries?
3. Plan a week's diet for Mr. Pasha which he can either carry with him or secure "on the road." What foods, typical in the Italian family's menu, must Mr. Pasha learn to avoid?
4. Discuss the use of patent "stomach medicines" by patients with mild chronic gastric symptoms. What is the principal ingredient of these drugs? What complication can occur from overuse of these drugs? What is the chief disadvantage of their use?
5. Describe the "continuous drip therapy," including the purpose, equipment, solutions used and the nursing care of the patient.
6. Mr. Pasha handed a piece of paper to the nurse on which was written "amino acids and dextrimaltose." He then said, "Some fellow told me if I took this, it would cure my ulcers. Is this true?" What has been reported in the literature concerning this combination of drugs? What should the nurse do about Mr. Pasha's question?

THE TRUCK DRIVER WITH INDIGESTION—PATIENT STUDY—(*Continued*)

After discharge from the hospital, Mr. Pasha felt well and did not have pain for about 5 months. Then one morning when he returned from work he felt weak and dizzy. He lay down for a while and was awakened when he suddenly vomited a considerable amount of dark fluid. Shortly thereafter, he passed a tarry stool and had four more before returning to the hospital. His diagnosis was "upper G.I. hemorrhage, probably on basis of peptic ulcer although esophageal varices are to be considered." Shortly after his admission, he became more pale, pulse increased and blood pressure dropped. An emergency operation was scheduled.

At 7 P.M. Mr. Pasha was put on nothing P.O. and received a transfusion of 500 cc. of whole blood and an infusion of 500 cc. of normal saline. Atropine and morphine were given and he was taken to the O.R. at 10:30 P.M. A subtotal gastrectomy and gastrojejunostomy were done under general anesthesia. Following the anastomosis, the abdominal cavity was irrigated to remove the blood and 1 Gm. of streptomycin and 200,000 units of penicillin were instilled in the peritoneal cavity. During surgery, Mr. Pasha received 5 pints of blood. At the closing of his abdomen, his blood pressure was 110/70.

Mr. Pasha's orders postoperatively included continuous gastric suction which was continued for 3 days, when he gave evidence of retaining fluids by mouth. Thereafter, his postoperative convalescence was satisfactory. He was discharged with specific instructions regarding diet, emotionally disturbing situations, work and other activities.

References

Merrill, I., and Morris, M.: Nursing care in gastric surgery, Trained Nurse and Hosp. Rev. 115:248, 1951.
McLaughlin, Mary Frances: Perforated gastric ulcer, Am. J. Nursing 50:53, 1950.

Questions Relating to the Patient Study

1. The most dangerous complication of peptic ulcer is

   a.____cancer.   d.____hemorrhage.
   b.____acute perforation.   c.____pyloric stenosis.
   c.____coronary thrombosis.

2. The general appearance of a patient in the initial stage of gastric hemorrhage will be

   a.____flushed, lethargic.   d.____jaundiced, comatose.
   b.____grayish, pallid, apathetic.   e.____flushed, restless.
   c.____pallid, drawn, apprehen-
         sive.

3. Plication of the ulcer is a common surgical procedure. In this operation

   a.____the ulcer and immediate area involved are removed.
   b.____a tube is placed in the stomach through the abdomen and feedings are administered in this way.
   c.____the ulcer is closed by a purse-string suture.
   d.____the stomach is anastomosed to the jejunum, thereby by-passing the ulcer.

4. Esophageal varices were considered in the tentative diagnosis because of the presence of

   a.____pain.   c.____abnormal respirations.
   b.____hemorrhage.   d.____tarry stool.

5. The immediate actions of the preoperative adult dosage of morphine sulfate are

   a.____decrease of heart beat.
   b.____no alteration of blood pressure.

    c._____decrease of blood pressure.
    d._____dilatation of peripheral vessels.
    e._____increase of heart beat followed by decrease.

6. Prolonged actions of preoperative morphine are

    a._____decrease of anxiety.
    b._____check of secretions.
    c._____dilatation of the pupils.
    d._____lessening of excitement during anesthetic induction.

7. The technic usually practiced in the O.R. for gastro-intestinal surgery includes:

    a._____A separate set of instruments is used when the intestine or stomach is opened in order to prevent peritoneal contamination.
    b._____The contents of the stomach are considered sterile; therefore, no modification in technic to prevent abdominal contamination is necessary.
    c._____The cutting edge of needles of the straight or curved variety is used in gastro-intestinal surgery.
    d._____Round-bodied needles of the straight or curved variety are used in gastro-intestinal surgery.
    e._____Rubber-shod instruments are used most commonly when an anastomosis is done.
    f._____Kocher and Allis clamps are used most commonly when an anastomosis is done.

8. Gastric lavage operates on the principle of

    a._____the lever.   c._____air pressure.
    b._____the siphon.   d._____gravity.

9. A Miller-Abbott tube is a

    a._____single-lumen tube with a mercury-weighted bag.
    b._____double-lumen tube with a mercury-weighted bag.
    c._____single-lumen tube with an inflatable balloon at the end.
    d._____double-lumen tube with an inflatable balloon at the end.

10. The Miller-Abbott tube is used for

    a._____suction and feeding.
    b._____irrigation and suction.
    c._____irrigation and feeding.

11. The inflatable bag of a gastro-intestinal tube should be injected with air

    a._____when it reaches the esoph-   c._____when it reaches the duo-
        agus.   denum.
    b._____when it reaches the py-   d._____before it is inserted.
        lorus.

12. When a drug is given through a gastro-intestinal suction tube

    a. it is necessary to clamp off the suction for about an hour

        (1)_____prior to its administration to allow for more rapid absorption of the drug.

        (2)_____after the drug is administered to prevent its being suctioned into the drainage bottle.

    b. it is

        (1)_____unnecessary to dissolve a small tablet which can slip through the tubing.

        (2)_____necessary to dissolve all tablet medications in a small amount of warm water.

13. When a gastro-intestinal suction tube is irrigated or aspirated it is important to

    a._____aspirate the same amount of fluid as was injected.

    b._____use force because the small perforations in the proximal end are small and may be clogged.

    c._____withdraw the tube if the patient vomits during the procedure.

    d._____measure every cubic centimeter of fluid that is either inserted or aspirated.

14. A gastro-intestinal tube should be pinched during withdrawal to

    a._____cut off air pressure on any fluid that remains in the tube.

    b._____prevent trauma to mucous membranes by the force of suction.

    c._____prevent pressure noises which might be upsetting to the patient.

    d._____prevent the transfer of organisms from a relatively "dirty" area to a cleaner area.

15. To maintain fluid balance during gastric suction, it may be necessary to administer

    a._____sodium bicarbonate

    b._____dilute hydrochloric acid

    c._____infusions of salt solution

    in order to replace

    a._____chlorides.   b._____sodium ions.   c._____hydrogen ions.

16. Check those foods which may be offered to Mr. Pasha while he is on a bland diet:

    a._____strained peas.   f._____Spam.

    b._____diluted tomato juice.   g._____steamed oysters.

    c._____corn (removed from the   h._____canned tuna fish with the cob).   oil drained off.

    d._____grapefruit juice.   i._____weak tea.

    e._____salt pork.   j._____whole wheat bread.

17. Marginal ulcers may develop in Mr. Pasha. These are described as ulcers which occur

a.____prior to surgery at the gastro-intestinal juncture.
b.____in an organ adjacent to the stomach or duodenum, e.g. the pancreas.
c.____at the site of the anastomosis of the jejunum and stomach.
d.____at the cardiac end of the stomach near the esophagus.

18. Duodenal fistula may occur after a gastro-jejunostomy. The nurse's responsibility is to anticipate and care for the following problems:

a.____distention, borborygmi, constipation.
b.____loss of chlorides, skin digestion, duodenal obstruction.
c.____marginal ulcers, acidosis, dehydration.
d.____skin digestion, alkalosis, peritonitis.

19. Match the following:

a. Gastric ulcer

A. Areas of stomach most commonly affected:
(1)____greater curvature.
(2)____lesser curvature.

b. Gastric carcinoma

B. Acidity:
(1)____lower than normal (achlorhydria).
(2)____higher than normal.
C. Size:
(1)____up to 1 cm. usually.
(2)____over 1 cm.
D. Ability to heal:
(1)____does not heal.
(2)____may heal.

Questions for Discussion and Student Projects

1. Nonoperative treatment of perforated duodenal ulcer has been tried and recommended. What could be anticipated as the likely treatment, possible complications and required nursing care of such a patient?
2. Explain the principles of pressure involved when fluids are aspirated from the gastro-intestinal system via Wangensteen suction.
3. What is meant by the "dumping syndrome" in postgastrectomy patients? Is this a serious problem? How can it be remedied or prevented?
4. From the list below, check the items you think should have been thoroughly discussed with Mr. Pasha with a view to preventing the acute recurrence of ulcers followed by perforation:

a.____Habits of mastication.
b.____Amount of time usually spent at meals.
c.____Addiction to patent medicines.
d.____Use of cathartics.
e.____Family relationships.
f.____Semi-annual physical examination.

What specific points would you include in your discussion?

5. Prepare 6 menus for a noon lunch box for Mr. Pasha to demonstrate that variety can be offered while maintaining a bland diet.

6. Would it be advisable for Mr. Pasha to return to his former job as a truck driver? Support your answer with specific reference to (a) dietary modifications and (b) emotional demands which may result from this work.

7. Discuss the action of Banthine* as it relates to action on

a. the vagus nerve.
b. hydrochloric-acid secretion.
c. gastroduodenal motility.
d. ulcer pain.
e. ulcer healing.

How does the action of this drug compare with that of atropine sulfate? How does it differ?

8. Consult the most recent volume of *Vital Statistics of the United States,* U.S. Dept. of Commerce, Bureau of Census, Washington, D.C., and compare the mortality rate of carcinoma of the stomach with that of carcinoma of the breast. What is being done in your hospital and community to encourage patients to secure an early diagnosis? How can this program be improved?

9. Esophageal varices have been treated by producing a shunt of the portal blood into the systemic venous system either by anastomosis between the splenic vein (after splenectomy) and the left renal vein or by direct anastomosis between the portal vein and the vena cava. Explain the rationale of such surgery.

THE JEALOUS BROTHER

Background Review Questions

1. The primary function of the large intestine is to absorb

a._____fatty acids and glycerol.
b._____amino acids.
c._____water and inorganic salts.
d._____glucose and fructose.

2. Principles which illustrate normal functioning of the intestinal tract are that

a._____local distention of the intestinal wall is an integral part of abnormal peristalsis.
b._____pressure applied to an enclosed gas or liquid is transmitted without diminution in all directions.
c._____voluntary muscle tissue relaxing and contracting produces peristalsis which moves the contents of the intestine in a downward direction.
d._____the process of digestion is continued although no digestive glands are in the colon.

3. Mucous membrane of the large intestine is

a._____more sensitive to changes of temperature than skin.
b._____less sensitive to changes of temperature than skin.

* Searle product.

4. In an abnormally distended intestinal tract, the absorption of gas is

    a._____increased, blood supply is increased, peristaltic action becomes inefficient and non-existent.

    b._____increased, blood supply is reduced, peristaltic action becomes increased.

    c._____diminished, blood supply is increased, peristaltic action becomes increased.

    d._____diminished, blood supply is reduced, peristaltic action becomes inefficient and non-existent.

5. A milk-and-molasses enema acts as follows:

    a._____The solution is retained and coats the mucous membranes so that irritation is lessened.

    b._____Molasses lowers the surface tension of the milk which in turn combines more quickly with feces.

    c._____Carbon dioxide gas is formed which irritates the intestinal muscles and causes contractions.

6. Best support of a can of solution for an enema is given by holding the can

    a._____near the lower part of the handle.

    b._____near the middle part of the handle.

    c._____near the top part of the handle.

THE JEALOUS BROTHER—PATIENT STUDY

Ever since he could remember, Jasper Jones never was able to do things as well as his younger brother, Reginald. During his high school years he was inactive in sports, for he was thin, easily winded, and had frequent stomach upsets. Jasper was rejected as physically unfit for military service but he was pleased when Reginald was accepted, for now he would feel free to be an individual in his own right and would no longer be compared to his brother by his parents.

But then came the most upsetting episode in his life when he was 27 years old—a girl made light of his serious intentions toward her. The climax came when she belittled him at a dance. He had bought her a corsage and escorted her to the ball, but she refused to dance with him and went home with another boy. Jasper became quite ill that night and had to be hospitalized. This was the sixth hospitalization for practically the same set of symptoms: diarrhea, blood and mucus in the stools, abdominal cramps, loss of appetite and slight anemia. Heretofore, he had been able to get back to his more normal pattern of activity after 2 or 3 weeks of rest, proper diet, blood transfusions, etc. But this time, Jasper did not appear to respond so readily to medical treatment. Therefore a consultation was held with the surgical staff.

A sigmoidoscopy revealed a tender crater, approximately 3 cm. in diameter, on the anterior wall just inside the anus. Ulcerations were felt and terrific spasms were noted 2 inches above the anus. Roentgenograms showed that the terminal ileum and associated colon were involved as well as the transverse and descending colon. An ileostomy was done for his ulcerative colitis at this time.

He had some difficulty accepting this temporary procedure but tolerated it for 6 months when the ileum was closed.

At present, Mr. Jones is 30 years of age. About a month ago his brother came back to his home town, having received decorations for outstanding valor in the service. In addition, Reginald brought his war bride. The evening before Reginald arrived, Jasper had another attack. So much of the lower bowel was involved that a colectomy with permanent ileostomy was done. His postoperative recovery was slow but progressive even though he resented the fact that he now had a permanent abdominal opening.

Dressings and skin care were a real problem. Jasper often complained about being "bathed in feces." Upon several occasions he announced the desire to "quit living." With real tact and patience, over a period of time, the nurses were able to get him to change his dressings. When the good news reached him that a position as clerk in the local bank awaited his recovery, he began to eat better and took a greater interest in himself. He was discharged with a gratifying and optimistic outlook on life.

References

Goodman, M.: Colostomy deodorants, Surgery 28:550, 1950.

Green, J.: Psychogenesis and psychotherapy of ulcerative colitis, Psych. Med. IX:151, May–June, 1947.

Portis, Sidney A.: The clinical significance of emotional disturbances affecting the stomach, duodenum, and biliary tract, Psych. Med. VI:71–73, 1944.

Thompson, Bernice: Use of the Binkley colostomy irrigator, Am. J. Nursing 48:235, 1948.

Questions Relating to the Patient Study

1. The diagnosis of ulcerative colitis can be confirmed by

   a.____gastro-intestinal series.   d.____barium enema.
   b.____stool culture.   e.____biopsy.
   c.____sigmoidoscopy.

2. Factors predisposing to ulcerative colitis include

   a.____alcoholism.   d.____infection.
   b.____food allergy.   e.____emotional trauma.
   c.____dietary deficiency.   f.____malignancy.

3. Symptoms which most accurately describe ulcerative colitis are

   a.____nausea and vomiting, anoxemia, weight loss, abdominal cramps.
   b.____skin rash, fever, anoxia, anemia, nausea and vomiting.
   c.____leukocytosis, fever, diarrhea, nausea and vomiting, weight loss.
   d.____diarrhea, anemia, anorexia, weight loss, abdominal cramps.
   e.____anemia, intestinal mucosal hemorrhage, weight loss, purpura, skin rash.

4. The cause of chronic ulcerative colitis is

   a._____a deficiency in red blood   d._____improper dietary habits.
   cells.   e._____metal poisoning.
   b._____intestinal parasites.   f._____unknown.
   c._____alcoholism.

5. Chronic ulcerative colitis usually commences at

   a._____a lower portion of the colon and progresses upward.
   b._____the proximal segment and progresses to the distal end of the tract.
   c._____no specific area but spreads in both directions from the initial focus.

6. The characteristic stools in ulcerative colitis usually are

   a._____well formed but tinged with blood.
   b._____diarrheal with blood and mucus.
   c._____clay-colored with blood.
   d._____gray, foamy.
   e._____greenish watery.

7. A serious complication which may develop in patients with chronic ulcerative colitis is

   a._____gastric perforation.   d._____megacolon.
   b._____peritonitis.   e._____anal fistulae.
   c._____intestinal perforation.

8. When placed on nothing by mouth preoperatively, the only water available to Mr. Jones is from oxidation of

   a._____CHO.   c._____protein.
   b._____fat.   d._____minerals.

9. Symptoms of dehydration such as might be seen in ulcerative colitis are

   a._____weakness, anorexia, muscular twitching, fatigue.
   b._____clammy skin, subnormal temperature, pallor, anemia.
   c._____anxiety, dysphagia, tachycardia, nausea.
   d._____hunger pains, excessive salivation, lowered blood pressure, apprehension.

10. Which practices would be most effective in helping Mr. Jones to find a solution to his problems?

   a._____To devise recreational and diversional therapy for him so that he might forget those things which aggravate him.
   b._____To encourage him to talk of his family, ambitions, etc.
   c._____To use insistence when he refuses a treatment or medication, for he has probably had his own way long enough.
   d._____To recognize the fact that if medical therapy has failed, the last resort is surgery and that it is too late for psychotherapy.

11. The items which would be needed by the physician as he prepares to do a sigmoidoscopy on Mr. Jones are a sigmoidoscope with battery cord and lights plus

   a._____a local anesthetic, biopsy forceps, long cotton swabs, air insufflator.

   b._____germicide with sponge forceps, rubber gloves, lubricant, biopsy forceps.

   c._____lubricant, air insufflator, ordinary cotton applicator sticks, Nupercaine ointment.

   d._____rubber gloves, lubricant, air insufflator, long cotton swabs.

12. During his siege of chronic ulcerative colitis, the only menu which Mr. Jones would be able to tolerate is comprised of

   a._____consommé, french fried potatoes, creamed chicken, puréed peas, sponge cake.

   b._____bouillon, roast beef, mashed potatoes, carrots, prune soufflé.

   c._____clear meat soup, tuna fish, baked potato, string beans, apple pie.

   d._____fresh fruit salad, salmon, asparagus tips, spinach, applesauce.

13. It has been said that a patient with an ileostomy is one of the most difficult to nurse. The chief reason for this is that

   a._____they are subject to pathologic fractures and therefore require meticulous handling.

   b._____their prolonged illness makes them irritable, weak, and, at times, psychopathic.

   c._____for the most part, their problems are insoluble, which means that an ileostomy is only palliative.

   d._____ulcerative colitis often leads to carcinoma; most patients realize the hopelessness of their prognosis.

14. Aluminum paste used to protect the skin around an ileostomy should be mixed with

   a._____zinc oxide.   d._____water.
   b._____carbon tetrachloride.   e._____alcohol.
   c._____sweet oil.

15. Casec is effective in protecting the skin from fecal drainage because it

   a._____coats the skin.

   b._____neutralizes hydrochloric acid.

   c._____acts as an antiseptic.

   d._____acts as a counterirritant.

   e._____reacts with digestive enzymes.

16. Mr. Jones was ordered up in a chair on the second postoperative day. He complained of pain and swelling in his right leg and asked the nurse to rub it. She should

   a._____notify the physician and keep him in bed.

   b._____get him up but keep his leg elevated.

c._____rub his leg gently, apply heat, and keep him in bed.
d._____give the codeine order, notify the physician and keep him in bed.
e._____give the codeine order, notify the physician and get him up.

17. Following several catheterizations for retention, Mr. Jones developed a mild cystitis. Symptoms he complained of were

a.__✓__frequency of urination with tenesmus. *straining*
b._____pain, most severe just before urination began.
c._____inability to begin micturition.
d._____pain in the hollow of the back.
e._____pain over the kidney area.
f._____pain in the region of the bladder.

18. A bladder instillation of 10 cc. of 10 per cent Argyrol was ordered for Mr. Jones' cystitis. The bottle labeled "Argyrol" was not in the medicine closet. The nurse should select one with a label reading

a._____silver chloride.
b.__✓__silver protein.
c._____silver nitrate.
d._____silver lactate.
e._____silver picrate.

19. Potassium permanganate often is used as an irrigating fluid for the bladder in cystitis. This compound releases O_2 and the brown precipitate of

a._____K_2O.   b._____N_2O.   c.__✓__MnO_2.   d._____$KMnO_2$.

20. In using $KMnO_4$, the following precautions should be observed:

a._____The solution is most effective when it is brown.
b.__✓__The solution is no longer effective when it has turned brown.
c._____1:1,000 is the most effective dilution for lavage.
d.__✓__It should not be used for lavage in strength greater than 1:5,000.

21. Gantrisin is a drug effective in combatting and preventing cystitis. It is a member of which group of drugs?

a._____Aureomycin, terramycin, erythromycin, etc.
b._____Penicillin, duracillin, etc.
c.__✓__Sulfa drugs.
d._____None of the above.

22. Match the following:

a. ileostomy.
b. colostomy.

(1)__b__discharge can be regulated.
(2)__a__discharge is continuous.
(3)__a__liquid drainage.
(4)__b__soft and/or formed discharge.
(5)__a__a bag must be worn.
(6)__b__a bag is not necessary.

23. Colostomy irrigations are done most satisfactorily by using a
    a.____Dakin's syringe and rectal tube.
    b.__✓__irrigating can and catheter.
    c.____funnel and catheter.
    d.____irrigating can, rubber tubing with glass tapering tip.

24. During a colostomy irrigation, if the patient complains of cramps, the nurse should
    a.____raise the irrigating can so that the irrigation can be completed quickly.
    b.____reassure the patient by telling him that this can be expected; continue the irrigation.
    c.____pinch the tubing so that less fluid enters the colon.
    d.__✓__discontinue the inflow and allow the patient to rest.

25. When ureters have been transplanted into a colostomy (as a result of a combined abdomino-perineal resection and cystectomy), an irrigation is
    a.__✓__never done.
    b.____done less frequently than for an ordinary colostomy.
    c.____done only when the patient has an urge to defecate.
    d.____done more frequently than for an ordinary colostomy.

26. The reason for the decision reached in the preceding question is that
    a.__✓__an ascending urinary infection may result.
    b.____the nature of the drainage (urine and feces) does not warrant frequent irrigations.
    c.____an irrigation assists nature to perform a natural function.
    d.____contamination is kept at a minimum.

27. The tubing used in a colostomy irrigation should be
    a.____of hard rubber to facilitate the displacement of masses of formed stool.
    b.____made of glass so that the return flow may be observed clearly.
    c.__✓__a No. 16 or 18 soft rubber catheter because it is least harmful and most effective.
    d.____a No. 30 rectal tube since ordinarily this is used in giving an enema.

28. The irrigating can should be not higher than 2 feet above the level of the colostomy opening because
    a.____there is less chance for the solution to become cold, thus chilling a sensitive patient.
    b.____the maximum pressure is achieved at this level, therefore it is unnecessary to increase the height.
    c.____pressure is at its optimum level at this height; increasing it would be harmful to the bowel.

d._____most patients do not have irrigating poles, hence the compromise of keeping the can at approximately the level of the flushing reservoir.

Questions for Discussion and Student Projects

1. Describe the movements of the small intestine as it acts on chyme. What prevents food from being moved in the opposite direction?
2. Describe the mass action of the large intestine. Translate these activities into understandable language for patients having an ileostomy or colostomy.
3. What styles and types of ileostomy bags are on the market? Collect literature and price lists. How effective are those which can be "cemented" to the skin?
4. What equipment which is found in most homes can be utilized in improvising

   a. an ileostomy bag with belt.
   b. an irrigation set for a colostomy patient.

5. Attempts have been made to control objectionable odors from a colostomy and ileostomy. How effective are the following deodorants?

   a. Powdered chlorophyll.   b. Powdered charcoal.

6. What are some of the common reactions of patients to a permanent colostomy? Consider your own reactions to the procedure. Why is this important?
7. Some surgeons do not recommend irrigations for colostomies and others make it a routine. Review the recent literature for the results reported by the two groups. How does this affect the kind of teaching which the nurse carries out both in the hospital and in the field of public health nursing?
8. In a colostomy, the proximal end of the intestinal tract can be kept clean easily and in good function. How is the distal portion taken care of in this respect? (This is a situation in which the distal portion has not been removed as in an abdominoperineal resection.)
9. It has been reported in medical literature that following a complete colectomy, the ileum was sutured to an intact anal sphincter. What difficulties might be anticipated and what can the nurse do about these?
10. Mr. Ambrogia was ready for discharge from the hospital following surgery resulting in a permanent colostomy. At this time, it was thought best to demonstrate the care of this new outlet to his wife even though Mr. Ambrogia was successful in caring for himself. Mrs. Ambrogia was shocked by the procedure and Mr. Ambrogia was embarrassed as well as upset emotionally over her reaction. What could have been done to avert such a reaction? What can be done now to ease the situation?
11. An elderly gentleman had a colostomy who was not able to speak English or understand it very well. On the third postoperative day he insisted on having a bedpan because he had not had a defecation

for several days and wanted to try. How would you handle this situation since it is obvious that he did not know the nature of the operation?

12. Mr. Flavius is about to be discharged from the hospital following a colostomy. Prepare a list of foods for a constipating diet, using the following classifications:

a. Vegetables.   e. Meats.
b. Fruits.   f. Desserts.
c. Breads and cereals.   g. Miscellaneous.
d. Dairy products.

Using the same classifications, list the foods which Mr. Flavius should avoid.

13. The Binkley irrigator is a favorite type of equipment which a colostomy patient may find useful if he has to irrigate his colostomy. What advantages does this outfit have as compared with ordinary hospital equipment used for irrigation? How expensive is it? How can it be kept clean?

THE LAW OFFICE SECRETARY—PATIENT STUDY

Miss Andrews was near collapse when the taxi driver brought her to the hospital. She had been sick all night in her room in the residence club and had been unable to secure any help until morning.

Miss Andrews, a secretary in a law office, had lived in the club for years. Although she usually took her meals at the club, recently she had been eating her lunch at quick-lunch counters and drugstores in order to go shopping during her lunch hour.

She realized that she had had some "indigestion" for several days, but did not become concerned until the night before admission. Then she had severe abdominal cramps and frequent bloody stools.

Her temperature on admission was normal, but she appeared dehydrated. Parenteral fluids were given and a stool specimen was obtained.

A diagnosis of amebic dysentery was established. Diodoquin 0.25 Gm. t.i.d. for 21 days and carbarsone 0.5 Gm. for 10 days were ordered. She was placed on stool precautions and given intravenous feedings until ready for a light bland diet.

After 2 weeks Miss Andrews returned to the residence club and to work, with instructions to return to her physician for follow-up.

References

Editorial: The problems of amebiasis, J.A.M.A. 134:1095, 1947.
Editorial: Building our defenses against influenza, Am. J. Pub. Health 39:221, 1949.
Johnson, Thomas A., ed.: Management of Common Gastro-intestinal Diseases, pp. 253–275, Philadelphia, Lippincott, 1948.
Mayo, Merle: Nursing care in bacillary dysentery, Am. J. Nursing 50:304, 1950.
Most, Harry, et al.: Terramycin 100% effective against amebiasis, Public Health Rep. 65:1684, 1950.

Questions Relating to the Patient Study

1. Amebic dysentery is characterized by its

   a._____short course.
   b.__✓__chronicity.
   c.__✓__intermittent attacks.
   d._____persistent severity.
   e._____rapidly fatal termination.

2. Common methods of infection by amebic dysentery are by

   a._____dust.
   b.__✓__water.
   c._____insect carriers.
   d._____droplets.
   e.__✓__carriers.

3. The chief symptoms of acute amebic dysentery are

   a._____slight fever, weight loss, dyspepsia.
   b._____high fever, dehydration, vomiting.
   c.__✓__weight loss, slight fever, diarrhea.
   d._____frequent, small, mucopurulent stools.
   e.__✓__frequent, small stools with blood and mucus.

4. The complications of amebic dysentery are

   a._____peritonitis.
   b._____liver abscesses.
   c._____hepatitis.
   d._____cirrhosis of the liver.
   e._____chronic ulcerative colitis.

5. Miss Andrews' dietary pattern should be

   (place the letter of correct diet in front of appropriate line indicating the period at which the diet is appropriate):

   a. withhold food, giving glucose intravenously.
   b. diet of boiled skim milk.
   c. diet of barley water, chicken broth, egg albumin and milk with lime water.
   d. diet of mashed baked bananas and skim milk.
   e. diet of milk toast, custard, gelatin, tapioca, rice and bread puddings.
   f. diet of lean chicken, fish and fowl.

   (1)__a__first few days.
   (2)__c__following the period when the attack is still severe.
   (3)__e__convalescent period when the symptoms lessen.

6. Diodoquin may be used satisfactorily   *Anti -parasite*

   a._____on bed patients only.
   b.__✓__on ambulatory patients.
   c._____as a supplement to other amebicides.
   d._____as the only medication in severe cases.
   e.__✓__on the symptomless cyst-carrier.

7. Significant precautions in the nursing care of patients with amebic dysentery

   a. for hospital personnel are

    (1)_____care of nasal secretions.
    (2)_____sterilization of dishes.
    (3)_____care of stools and bedpan.
    (4)_____care of urine.
    (5)_____sterilization of linens.

  b. for the patient are

    (1)_____care of the hands.
    (2)_____care of stools.
    (3)_____care of urine.
    (4)_____handling of food.
    (5)_____care of nasal secretions.

8. A patient with severe diarrhea should be

  a._____allowed the freedom of his room, without contact with other patients.
  b._____confined to bed.
  c._____prohibited the use of cigarettes and alcohol.
  d._____moved to a cooler climate when possible.
  e._____prohibited from having visitors.

9. Acute amebic hepatitis occurs in 5 per cent of all cases of amebic dysentery. Symptoms of its onset would be

  a._____chills and fever.
  b._____intense pain over an enlarged liver.
  c._____vomiting and nausea.
  d._____shoulder pain.
  e._____cramps in the limbs.

10. Liver-abscess formation is characterized by

  a._____an increase in daily temperature with chills and sweating during the morning.
  b._____an increase in daily temperature with elevation in the morning.
  c._____anorexia, pain.
  d._____tenderness and enlargement of the liver.
  e._____muscular flabbiness over the liver.

11. Constipation following the elimination of the amebic infection may be treated with

  a._____milk of magnesia.
  b._____mineral oil.
  c._____suppositories.
  d._____saline enemas.
  e._____soapsuds enemas.

12. Amebic cysts are destroyed by

  a._____heating water to 120°F.
  b._____soap and water.
  c._____pasteurizing milk.
  d._____exposure to air.
  e._____prolonged exposure to sunlight.

Questions for Discussion and Student Projects

1. How long should the stools be checked before Miss Andrews is dismissed from the hospital? How often should the stools be checked after discharge, and when would the disease be considered cured?
2. How may Miss Andrews be assisted in accepting this chronic and frequently recurring illness with its debilitating effects? How would you encourage her as you care for her each day?
3. What instructions should Miss Andrews receive in relation to diet, medications and preventive aspects before discharge? What should she be told about her prognosis? Will this condition interfere with her plans to be married?
4. What measures would the local public health department use to prevent further incidence of amebic dysentery after Miss Andrews' case was reported? Why is it essential that all cases of this disease be reported? If you were a public health nurse and Miss Andrews returned to your district with referral for follow-up, what would be your responsibilities?

Questions Relating to Dysentery in General

1. Symptoms of bacillary dysentery include

   a._____chills and general chilliness.
   b._____urticaria.
   c._____aching and occasional convulsions.
   d._____abdominal cramp and diarrhea.
   e._____lack of fever.

2. Complications of bacillary dysentery include

   a._____arthritis, usually in the knees.
   b._____leukocytosis.
   c._____secondary anemia.
   d._____soreness in the lymph glands.
   e._____ulcerative colitis.

3. A patient with bacillary dysentery probably would give the following history:

   a._____stopping at a motel.
   b._____eating at a quick-lunch counter.
   c._____radical change of climate.
   d._____shortness of breath.
   e._____overwork.

4. The bacillus of dysentery thrives under

   a._____moisture.
   b._____cold or freezing.
   c._____phenol solution.
   d._____mercuric chloride.
   e._____sunlight.

5. Relapse in bacillary dysentery may cause a chronic condition. The nurse should guard against

a._____unusual physical exertion.
b._____keeping the patient too warm.
c._____occurrence of frequent stools.
d._____rapid increase in diet.

Questions for Discussion and Student Projects

1. How would amebic dysentery be distinguished from bacillary dysentery? Why is it important to make the distinction?
2. As a student nurse assigned to give a retention enema, how would you explain the technic to the patient? How would you secure her co-operation if she had a great dislike for enemas? Can you suggest adequate distractions for the period when she had to lie in one position?
3. Discuss the incidence and increase of amebic dysentery in this country during the past 20 years. Is there a climate or temperature relationship to the incidence? Are there other factors?
4. Describe the incidence of amebic dysentery at the Chicago World's Fair in 1933. What was typical about the occurrence of the disease? What public health measures were necessary to control the epidemic?
5. Discuss the therapeutic effects of the various drugs used in the treatment of amebic dysentery. What are the toxic effects of each?
6. From your clinical experience with amebic dysentery, what precautions would you take in ordering food in a public restaurant? If you were traveling in Mexico, what type of restaurant would you select? What type of food would be safe to eat in a native village?
7. What would the City Health Department advise the citizens to do if intestinal influenza reached epidemic proportions in a community?
8. How would you distinguish intestinal influenza from bacillary or amebic dysentery? Discuss the course, treatment, precautions and nursing care of intestinal influenza.

References

Elman, Robert: Fluid balance from the nurse's point of view, Am. J. Nursing 49:222, 1949.
Peters, J. P.: Effect of injury and disease on nitrogen metabolism, Am. J. Med. 5:100, 1948.

Nursing Care of Patients with Other Disorders of the Alimentary System

A. Appendectomy

Jack Donay had abdominal pain for 2 days; thinking it was due to constipation, he took a cathartic. However, the pain became more severe, and upon the advice of a physician he came to the hospital. A diagnosis of ruptured appendix and peritonitis was made. A white cell count of 14,000 with 86 per cent polyneutrophils was reported. An appendectomy with Penrose drainage was done under spinal anesthesia.

1. The purpose of placing Mr. Donay in Fowler's position as soon as he returned to the ward was to

   a._____aid drainage toward the pelvic region.
   b._____aid drainage toward the diaphragm.
   c._____relax the abdominal muscles.
   d._____minimize the loss of fluids by drainage.
   e._____minimize postoperative shock.

2. The laboratory report indicated

   a._____a severe infection; good resistance.
   b._____a severe infection; poor resistance.
   c._____a moderate infection; good resistance.
   d._____a moderate infection; poor resistance.
   e._____slight infection; good resistance.
   f._____slight infection; poor resistance.

3. The gridiron incision for an appendectomy usually is made in the following region of the abdomen:

   a._____right hypochondriac.   d._____umbilical.
   b._____right lumbar.   e._____pubic.
   c._____right iliac.

4. When acute abdominal distress is experienced, it is wise to consult a physician. Meanwhile, relief may be obtained by doing the following:

   a._____Apply heat to the abdomen, take an enema, take nothing by mouth.
   b._____Apply an ice bag to the abdomen, rest in bed, take no cathartic.
   c._____Take a mild laxative, limit intake to water only, keep quiet.
   d._____Take the temperature, stay in bed, apply a hot-water bottle to the abdomen, prevent chilling.

5. Symptoms indicating a rupture of the appendix are

   a._____sudden sharp, excruciating pain, drawing up of the right leg, rise in temperature and pulse followed by a drop in both.
   b._____boardlike rigidity of the abdomen, spiking temperature, cold clammy skin.
   c._____apprehension, a sensation of something having "given way" in the abdomen, labored respirations.
   d._____a rapid rise in pulse, respirations and temperature, an increasing pulse pressure, sharp pain in the R.L.Q., nausea, vomiting.

B. Paralytic Ileus

1. Occasionally, following a surgical abdominal procedure, paralytic ileus occurs. This is because of

   a.____an inhibition of intestinal peristalsis brought about by over-activity of the sympathetic nervous system.
   b.____an inflation of the lower intestinal tract due to an interference with the mucosal absorption of nitrogen.
   c.____stimulation of the intestinal muscles of contraction during exploration and palpation of the intestinal tract.

2. The chief symptom of paralytic ileus is

   a.____flaccid abdomen.   c.____diarrhea.
   b.____acute pain.   d.____distention.

3. The best treatment for paralytic ileus is

   a.____Prostigmine.   d.____colonic irrigation.
   b.____turpentine stupes.   e.____rectal tube.
   c.____gastro-intestinal suction

C. 1. Femoral hernia occurs most frequently in the

   a.____adult male.   c.____female child.
   b.____adult female.   d.____male child.

2. The chief danger of abdominal hernia is the possibility of

   a.____rupture.   d.____peritonitis.
   b.____perforation.   e.____strangulation.
   c.____cicatricial formation.

3. The nurse's chief responsibility in the postoperative care of a patient who has had an inguinal herniorrhaphy is to

   a.____insist that he remain flat in bed for at least a week; longer if the physician so orders.
   b.____prevent pulmonary stasis by turning him frequently and encouraging deep breathing.
   c.____avoid undue strain on the wound.
   d.____ambulate this individual as soon as possible (depending upon the anesthetic used).
   e.____teach him the proper use of a truss and how it can be readjusted to meet his personal needs.

D. Intestinal Obstruction

1. Number in order of frequency the causes of intestinal obstruction:

   a._4_intussusception.
   b._1_adhesions.
   c._3_tumor.
   d._5_volvulus.
   e._2_hernia.

2. Symptoms of an intestinal obstruction are described most clearly as
   sound of flatus is intestino
   a._____regurgitation, tympanitis, nystagmus, borborygmus.
   b.___✓__colicky pain, constipation, fecal vomiting, borborygmus.
   c._____diarrhea, increased pulse rate, nausea, abdominal tenderness.
   d._____fecal impaction, intense, knifelike abdominal pain, temperature elevation.

E. Rectal Surgery

1. Match the symptoms which are associated most frequently with

   a. hemorrhoids.
   b. fissure-in-ano.
   c. anal fistula.
   d. ischiorectal abscess.

   (1)__c__little pain.
   (2)__d__severe local pain.
   (3)__d__chills.
   (4)__b__purulent discharge.
   (5)__ac__itching.
   (6)__a__bleeding at stool.
   (7)__d__fever.
   (8)__b__crack in lining.
   (9)__a__excruciating pain on defecation.

2. Hemorrhoids are brought about by

   a._____non-support of the hemorrhoidal arteries.
   b.___✓__high venous pressure within the abdominal cavity.
   c._____hereditary weakness in the arterial walls.
   d.___✓__hereditary weakness in the venous walls.

F. Tumors

1. Match the following types of tumors:

   a. fibroma.
   b. chordoma.
   c. lipoma.
   d. chondroma.
   e. lymphoma.
   f. angioma.
   g. osteoma.
   h. neuroma.
   i. glioma.
   j. adenoma.
   k. teratoma.

   (1)__f__blood vessels.
   (2)__h__nerve fibers.
   (3)__g__bone tissue.
   (4)__j__glandular epithelium.
   (5)__b__chorda dorsalis.
   (6)__k__more than one germinal layer.
   (7)__i__glia tissue.
   (8)__a__connective tissue.
   (9)__c__fat tissue.
   (10)__e__lymphatic tissue.
   (11)__d__cartilage tissue.

Questions for Discussion and Student Projects

1. What is meant by a "nitrogen balance" in the body? How is it achieved and of what significance is it? What are the implications of a "positive" or "negative" nitrogen balance?
2. Express diagrammatically the physiologic phenomenon which takes place in the tissue when electrolytes are lost as a result of vomiting.

Demonstrate the reverse process when proper electrolyte balance is restored.

3. Describe the symptoms which will be displayed when each of the following electrolytes is lost or lowered:

   a. sodium.
   b. potassium.
   c. calcium.

   Give examples showing how these electrolytes can become insufficient for normal functioning.

4. Discuss hypoproteinemia as it relates to its effect on the following surgical situations:

   a. an anastomosis in the gastro-intestinal tract.
   b. peristaltic action in the stomach and ileum.
   c. incidence of shock.
   d. incidence of infection.
   e. tissue following a general anesthetic.

5. pHisoderm* is a synthetic skin detergent. Describe the effectiveness of this agent by comparing it with Ivory soap as an adjunct in the scrub-up procedure for surgical operations.

6. Why is the surgeon concerned about an individual who has swallowed lye when it is known that caustic burns heal readily?

7. In laxative advertisements, one's attention is often called to "middle-age irregularity." Is there such an ailment? Is the taking of a laxative the answer? Comment.

8. What is meant by Alvarez' aphorism, "The stomach is the fire alarm of the body; do not treat the fire by pouring water on the fire alarm."

9. Consult the last 10 volumes of *Vital Statistics of the United States* and determine the number of deaths attributed to appendicitis within these 10 years. What seems to be the trend? What may be the reason?

10. How has the emphasis on early P.O. rising affected the convalescence of the patient who has had a herniorrhaphy? What precautionary measures should such a patient follow? Prepare a list of questions which you believe such a patient should ask the doctor following an inguinal herniorrhaphy.

11. Describe perineal care following an abdominoperineal resection, insofar as dressings, irrigation and control of odors is concerned. How does such a wound heal? Describe the care of the perineum after the wound has healed.

12. Some surgeons insist that a patient with cancer of the intestinal tract should have either no protein or a very low protein diet preoperatively. What is the reasoning behind this?

13. What is (are) the function(s) of the American Cancer Society? How is it financed? Of what value is this organization to a particular cancer patient for whom you are caring? How can this aid be secured?

14. What facilities for cancer detection exist in your community? How

* Winthrop-Stearns, Inc., product.

effective was this program during the past year? How expensive is it? How can it be improved?

15. In some communities, general hospitals are so crowded that they are unable to keep cancer patients over a long-protracted illness. It is against the policy of most general hospitals to care for the terminal cancer patient even if there are no financial limitations. Investigate provisions for these patients in your community. What can be done to meet this need?

16. Investigate the reported results on the use of radioactive colloidal gold in treating malignant tumors. What are the nursing implications with regard to the use of this substance?

17. How can you raise a patient's morale when he knows he has cancer of the esophagus and a short time to live?

THE PATIENT WITH THE "MISERY"

Background Review Questions

1. The chief function of the gallbladder is to

   a._____manufacture bile and insulin.
   b._____manufacture bile and destroy red blood cells.
   c._____concentrate and store bile.
   d._____store bile, amino acids and fats.

2. The total capacity of the gallbladder is approximately

   a._____10 cc.   c._____50 cc.   e._____500 cc.
   b._____30 cc.   d._____100 cc.

3. The passageway from the gallbladder to the intestinal tract is

   a._____cystic duct→joins the hepatic duct→common duct→empties into the ampulla of Vater with the pancreatic duct.
   b._____biliary duct→joins the hepatic duct→common duct→duodenal duct.
   c._____common bile duct→unites with the hepatic duct→empties into the duodenum with the pancreatic duct.

4. Bilirubin is a waste product derived from destruction of worn-out

   a._____erythrocytes.   c._____macrophages.
   b._____leukocytes.   d._____muscle cells.

5. Normally the plasma bilirubin level remains markedly constant because the

   a._____hepatic cells remove bilirubin from the blood passing through the liver.
   b._____macrophages of spleen remove bile from the blood passing through that organ.
   c._____macrophages of lymph nodes remove bile from the lymph passing through the sinuses.
   d._____glomeruli of the kidneys eliminate bilirubin in the urine.

6. The stimulus which is specific upon the gallbladder causing it to contract, releasing bile into the cystic duct, is the hormone

   a.____cholecystokinin.   c.____enterokinase.
   b.____secretin.   d.____histamine.

7. The purpose of duodenal drainage is to examine the intestinal fluid for

   a.____gastric juices and chyle.
   b.____gastric juices and pancreatic juices.
   c.____pathogenic organisms.
   d.____bile salts and pancreatic juices.
   e.____bile salts and gastric juices.

8. A patient with obstruction of the common bile duct may show a prolonged bleeding and clotting time because when bile salts are absent from the small intestine

   a.____the extrinsic factor is not absorbed.
   b.____vitamin K is not absorbed.
   c.____the ionized calcium level falls.
   d.____bilirubin accumulates in the plasma.

THE PATIENT WITH THE "MISERY"—PATIENT STUDY

"I'se got misery," moaned Mamie Johnson, as she held her abdomen, and looked at the nurse pitifully from her hospital bed.

Mrs. Johnson is a "story-book" picture of a Southern Negro "mammy." She is 40 years old, 5 feet tall and weighs 210 pounds.

Her history of indigestion dates back to when she was 6 years old, when she experienced distress after eating fried foods. However, by simply avoiding these foods she prevented unpleasant episodes.

After her last baby was born, 8 months ago, Mrs. Johnson noticed that her symptoms after meals become more severe. When she experienced an unusually sharp attack of pain in the R.U.Q., which soda bicarbonate did not alleviate, she came to the hospital.

Mr. Johnson, who seemed very devoted, accompanied her. He stated that he was employed in a shirt factory. The seven children had been left in the care of his sister, who seemed to be glad to have them.

After a series of diagnostic tests, the usual preparation for surgery was carried out. A cholecystectomy was performed. A Penrose tube was placed in the foramen of Winslow. A second drain was a T tube connected to a sterile rubber tubing.

Mrs. Johnson was reluctant to move and did so only at the urging of the nurse. When she got out of bed she had a wound disruption which necessitated re-suturing of the wound.

Following recovery from this complication, Mrs. Johnson's convalescence was uneventful and she was discharged on the tenth postoperative day.

References

Buckley, M. E., and Crenshaw, V. P.: Nursing care of a patient with cholecystitis, Am. J. Nursing **46**:812, 1946.

Davis, A., and Dollard, J.: Children of Bondage, Washington, D.C., American Council on Education, 1940.

Koos, Earl Loman: Sociology of the Patient, pp. 41–112, "Patient and His Groups," New York, McGraw-Hill, 1950.

Mann, G. V.: Dietary aspects of cholesterol metabolism and disease, J. Am. Dietet. Assoc. 21:341, 1945.

Myrdal, Gunnar: American Dilemma, New York, Harpers, 1944.

Questions Relating to the Patient Study

1. Mrs. Johnson experienced distress after ingesting fatty foods because

   a.____ obstruction of the bile duct prevented emptying of the bile into the intestine.
   b.____ the liver was manufacturing inadequate bile.
   c.____ fatty foods usually are indigestible.
   d.____ she had a dislike of fatty foods, resulting from childhood illnesses.

2. Fats are better tolerated if they are

   a.____ cooked.   c.____ neither (a) nor (b).
   b.____ uncooked.   d.____ either (a) or (b).

3. The chief purpose of a cholecystography is to

   a.____ note whether the gallbladder contains stones.
   b.____ determine the concentration ability of the gallbladder.
   c.____ observe the patency of the common bile duct.
   d.____ detect obstruction at the ampulla of Vater.

4. For a Graham-Cole test, Mrs. Johnson would have the following experience:

   a.____ The fasting patient empties her bladder and drinks 500 cc. of water containing 40 Gm. of galactose. A specimen of urine is collected before the ingestion of galactose and hourly thereafter for 5 hours.
   b.____ A duodenal tube is passed and a sample of fluid is obtained; the lack of bile would indicate an obstruction somewhere in the common duct.
   c.____ Bromsulphalein 2 mg. per kilogram of body weight is injected intravenously. Serum is obtained 30 minutes later, made alkaline and compared with the bromsulphalein standard series.
   d.____ Dye is taken after a nonfat evening meal; a roentgenogram is taken the next morning before eating. The patient then has a fatty meal which is followed by a roentgenogram.

5. Mrs. Johnson also had an icterus index determination. This is done to test for

   a.____ bilirubin.   c.____ bile salts.
   b.____ urobilin.   d.____ cholesterol.

6. A marked jaundice would be indicated by an icteric index of

  a._____5–15 units/100 cc. of serum.
  b._____15–25 units/100 cc. of serum.
  c._____25–40 units/100 cc. of serum.
  d.___✓___40–50 units/100 cc. of serum.
  e.___✓___50–75 units/100 cc. of serum.

7. A duodenal drainage is done so that intestinal fluid in the region of the duodenum can be examined for

  a.___✓___bile salts.
  b._____gastric juices.
  c.___✓___pancreatic juices.
  d._____*Bacillus coli.*
  e._____pathogenic organisms.
  f._____chyle.

8. Principles to remember which make the passing of a duodenal drainage tube more pleasant are that

  a._____passing the tube through the nose prevents gagging.
  b.___✓___the tube may be made smooth by dipping the end in water.
  c._____having the patient lie on his left side after the tubing has entered the stomach will facilitate its passage into the duodenum.
  d._____ice-cold substances are irritating to the lining of the stomach, therefore rubber tubing should not be chilled before passing.

9. The usual incision made in biliary surgery is

  a._____midline.
  b._____transverse.
  c._____right rectus.
  d.___✓___subcostal.
  e._____gridiron.

10. Symptoms of surgical jaundice for which the nurse must be on the alert in biliary patients are

  a._____black stools, concentrated dark urine, yellow "whites" of the eyes.
  b.___✓___itchy skin, clay-colored stools, dark-colored urine.
  c._____"yellow" skin, dark brown stools, light amber urine.
  d._____yellow sclera, straw-colored urine, putty-colored stools.

11. In jaundiced patients severe postoperative hemorrhage may occur because

  a._____liver damage decreases the manufacture of prothrombin.
  b._____liver damage decreases the synthesis of vitamin K.
  c.___✓___vitamin K, necessary for the manufacture of prothrombin, is not absorbed in the absence of bile salts.
  d._____increased bile in the blood stream lengthens the clotting time of the blood.

12. Upper respiratory complications are more common in patients with biliary surgery than in other types of surgery because of the

  a._____lowering of resistance due to bile in the blood.
  b.___✓___proximity of incision to the diaphragm.
  c._____invasion of the blood stream by infection from the biliary tract.

13. Prevention of pulmonary complications is particularly important for Mrs. Johnson because of the

    a.✓ obesity of the patient.
    b.___tendency of the Negro race to upper respiratory disease.
    c.___racial inertia of the patient.
    d.✓ proximity of the wound to the diaphragm.

14. Pulmonary complications can be prevented by

    a.✓ encouraging her to blow into a paper bag for 5 minutes every hour.
    b.___massaging her extremities and back.
    c.___keeping her heavily sedated for the first 2 postoperative days.
    d.___limiting her movements to prevent wound evisceration.
    e.✓ getting her out of bed and ambulating as soon as possible.

15. A wound disruption or evisceration often can be prevented by

    a.___suturing the skin with steel wire instead of black silk.
    b.✓ applying a supporting scultetus binder.
    c.✓ postponing surgery of patients with a persistent cough.
    d.___bed rest for at least 2 days postoperatively.

16. Mrs. Johnson does not like to move or take deep breaths because she says she has pain. This is due to

    a.___trauma of the tissues incurred during surgery.
    b.✓ the proximity of the diaphragm to the incision.
    c.___the pain she had before her operation.
    d.___a psychologic reaction commonly experienced by biliary patients.
    e.___the sutures which act as invading foreign bodies in tissue.

17. If Mrs. Johnson is getting out of bed and suddenly feels that something has given way in her incision, the nurse should

    a.___disregard it unless it is accompanied by pain.
    b.✓ get her back into bed and examine the wound.
    c.___reassure her but insist that she get out of bed to prevent postoperative complications.
    d.___recognize that this can be expected in gallbladder patients.

18. If on examination of the wound the nurse discovers extensive wound disruption, she should immediately place an emergency call for the surgeon, reassure the patient and

    a.___raise the head of the bed, instruct the patient to breathe deeply, prepare a tray for suturing.
    b.___lower the head of the bed, don sterile gloves, push back the viscera with a dry sterile dressing, instruct the patient not to cough.
    c.___raise the head of the bed, apply a sterile dressing moistened with saline to the viscera, instruct the patient to breathe deeply.

    d._____raise the head of the bed, don sterile gloves, push back the viscera with a dry sterile dressing, instruct the patient to breathe deeply.

    e.__✓__lower the head of the bed, apply a sterile dressing moistened with normal saline, instruct the patient not to cough.

19. If the head nurse asked you to give Mrs. Johnson "surgical fluids," you would give her

    a._____milk, eggnog, broth.
    b.__✓__tea, broth, orange juice.
    c._____tea, cream soup, ginger ale.

Questions for Discussion and Student Projects

1. Explain the physiologic and pathologic basis of pain experienced after the ingestion of fat by a patient with gallbladder disease. Why may this pain persist for several months postoperatively?
2. Pulmonary and circulatory postoperative complications occur more frequently in surgical patients with biliary problems than in most other conditions. Why is this so? What can be done by the nurse to reduce such complications?
3. Plan a low-fat menu for Mrs. Johnson for a week. List those foods which she should avoid. (Plan this diet in such a way that it can be realized with a low income.)
4. Will Mrs. Johnson be able to assume full care of her 7 children when she returns home? What assistance can you offer in helping her to plan her domestic chores so that she will not be dependent on her sister-in-law?
5. In a 6-month follow-up visit to the out-patient department, Mrs. Johnson weighed 225 pounds and was "feeling fine." Did it appear that she was convalescing according to the hopes of the surgical staff? Does she need any further instructions or follow-up visits? Why?
6. What advantages does the new Telepaque* for oral cholecystography have over Priodax and other opaque gallbladder dyes?
7. How are colored patients cared for in your institutions? Are there any problems of adjustment?
8. Do you think Mamie Johnson's experiences as a member of a minority group would affect her attitude in the hospital? How?
9. Compare the experiences of a Negro of Mrs. Johnson's socio-economic group with those of a highly educated professional Negro worker. Which do you think would have the most difficult adjustment problems? Why?
10. How might experiences in being a member of a minority group affect an individual's behavior toward the majority group? Why?

THE STUDENT NURSE WITH JAUNDICE—PATIENT STUDY

Patsy Hall, a second-year student nurse, had just returned to duty after a long illness and convalescence. Patsy had been in an automobile accident

* Winthrop-Stearns, Inc., product.

a month ago, receiving a severe head injury. She had bled profusely from deep lacerations and had required several blood transfusions. Following several weeks' convalescence at home, which was prolonged slightly by a mild upper respiratory infection. Patsy was eager to resume her experience in pediatrics. She told her classmates enthusiastically that she would be a much better nurse now, for she *knew* how frightened patients were when they saw flasks of blood at the bedside.

Patsy's classmates noticed that their pal seemed exhausted each evening when she returned to the dormitory, but thought it was due to her previous illness. However, after a week she developed anorexia, nausea and heartburn and her roommate noticed a slight yellowish tinge to her skin. She was persuaded to go to the student health service and was immediately readmitted to the hospital where, after a series of examinations, a diagnosis of viral hepatitis was made.

Her orders included bed rest, forced fluids, vitamin-B complex and casein hydrolysate.

The jaundice cleared up in 2 weeks, but she remained in the hospital several weeks longer with very gradually increased activity. As her parents live in the city she returned home, and reported to the student health service periodically for follow-up.

References

Baxter, Ola V.: Nursing care of patients with infectious hepatitis, Am. J. Nursing 46:385, 1946.

Brown, Amy Frances, and Franklin, Murray: Viral hepatitis, Am. J. Nursing 50:439, 1950.

Capps, Richard: Infectious hepatitis, Am. J. Nursing 46:383, 1946.

Questions Relating to the Patient Study

1. The causative organism of viral hepatitis is

   a.____streptococcus.   c.__✓__filtrable virus.
   b.____staphylococcus.   d.____ameba.

2. Miss Hall probably was infected by

   a.____contaminated water supply.
   b.__✓__blood from a carrier of the disease.
   c.____cross-infection from a patient in the double room.
   d.____blood infection from her head lacerations.

3. Drugs which would be used with caution for Miss Hall because of the inability of the liver to detoxify them would be

   a.__✓__morphine.   d.____sulfonamides.
   b.____salicylates.   e.____penicillin.
   c.____barbiturates.

4. Drugs which would be contraindicated because of their hepatotoxic effect would be

a.___✓___ether.
b._____penicillin.
c.___✓___sulfonamides.
d._____liver extract.
e._____arsenic salts.

5. Miss Hall would be interested in the reasons for dietary restrictions. The hospital dietitian would explain that

   a.___✓___she needed a large amount of lean meat to regenerate the liver tissue.
   b.___✓___the protein in meat and eggs converts fat to lecithin, which avoids congestion of fats in the liver.
   c._____she could have as many eggs as she desired because they are a pure form of protein.
   d._____she could have cream and butter because she needed extra nourishment.
   e.___✓___she could have starchy foods and desserts because they have a protective effect on the liver.
   f._____she could have starchy foods because they have a protein-sparing effect.
   g._____extra vitamins must be included because the food nutrients are leached out by loose stools.
   h.___✓___extra vitamins are needed because the bile supply is low and fat-soluble vitamins are poorly assimilated.
   i.___✓___thiamine helps prevent fatty liver, so B-complex vitamins are important.
   j._____alcohol has little effect on the liver or bile flow.

6. The itching of jaundice may be relieved by use of

   a._____adrenalin.
   b.___✓___starch baths.
   c._____wet compresses.
   d.___✓___oil inunctions.
   e._____saline injections.

7. Compare infectious hepatitis with homologous serum hepatitis by filling in the following table.

	Infectious Hepatitis	Homologous Hepatitis
Causal organism	*Virus*	*Virus*
Modes of transmission	*Fecally contam. food or H₂O*	*Contaminated blood, needles, egair*
Prevention and control		
Clinical picture	*anorexia, nausea, fever, malaise, tenderness - enlarged liver*	*pain RUc*
Treatment and nursing care		

Questions for Discussion and Student Projects

A. Related to Patient Study

   1. Discuss the use of parenteral fluids and maintenance of water balance for patients with hepatitis. What intake is desirable and what solutions are used?
   2. What explanation would you give Miss Hall in relation to bed rest after she feels better and is eager to be up and discharged? Why are prolonged bed rest and restricted activity important?

3. As a medical nursing instructor, how could you use this case to illustrate the importance of sterile technic?
4. How would the student nurse prevent the recurrence of this situation for herself or a patient? What preventive measures may be taken?
5. What teaching should Miss Hall have before discharge? How would you explain to her the actual changes in the liver and the measures necessary to assure recovery?

B. Related to Hepatitis in General

1. How may toxic hepatitis, as a sequel to other infections, be distinguished from infectious hepatitis? How do the history and treatment differ?
2. Discuss the incidence of drug injury in the development of toxic hepatitis. What part do common chemicals, such as carbon tetrachloride, play in this disease?
3. Discuss the problem of viral hepatitis in the fields of public health and military medicine and its increasing importance in civilian medicine.
4. As a public health nurse assigned to follow up a case of infectious hepatitis, what would you do if you found the patient, a 9-year-old girl, playing around the house with a chocolate nut candy bar in her hand? If a Jewish grandmother was in charge of the child while the mother worked, how would you explain the necessary convalescent care to her?
5. What precautions in the use of a needle and syringe are indicated to avoid infectious hepatitis? Why is it impractical to use a single syringe with a change of needle for each patient?

decreased serum Albuminum + cholesterol

Section 4. Nursing Care of Patients with Disorders of the Genitourinary System*

STUDY SUGGESTIONS: Before beginning the study of this Section, the student will find it helpful to

A. Review

    1. Anatomy and physiology: the urinary tract.
    2. Chemistry: blood chemistry, urinalysis.
    3. Nursing arts: collection of specimens, catheterization.
    4. Physics: pressure in liquids.

B. Study

    1. In medical nursing texts: diseases of the urinary system.
    2. In nutrition texts: diet therapy in kidney disease.
    3. In pharmacology texts: drugs which affect the urinary tract, drugs used in the treatment of bacterial infections.
    4. In surgical nursing texts: surgery of the urinary tract and the male reproductive organs.

C. Read the additional References listed before attempting to answer the questions relating to each patient study.

THE MAN WITH THE SWOLLEN FACE

Background Review Questions

1. Secretion of urine takes place in the portion of the kidneys known as the

    a._____pelvis.
    b._____cortex.
    c._____calyx.
    d._____renal vein.

2. In addition to the excretion of waste products, another equally important function of the kidney is the

    a._____manufacture of insulin for glucose metabolism.
    b._____maintenance of the reaction (pH) of plasma within normal limits.
    c._____elimination of excess bile from the blood.
    d._____manufacture of an enzyme for the stimulation of bladder evacuation.

3. The amount of blood flowing through the kidneys is

---

* Genitourinary conditions in children are considered in the pediatric section.

118

a._____greater than the amount flowing through other organs.
b._____less than the amount flowing through other organs.
c._____not essentially different from the amount flowing through other organs.

4. Urine formation in the kidney consists of three phases. These are (fill in blank spaces)

a. (1) *Filtration* through the _glomerulus_ of _majority of fluid_ *protein free filtrate* from the blood plasma.
(2) *Absorption* of the _majority_ consisting of _G/a_ *of fluid* in the tubules.
(3) *Secretion* by the tubule cells of _creatinine_ and ____urea____.

b. The glomeruli filtrate contains all of the substances found in the blood plasma, except_____ _protein_ .

5. If the filtration pressure within the glomeruli of the normal kidney falls below the average level, the result will be a (an)

a._____increase in the albumin content of the urine excreted.
b._____increase in the volume of urine excreted.
c._____decrease in the volume of urine excreted.
d._____decrease in the specific gravity of the urine excreted.

6. A fall in plasma osmotic pressure tends to influence kidney function by

a._____decreasing the volume of urine excreted.
b._____increasing the glucose content of the urine excreted.
c._____increasing the albumin content of the urine excreted.
d._____increasing the volume of urine production.

7. The primary function of the kidney tubules is to

a._____return plasma proteins to the blood.
b._____reabsorb urea and creatine from the protein-free filtrate passing through them.
c._____reabsorb water, glucose and chlorides from the protein-free plasma filtrate passing through them.
d._____act as a filter preventing plasma proteins from leaving the blood.

8. When a diabetic patient shows a "4 + sugar" on urinalysis, it probably indicates that the

a._____kidney tubules are damaged.
b._____glucose level of the protein-free filtrate is so far above threshhold levels that the tubules cannot remove it all.
c._____glomerular walls have been damaged, making them permeable to this excessive amount of glucose.
d._____hormone pituitrin is not being secreted in normal amounts.

9. Which of the following substances is *not* found in normal urine?

    a._____acetone.
    b._____urea.
    c._____chlorides.
    d._____creatine.

10. The posterior pituitary gland secretes a hormone which influences normal kidney function because it stimulates the

    a._____glomeruli to withhold proteins from the urine.
    b._____kidney tubules to reabsorb water from the fluid within them.
    c._____glomeruli to control the quantity of fluid passing through them.
    d._____kidney tubules to reabsorb glucose from the fluid within them.

11. If you have a patient whose urinalysis shows marked albuminuria, you would suspect that

    a._____the kidney tubules are impaired.
    b._____the walls of the glomeruli are impaired.
    c._____the pressure within Bowman's capsule approximates that of the glomeruli.
    d._____something is obstructing the flow of fluid through the tubules.

12. Albuminuria is the most common symptom of kidney damage. It may also occur, without indicating kidney damage, after

    a._____consuming large amounts of protein.
    b._____strenuous exercise.
    c._____imbibing alcoholic beverages.
    d._____emotional disturbances.
    e._____the use of vasodilator drugs.

13. The specific gravity of urine will depend upon the (check the true items)

    a._____water content.
    b._____bile content.
    c._____salt content.
    d._____solid content.
    e._____total volume.

14. The normal specific gravity of 24 hours' total mixed urine is between

    a._____1.005–1.010.
    b.___✓__1.010–1.015.
    c._____1.015–1.020.
    d._____1.020–1.025.
    e._____1.025–1.030.

15. The amount of urea in the urine depends on the quantity in the blood and the ability of the kidneys to excrete. Normal blood urea is within the following limits:

    a._____20–40 mg. per 100 cc. of blood.
    b._____40–60 mg. per 100 cc. of blood.

   c._____60–80 mg. per 100 cc. of blood.
   d._____80–100 mg. per 100 cc. of blood.
   e._____100–120 mg. per 100 cc. of blood.

16. The normal limits of non-protein nitrogen are

   a._____10–20 mg. per 100 cc.
   b._____25–40 mg. per 100 cc.
   c._____40–60 mg. per 100 cc.
   d._____60–80 mg. per 100 cc.
   e._____80–100 mg. per 100 cc.

17. The normal limits for phenolsulfonephthalein excretion in 2 hours is

   a._____15–30 per cent.
   b._____30–50 per cent.
   c._____60–85 per cent.
   d._____75–90 per cent.
   e._____85–100 per cent.

18. The non-protein nitrogen content of the blood is important because it indicates

   a._____whether the patient has had adequate protein intake which is essential for wound healing.
   b._____the concentration of creatinine, urea, and uric acid which is significant for proper drug therapy.
   c._____the amount of waste products in the blood which in turn reflects kidney function.
   d._____the nitrogenous constituents of the blood which remain after precipitation of the minerals.

19. A non-protein nitrogen (N.P.N.) content of the blood which is considered to be elevated is

   a._____10 mg./100 cc. of blood.
   b._____20 mg./100 cc. of blood.
   c._____40 mg./100 cc. of blood.
   d._____60 mg./100 cc. of blood.

20. The nurse may help in reducing the N.P.N. of her patient by

   a._____having him exercise more.
   b._____encouraging him to take fluids.
   c._____limiting his fluid intake.
   d._____serving him more protein-containing foods.
   e._____increasing his vitamin and mineral intake.

21. A quantitative test for recording the formed elements in urine is_____
_____.
A test to measure the concentration or dilution of urine is_____.
A test to determine the ability of the tube cells to secrete dye is_____.
A test to measure the rate of excretion of the principal nitrogenous waste is_____.

22. Acute glomerulonephritis is associated with infections. The causal organism of the infection most commonly associated with this disease is:

    a._____streptococcus.
    b._____colon bacillus.
    c._____virus.
    d._____staphylococcus.
    e._____tubercle bacillus.

23. The renal lesion is the result of

    a._____invasion of the kidney by the causal organism.
    b._____immunologic response to infection.
    c._____invasion of the blood stream by the causal organism.
    d._____ascending infection following cystitis.

24. Symptoms of acute glomerulonephritis usually occur

    a._____during the height of the infection.
    b._____immediately following the infection.
    c._____2 to 3 weeks after the infection.
    d._____6 to 12 months after the infection.

25. The resulting kidney pathology is

    a._____abscesses of the kidney pelvis.
    b._____urinary calculi.
    c._____narrowing or closing of the capillaries.
    d._____abscesses of the kidney cortex.

26. The most typical urinary findings are

    a._____albumin, casts, red cells.
    b._____albumin, casts, white cells.
    c._____bile, white cells, red cells.
    d._____albumin, bile, casts.

27. The most typical physical findings include

    a._____elevated blood pressure.
    b._____reduced blood pressure.

    a._____edema of the face.
    b._____dependent edema.

    a._____increased pulse rate.
    b._____decreased pulse rate.

28. Place the number of the phrase which relates to it before the condition named:

    a._____anuria.
    b._____polyuria.
    c._____oliguria.
    d._____lithuria.

    (1) presence of bile in urine.
    (2) presence of albuminoid in urine.
    (3) presence of blood in urine.

e._____phosphaturia.
f._____oxaluria.
g._____glycosuria.
h._____albuminuria.
i._____acetonuria.
j._____hematuria.
k._____hemoglobinuria.
l._____indicanuria.
m._____choluria.
n._____chyluria.
o._____pyuria.

(4) presence of pus in urine.
(5) increased flow of urine.
(6) increased amount of indican in urine.
(7) increased flow of saliva.
(8) excess of oxalic acid in urine.
(9) suppression of thirst.
(10) decreased quantity of urine.
(11) suppression of urine.
(12) presence of albumin in urine.
(13) presence of fat in urine.
(14) presence of cancer cells in urine.
(15) excess of uric acid in urine.
(16) excess of acetone bodies in urine.
(17) excess of phosphates in urine.
(18) presence of sodium chloride in urine.
(19) presence of sugar in urine.
(20) presence of hemoglobin in urine.

29. Distinguish between suppression and retention by filling in the following table.

	Definition	Symptoms	Possible Results
Retention............			
Suppression.........			

THE MAN WITH THE SWOLLEN FACE—PATIENT STUDY

Mr. Keller was admitted to the male medical ward from the emergency ward with complaints of puffiness about the eyes and face for the past 4 days. He said that he had had a sore throat 2 weeks before admission which had lasted for 2 days. Three days before admission he awakened with a headache of a "pulsating" type which seemed to localize over the right parietal region. At work that day he lifted some heavy pipes, and noticed what he described as small tender lumps in each groin. Because of general malaise, he did not work the next day. On Saturday and Sunday the headache was very severe and the edema more prominent. He became concerned by Sunday evening, and came to the hospital seeking relief.

Preliminary examination in the admitting ward disclosed an elevated blood pressure and hematuria. He was admitted to the medical ward with the tentative diagnosis of acute glomerulonephritis.

On physical examination Mr. Keller was found to be a well-developed, well-nourished individual, not appearing acutely ill. His pharynx appeared slightly congested (tonsils had been removed at the age of 5). His blood pressure readings were: left arm 160/94, right arm 170/98, pulse 80, respirations 20, temperature 36.8° centigrade. His admission weight was 140 pounds. (He stated that he usually weighed 130–135 pounds.) There was a question of slight cardiac enlargement.

Mr. Keller stated that he was a widower with two young children. He and his children live in a 5-room apartment with his brother, sister-in-law and their two older children. He completed the eleventh grade in school, and is now employed as a laborer with a utilities construction company. He boasts of drinking one case of beer a day, and smokes about one pack of cigarettes daily. He indicates no particular recreational interest.

Upon admission Mr. Keller seemed very resentful and cynical toward his condition. He said that he had not come to the hospital to stay and that he "felt foolish and disgusted with so much fuss."

The first day in the hospital Mr. Keller was given a phenolsulfone-phthalein test; urine was sent to the laboratory for examination; a throat culture and blood for chemistry and blood count were taken. Following the results of the test, the physician's notes included: "kidney function markedly impaired: throat culture positive for hemolytic streptococcus."

On the second day of hospitalization, Mr. Keller complained of difficulty in breathing. Examination disclosed incipient cardiac failure and pleural effusion. Intravenous aminophylline was given, which relieved the dyspnea.

The following orders were written:

> Low-protein, low-sodium diet.
> Fluids—restrict to 1,200 cc./day.
> Penicillin 300,000 units daily.
> Digitalis gr. 1½ b.i.d.
> Weigh daily.

After 1 week of hospitalization the following changes were noted in the progress record:

Pleural effusion—decreasing.
Urinary output—increasing.
Weight—138.9 pounds.
Urine—chlorides decreased.
Edema—absent.
B.P.—180/115–150/70.

Three weeks after admission, Mr. Keller was symptom-free, with the exception of large numbers of red blood cells in the urine. Medications were canceled, and he was placed on a regular diet without free salt.

After he had been in the hospital for 5 weeks, the nurse reported symptoms of coryza, and penicillin was re-ordered. These symptoms subsided in a few days. One week later, when examination confirmed the fact that he was symptom-free, except for occasional red blood cells in the urine, Mr. Keller was discharged. He was instructed to remain on bed rest, and provisions were made for follow-up medical supervision.

Questions Relating to the Patient Study

1. Mr. Keller was given phenolsulfonephthalein intravenously at 10:00 A.M. the day following admission. The nurse's responsibility following this injection is to

   a._____collect all urine voided for a 24-hour period and label it "24-hour specimen."
   b._____collect all urine voided for a 12-hour period and label it "12-hour specimen."
   c._____collect urine specimens a.c. and p.c. and label them accurately with the time of collection.
   d._____collect urine specimens q. 2 hours for an 8-hour period and label them accurately with the time of collection.
   e._____collect urine specimens q. 15 minutes and label them accurately with the time of collection.

2. In order for the p.s.p. test to be carried out successfully, it is helpful to

   a._____urge the patient to void before the test.
   b._____have the patient refrain from voiding before the test.

   a._____restrict fluids before and during the test.
   b._____give fluids liberally before and during the test.

3. The most important single factor in the recovery of Mr. Keller is considered to be

   a._____chemotherapy.
   b._____bed rest.
   c._____diet therapy.
   d._____antihistaminic drugs.

4. Care of Mr. Keller's skin is of particular importance because

   a._____the excretory function of the skin can relieve the kidney, providing rest.
   b._____the skin can excrete enough waste products to prevent uremia.
   c._____edematous patients are more susceptible to decubitus ulcers.
   d._____the medical treatment increases perspiration, which is irritating to skin.

5. Mouth care for Mr. Keller is

   a._____important because sore tongue and gums frequently are associated with his condition.
   b._____no more or less important than good oral hygiene for all
   patients.
   c._____important because it may assist him in restricting fluid intake.
   d._____important because of the characteristic halitosis associated with
   this condition.

6. Mr. Keller's weight loss probably was due to

   a._____lack of adequate food intake.
   b._____the debilitating effects of disease.
   c._____improvement in urinary output.

   This would indicate the

   a._____need for increased caloric intake.
   b._____need for continuing chemotherapy.
   c._____encouraging results of treatment.

7. Penicillin during the first stages of Mr. Keller's hospitalization was
   ordered primarily for

   a._____urinary antisepsis.
   b._____the control of blood-stream infection.
   c._____the control of foci of infection.

8. Mr. Keller's laboratory report follows below:

   Directions: Indicate in the appropriate columns whether each item is
   normal, below normal or above normal by using a check
   (✓). In the spaces at the extreme right of the page, write
   the normal figures or results for those items which are
   below normal or above normal.

a.	*Urine*	*Below*	*Normal*	*Above*	*Normal Figure*
	(1) Reaction slightly acid	___	___	___	___
	(2) Amount 200 cc. for 24 hours	___	___	___	___
	(3) Specific gravity 1.032	___	___	___	___
	(4) Albumin large quan-tity	___	___	___	___
	(5) Sugar negative	___	___	___	___
	(6) Bile negative	___	___	___	___

	Urine	*Below*	*Normal*	*Above*	*Normal Figure*
(7)	Color dark				
(8)	Appearance cloudy				
(9)	Leukocytes many				
(10)	Red blood cells many				
(11)	Casts many				
(12)	P.S.P. 30 per cent (total specimen)				

b.   *Blood*

(1)	Wassermann negative				
(2)	Kahn negative				
(3)	Erythrocytes 2,500,000/cu. mm.				
(4)	Hemoglobin 52 per cent				
(5)	Leukocytes 20,000				
(6)	Non-protein nitrogen 55 mg. per cent				
(7)	Urea nitrogen 50				
(8)	Uric acid 5 mg.				
(9)	Creatinine 4 mg.				
(10)	Sodium chloride 800 mg. per 100 cc.				
(11)	Blood pressure $\frac{170}{98}$				

9. By inserting a check in the proper blanks below, indicate the conclusions that reasonably may be drawn from the laboratory report as given for Mr. Keller:

   a. In appearance Mr. Keller has

   (1)_____a flushed skin.
   (2)_____normal skin color.
   (3)_____slight pallor of the lips and cheeks.
   (4)_____marked pallor of the lips and cheeks.
   (5)_____severe cyanosis of the lips and cheeks.

   b. The kidney infection is

   (1)_____severe.
   (2)_____moderate.
   (3)_____slight.

10. Aminophylline has the following physiologic effects:

    a._____stimulation of the myocardium, improvement of the circulation, dilation of the bronchi.
    b._____irritation of the kidney tubules, cardiac depressant, respiratory stimulant.
    c._____central nervous system depressant, kidney stimulant, circulatory stimulant.

d._____central nervous system stimulant, kidney irritant, cardiac depressant.

11. When aminophylline was administered to Mr. Keller the physician would expect the following effects:

   a._____restlessness and irritability, increased urinary output, decreased pulse rate.
   b._____increased urinary output, decreased dyspnea, decreased pleural effusion.
   c._____extreme drowsiness, no change in urinary output, decreased dyspnea.
   d._____increased hematuria, increased urinary output, restlessness and irritability.

12. Aminophylline may be administered orally, intravenously or intramuscularly, or by rectal suppository. The average adult dosage is:

   a. Orally:

      (1)_____0.1–0.2 Gm.
      (2)_____0.5–0.8 Gm.

   b. Intravenously or intramuscularly:

      (1)_____0.25 Gm.
      (2)_____0.5 Gm.

   c. Rectally:

      (1)_____0.36 Gm.
      (2)_____0.63 Gm.

References

Elman, Robert: Fluid balance from the nurse's point of view, Am. J. Nursing 49:222, 1949.
Hlohinec, Eileen M.: Nursing care in nephritis, Am. J. Nursing 48:689, 1948.
Leaf, Alexander: Nephritis in the adult, Am. J. Nursing 48:687, 1948.

Questions for Discussion and Student Projects

A. Related to Patient Study

   1. Outline the procedure to be followed if an intern told you he had given Mr. Keller phenolsulfonephthalein dye at 10 A.M.
   2. What type of mouth care would be provided for Mr. Keller? How often would it be given and why? Why is skin care important in nephritis? Explain the relationship between drafts, chilling, upper respiratory infections and nephritic patients?
   3. How may accurate weight recordings be taken of Mr. Keller? Discuss this nursing problem for the bed patient.
   4. Mr. Keller threatened to sign his release on the basis of his dissatis-

faction with his diet (low sodium, low protein). What explanation would you give him and how would you handle the problem? What would you, as a student, do if you found Mr. Keller or another similiar patient, accepting food from other patients or from his family?

5. How may you help Mr. Keller adjust to his illness? What evidence was noted of his apprehension and insecurity? What approaches were necessary to convince him of the seriousness of his condition? What is his prognosis?

6. How would you handle the situation when Mr. Keller became upset when he was required to use the bedpan instead of making the long trip to the bathroom for his stools? What might be done if he were un-co-operative and was discarding urine with the stools? What technics are used at your hospital to insure recording of intake and output?

7. What instruction should Mr. Keller have during hospitalization to prepare him for home care? What assistance might be given to his family in preparing for his discharge? What community resources are available in your locality to care for convalescent and chronic patients? What medical resources are available for continued supervision of Mr. Keller?

B. Related to Nephritis in General

1. Discuss the theories of high- and low-protein diets, low-sodium intake and limited and forced fluids in relation to the management of patients suffering with nephritis.

2. Review the renal function tests used in your hospital. Discuss insulin and PAH tests (para-aminohippurate). Which tests are used to measure total renal blood flow, filtration rate, tubular absorption and tubular excretion? What preparation and explanation does the patient require? What are the nurse's responsibilities?

3. Where does nephritis stand statistically as a direct or indirect cause of death in the United States? What is the life expectancy of a nephritic? What effect does this have on patients attempting to secure life insurance? What is the social and economic significance of the prolonged convalescence and continued ill health of nephritics?

4. What would you do if you discovered that a patient with chronic nephritis who understood the importance of limited activity when he returned home was worried about the inevitable demands of his family?

5. Discuss the management of a patient suffering from uremia.

6. Discuss the management of a person suffering from mercury poisoning. Give recent reports on the use of BAL (British anti-Lewisite) in mercury poisoning. Discuss the use of "artificial kidneys."

7. If, after returning home, a patient convalescing from nephritis developed an upper respiratory infection, what instructions should he have?

THE PRIMIPARA WITH "KIDNEY TROUBLE"

Background Review Questions

1. Urinary calculi are of two main types. Match the following classifications:

   Those formed in   *Calculi*

   a. alkaline urine.   (1)_____oxalate.
   b. acid urine.   (2)_____cystine.
                               (3)_____phosphate.
                               (4)_____xanthine.
                               (5)_____carbonate.
                               (6)_____uric acid.

2. Kidney stones are found most frequently

   a._____high in the calyx.
   b._____low in the calyx.
   c._____in the pelvis.
   d._____at the ureteropelvic junction.

3. A vitamin deficiency which is often held responsible for the development of renal calculi is of

   a._____vitamin A.   d._____vitamin D.
   b._____vitamin B.   e._____vitamin E.
   c._____vitamin C.   f._____vitamin K.

4. Factors which may be influential in preventing the recurrence of renal calculi are

   a._____elimination of remote pyogenic foci of infection in the tonsils, teeth, sinuses, etc.
   b._____administration of massive doses of vitamins B and D.
   c._____surgical correction of abnormal conditions of the thyroid gland.
   d._____regulation of the pH of the urine by diet, medications and fluids.

5. If a stone is of a type formed in alkaline urine, the following acidifying agents are employed:

   a._____alkaline-ash diet.   d._____sodium benzoate.
   b._____acid-ash diet.   e._____ammonium chloride.
   c._____sodium bicarbonate.

6. In general, the acid regimen is contraindicated in cases of renal calculi

   a._____when due to impaired function, because there is inability on the part of the kidney to excrete acid.
   b._____in the presence of a urinary infection due to urea-splitting organisms, producing an excessively acid urine.
   c._____in the presence of calcium oxalate stones, because acid therapy causes an increase in the amount of calcium excreted in the urine.

7. Those foods which would not be included on an acid-ash diet are

    a._____plain cookies, plain cake.
    b._____English walnuts.
    c._____bacon, ham.
    d._____American cheddar cheese.
    e._____salted butter, salted crackers.

8. Some of the more common theories which have been advanced as causing urinary lithiasis would include

    a._____racial predispositions; for example, the Negro since he lives more consistently in warmer climates.
    b._____kidney infections, particularly those due to the colon bacillus.
    c._____dietary deficiencies; this is true when there are often monotonous diets such as one in which cereals form the staple food.
    d._____hyperparathyroidism caused by parathyroid tumor; often this demonstrates a tendency to develop renal calculi because of a disturbance in Ca-P metabolism.

9. A litholapaxy is an operative procedure which accomplishes the following:

    a._____A stone(s) is (are) crushed in the bladder for easy removal.
    b._____A floating kidney is sutured to the lower ribs for reinforcement in nephroptosis.
    c._____A plastic operation is done to restore tissue function after a stone is removed.
    d._____Urinary-tract calculi are removed by means of a flexible ureteral bougie.

10. When a nephrolithotomy is done for a large calculus, the kidney incision usually is made

    a._____directly over the stone approaching the kidney laterally following the guide of the roentgenogram.
    b._____near the juncture of the ureter and kidney in an attempt to enter the pelvis.
    c._____into the kidney substance itself, opposite the side of the ureteral juncture.

THE PRIMIPARA WITH "KIDNEY TROUBLE"—PATIENT STUDY

Helen, who is now 30, felt she had a very deprived life because the social and economic position of her family was low. They were Russian, of the Greek Orthodox religion, and they attempted to impose upon Helen some of their strict beliefs. Her feeling of deprivation was further accentuated by an illness experienced at the age of 22, with attacks of pain in the costovertebral angles, more severe on the left side and radiating anteriorly.

These attacks continued intermittently for 2 years when she finally experienced a sudden and terrific attack of pain in the left flank which made her double up. Pain was so severe that it was accompanied by nausea, vomiting, chills and sweats; finally the pain radiated downward to the groin. She had a left ureterolithotomy and was told before she left the hospital that she must expect further "kidney trouble" because stones were found to be present in both kidneys.

After a satisfactory convalescence, Helen left home to get away from her family. She secured a job as a waitress and in a short while married a Jewish cab driver who had frequented her restaurant. Helen admitted she married for two reasons: to have a home of her own and to have a baby. They rented a pleasant 3-room apartment and bought some very nice furniture on the installment plan. Then Helen became pregnant, "before the kidneys got too bad."

After 4 months she was seen in the Obstetrical O.P.D. Her main problem was bilateral renal calculi and ensuing renal destruction, complicated by pregnancy. Her particular symptoms were generalized fatigue, nervousness and inability to work, recurrences of pain in the left costovertebral angle causing nausea and forcing her to lie down. She gave a urologic history of intermittent gross hematuria, cloudy urine and occasional dysuria, but had not passed any stones.

Pyelograms demonstrated tremendous bilateral hydronephrosis. Further films described the stones of the right side as numbering 20 and measuring 6–8 mm. in diameter, those on the left numbering 4 and measuring 1.5–3 cm. Helen was advised to have the pregnancy terminated and sterilization performed. Unable to reach a decision, she was discharged and asked to return to the Urology O.P.D.

Helen wanted the baby very much. Her husband was quiescent—he wanted the child for her sake. Helen's tenacity of purpose kept her from reaching a decision; she solved it by not returning to the O.P.D. for 3 months. Then a severe left abdominal pain forced her to return for admission. An induction was performed on her fourth hospital day and on the fifth day she was delivered of a dead fetus (about 6 months).

When transferred to the urology service, her laboratory findings were

Urine loaded with pus.
P.S.P. 5 per cent in 2 hours.
B.U.N. 35 mg.

Helen's temperature rose to 40.2°C. and she developed a left pleural effusion which was relieved in a few days. Attempts made to pass catheters into the left renal pelvis failed because of marked angulation in the ureteropelvic junction.

Her attitude was despondent; she repeated that the physical pain she had experienced made life seem not worthwhile; however, if the baby had lived, life would have assumed new meaning. With preliminary transfusions of blood, Helen had a right nephrostomy under general anesthesia. The kidney contained several hundred cubic centimeters of thick foul pus and was drained with a No. 40 catheter. No stones were removed, but, in 2 weeks, 7 stones came through the tube. The skin healed about the tube and at the time of her discharge she was draining 300–800 cc. of urine daily.

In another month, she was back for a permanent nephrostomy of the left side. Her general physical appearance had become changed by her long illness. Tall, but very thin, she lay in bed very quietly, drowsy and lethargic. She gave a picture of chronic illness. Her voice had developed a whining note. She became imperious in her demands and the nurses soon learned that most could be accomplished by allowing her to assume that she was dictating the procedure. Sedatives were many and frequent. She recognized medications and would become quite disgruntled if a mild drug such as aspirin were offered to her after she had asked for relief from pain.

Nursing care became a matter of irrigating each tube twice a day and changing dressings that were soaked by foul-smelling drainage. There was a danger of skin breakdown. Helen's ultimate prognosis is that of uremia through complete loss of kidney function. Although she now gets out of bed into a wheel chair, her back soon grows tired and the mechanical interference of Hubert and Humphrey (her names for the right and left drainage bottles) limits her enjoyment of this procedure. She may surprise us in her longevity, but to date no plan has been worked out for her.

References

Beck, Sr. M. Berenice: The Nurse, Handmaid of the Divine Physician, Philadelphia, Lippincott, 1945.

Flocks, R. H.: Renal stones, Am. J. Nursing 44:207, 1944.

Lowsley and Kirwin: Urology for Nurses, 2nd ed. Chapter 8, "Kidney," pp. 180–279, Philadelphia, Lippincott, 1948.

Schweishimer, W.: Kidney stones, Trained Nurse and Hosp. Rev. 120:40, 1948.

Questions Relating to the Patient Study

1. A retrograde pyelogram which Helen experienced is a test which is performed as follows:

   a.____a nontoxic shadow-forming iodine compound is injected intravenously or subcutaneously and when secreted unchanged by the kidneys, a roentgenogram is taken.

   b.____Hippuran is given orally in palatable form and roentgenograms are taken about 90 minutes after the ingestion of the drug.

   c.____a roentgenogram of the kidney pelvis and calyces is taken after these have been filled with radiopaque solution which has been injected through a catheter.

2. Helen had a B.U.N. (blood urea nitrogen) of 35 mg. per 100 cc. of blood. This is

   a.____below normal.   b.____normal.   c.____above normal.

3. A B.U.N. determination is significant because

   a.____urea nitrogen is entirely waste and is excreted by the kidneys; the normal concentration in the blood has a definite range.

   b.____a concentration above normal usually is due to irreparable bilateral renal destruction.

    c._____a concentration above normal is indicative of energy expenditure above normal.

    d._____an elevation in the urea-nitrogen estimation is a reliable prognostic maneuver, especially in advanced nephritis.

4. The purpose of straining all urine of patients who have a diagnosis of urinary calculi is to

    a._____determine how many stones still remain in the tract.

    b._____observe urinary contents other than stones which may be present.

    c._____note the size and shape of stones which may give a clue as to their origin.

    d._____keep the physician informed regarding the passage of stones.

    e._____save any stones, which may be passed, for chemical analysis.

5. During the passage of a kidney or ureteral stone, the patient may have acute renal colic. The nurse may expect the physician to order

    a._____acetylsalicylic acid 0.6 Gm.

    b._____codeine sulfate 0.03 Gm.

    c._____Demerol 50 mg.

    d._____morphine sulfate 0.03 Gm.

6. The usual position on the operating table for a patient who is to have kidney surgery is to lie on the

    a._____abdomen.   c._____involved side.

    b._____uninvolved side.   d._____back.

7. For better exposure during kidney surgery, it is often necessary to perform a rib resection. The following instruments will be necessary for such a procedure:

    a._____a bone rongeur, periosteal elevator, costatome, rib shears.

    b._____a bone rongeur, bone-holding forceps, chisel, rib shears.

    c._____rib shears, sequestrum forceps, periosteal elevator, osteotome.

    d._____rib shears, bone-holding forceps, costatome, chisel.

8. One of the dangers in doing a nephrostomy is the problem of bleeding because of the high vascularity of the organ. The most common method to control hemorrhage, before closing the wound, is to

    a._____swab the kidney incision line with compound benzoin tincture.

    b._____insert a pad or pads of fat into or along the kidney wound.

    c._____use interrupted mattress sutures which are tied in triple knots.

    d._____use chromic rather than plain catgut of about 3–0 or 4–0 size.

9. The amount of fluid ordinarily used to irrigate a kidney pelvis is

    a._____small in amount (10–15 cc.) because of the limited area of the pelvis.

    b._____1,000 cc. with about 100 cc. forced into the pelvis at a time before it is allowed to return.

    c._____500 cc. used as a continuous irrigation in and out of the kidney.

10. Special postoperative functions for which a nurse is responsible in the care of kidney surgical patients are to note

    a._____the temperature of the patient at least q. 4 hours because there is a tendency toward elevation brought about by increased waste products in the blood.

    b._____that the tendency toward infection is greater in kidney surgery than other types of abdominal surgery because of the presence of urine; therefore, urinary disinfectants should be used when changing surgical dressings.

    c._____that the tendency toward shock is greater in these patients than in other abdominal surgery. To prevent this complication, it is good foresight to maintain the Trendelenburg position for the first 6 hours P.O.

    d._____that she should be aware of any untoward symptoms suggestive of hemorrhage; such a complication may occur within 24 hours or several days after operation.

Questions for Discussion and Student Projects

1. Why was a nephrectomy not performed on Helen? How would you reassure a patient who fears that he will become an invalid if he has a nephrectomy?
2. Plan an alkaline-ash and an acid-ash menu for one day and point out the difference in each. When is each indicated? What medication supplements will facilitate the planning of such menus?
3. Discuss the use of Amphojel in the treatment of renal calculus. When indicated? Its mode of action? Wherein lies its usefulness? How long is a patient kept on this medication and what are the average doses?
4. Canvass the recent literature for the current thinking on the dissolution of stones. How and when is it effective? Qualify your statements.
5. What is the incidence of kidney problems in modern obstetric practice? What is being done to reduce it?
6. Of what significance is it to the nurse to know that a patient is a strict adherent of the Russian Greek Orthodox religion? (Dietary preferences, or any other factors.) Of what significance would the recommendation to terminate the pregnancy and perform a sterilization have been if Helen had been of the Roman Catholic faith?
7. What can be done to help Helen in the development of a more optimistic philosophy of life? How can her husband help her.
8. If Helen recovers sufficiently to return to her apartment, what restrictions will she have and what instructions should her husband have?
9. This young couple were able to afford the rent of their apartment because they were both working. What adjustments will have to be made with regard to their living quarters, continuing their installment payments on furniture and payment of hospital bills, etc.? How can this be approached most satisfactorily?

10. The fact that Helen referred to her drainage bottles as Hubert and Humphrey is indicative of a sense of humor even though she has sufficient reason to be despondent much of the time. How can this clue help the nurse in developing better rapport with Helen? In establishing a basis for a more optimistic attitude in Helen?

11. How can one encourage Helen to take care of herself? Set up a plan for

adequate skin care.   desirable diet intake.
control of odors.   intelligent observation of signifi-
exercise and rest.   cant symptoms, e.g. drainage,
proper fluid exchange.   toxic manifestations, etc.

Nursing Care of Patients with Other Kidney Disorders

A. Nephroptosis

1. The incidence of nephroptosis is greatest in

   a._____boys up to age 20.   c._____men between 20 and 40.
   b._____girls up to age 20.   d._____women between 20 and 40.

2. The common clinical picture of a patient having nephroptosis is

   a._____nausea and vomiting, dizziness, burning on urination, no significant pain.
   b._____pain, fatigue, hyperesthesia, insomnia, emotional upsets.
   c._____flatulence, constipation or diarrhea, no urinary symptoms, no nervous symptoms, no appreciable pain.
   d._____chronic pain, fatigue, lethargy, apathy, urinary frequency.

3. In nephroptosis, an acute attack of pain resembling renal colic due to kidney or ureteral stones is referred to as

   a._____Dietl's crisis.   c._____trabecula.   e._____renal toxicosis.
   b._____tenesmus.   d._____smegma.

4. The most desirable P.O. position after nephropexy is

   a._____Sims' lateral.   d._____prone.
   b._____Trendelenburg.   e._____dorsal recumbent.
   c._____semi-Fowler's.

5. The chief reason for the suggested position in question 4 is to

   a._____minimize the tendency toward shock and hemorrhage.
   b._____initiate a rehabilitative course early in the postoperative phase.
   c._____facilitate the formation of supporting adhesions and the healing of tissues in the position desired.

      d.———allow for needed rest and the assumption of the most desirable anatomic position.

  6. Occasionally a patient returns from the operating room with kidney pedicle clamps in place. Since the handle or handles should protrude from the dressings, the following nursing measures should be employed:

      a.———Place a bed cradle over the patient and do not allow him to turn from side to side.

      b.———Remove the clamps after 24 hours since they are there only to facilitate immediate postoperative hemostasis.

      c.———In turning the patient, turn him almost, but not quite, on his abdomen and support the abdomen by slipping a pillow under it.

      d.———If the clamps are in a right-sided incision, tell the patient he may lie on his left side; place a pillow against his back, taking care not to put pressure on the wound.

B. Ureteral Surgery

  1. Obstruction, other than calculus, may occur at the junction of the ureter and kidney pelvis. The treatment is usually a surgical plastic procedure, which means that the patient has a nephrostomy tube as well as a soft rubber splinting catheter in the reconstructed ureter. The nurse should anticipate the following postoperative problems:

      a.———The drainage tubes must be kept free of kinks to prevent undue pressure on the suture line.

      b.———The urine should be kept alkaline for an acid infection may lead to the deposition of calcium.

      c.———Fluid balance must be maintained for proper body function; hypotonic rather than hypertonic solutions should be used for catheter irrigation.

      d.———Infection must be controlled; the use of chemotherapy and proper dressing technic must be employed.

  2. When exstrophy, extensive trauma or cancer of the bladder makes it necessary to remove the bladder or to divert the urinary stream, transplantation of the ureters into the bowel is commonly done. The usual preoperative preparations for such an operative procedure include

      a.———fluid diet for from 1 to 3 days before surgery, nothing P.O. after midnight before the day of surgery.

      b.———the usual diet until 12 midnight before the day of surgery, thereafter nothing P.O.

      c.———a medication such as sulfaguanidine given for its high bacteriostatic action against intestinal bacteria.

      d.———an aqueous suspension such as aluminum hydroxide gel given for its mildly astringent and demulcent action.

3. Following a ureteral transplantation into the intestinal tract, the patient usually has a rectal tube in place. A physician may order that this be irrigated with saturated magnesium sulfate. The chief purpose of this is

  a._____for its mechanical action; it softens and increases the bulk of the intestinal contents.
  b._____to lessen edema which might block the small ureteral orifice.
  c._____to produce a cathartic effect which results from the osmotic action of the unabsorbed salt.

C. Male Sex Glands

1. The function(s) of the testicle is (are) to

  a._____produce spermatozoa.
  b._____secrete a fluid which lubricates and facilitates the passage of spermatozoa.
  c._____regulate the environmental temperature of the male sex glands.
  d._____produce an internal secretion which controls the secondary sexual characteristics of the male.

2. The spermatic cord serves to

  a._____support the testicle in the scrotum.
  b._____convey the nerves.
  c._____convey the vas deferens.
  d._____convey the blood and lymph vessels.

3. Cryptorchidism is the term applied to

  a._____a eunuch.   c._____a hermaphrodite.
  b._____an undescended   d._____an atrophied spermatic
       testicle.   cord.

4. Cryptorchidism may be repaired surgically by an

  a._____orchidectomy.   d._____orchidopexy.
  b._____orchotomy.   e._____orchectomy.
  c._____orchidotomy.

Questions for Discussion and Student Projects

1. Patients who have had a bilateral ureteral transplantation into the intestinal tract have the problem of regulating urinary output so that it is not a continuous dribble. Investigate the literature for suggestions which will help a nurse as she teaches such a patient. What can you add to this list?
2. List the ways in which a nurse may minimize infection in the postoperative care of patients with ureteral transplantation either to the abdominal skin or to the intestinal tract. What are the special hazards of such an infection?
3. What types of diet should be planned for the first 3 months after surgery for ureteral transplantation into the intestinal tract? Why?

THE PATRIARCH

Background Review Questions

1. The prostate is located

   a._____just below the bladder encircling the urethra.
   b._____just below the bladder behind the urethra.
   c._____in the bladder.
   d._____in the spermatic cord.
   e._____in the scrotum.

2. The function of the prostate gland is to

   a._____participate in the function of urination.
   b._____supply spermatozoa for ejaculation.
   c._____secrete seminal fluid at the time of ejaculation.
   d._____secrete a fluid which combines with other secretions to form seminal fluid.

3. The incidence of benign overgrowth of the prostate in men over 60 is about

   a._____10 per cent.
   b._____30 per cent.
   c._____60 per cent.
   d._____75 per cent.

4. Early symptoms suggesting a benign overgrowth of the prostate are

   a._____urinary frequency, nocturia, burning on urination, lethargy, anorexia.
   b._____overflow incontinence followed by complete retention, weight loss, dry skin and tongue.
   c._____urinary frequency, nocturia, pain in the inguinal regions or thighs, low W.B.C., ascites.
   d._____difficulty in starting the stream, pain in the lower back, suppression, low blood non-protein nitrogen.

5. Occasionally, a cystostomy is performed about 1 week or 10 days before a prostatectomy is done. The reason(s) for this 2-stage procedure is (are) that

   a._____the first stage (cystostomy) is often an emergency procedure to relieve a distended bladder.
   b._____a better surgical approach is made for a prostatectomy when the bladder has been decompressed by a cystostomy.
   c._____contamination is less when there is adequate bladder drainage; this is accomplished with a cystostomy.
   d._____there is an opportunity for optimum preparation of the patient, both physically and mentally, when a prostatectomy is not done immediately on hospital admission.

6. There are advantages and disadvantages to each of the 4 types of prostatectomy. By recognizing these, the nurse is able to anticipate likely postoperative complications and thereby aid in their prevention.

Match the letter of the operative procedure with its chief advantages or disadvantages:

a. Suprapubic prostatectomy.   c. Transurethral prostatectomy.
b. Perineal prostatectomy.   d. Retropubic prostatectomy.

(1)＿＿＿ it requires an abdominal incision.
(2)＿＿＿ it is easiest to perform.
(3)＿＿＿ there is a high incidence of shock postoperatively.
(4)＿＿＿ the approach is very vascular, and hemorrhage is often likely.
(5)＿＿＿ postoperatively, the wound is contaminated easily.
(6)＿＿＿ there is no incision.
(7)＿＿＿ cosmetically, it is a desirable incision.
(8)＿＿＿ skill is required to prevent injury to the rectum.

7. Many times it is customary to perform a bilateral vasectomy in conjunction with suprapubic prostatectomy. The reason for doing this is

   a.＿＿＿to repress the desire for sexual activity which often occurs postoperatively.
   b.＿＿＿to prevent the descent of infection from the seminal vesicles to the epididymis and testicles.
   c.＿＿＿as a matter of convenience. Otherwise, the patient would have to submit to this surgical procedure at another time.

8. If a patient has had a perineal prostatectomy, the nurse should remember the following:

   a.＿＿＿Always take a rectal temperature not only to determine body temperature but also to note the adequacy of perineal circulation.
   b.＿＿＿Under no conditions should a rectal temperature be taken.
   c.＿＿＿For his comfort, the patient should sit on a semi-inflated air cushion.
   d.＿＿＿Firm pressure is necessary for such a perineal wound, therefore the patient should sit on a hard surface.

9. The most important function of a Foley catheter (or any inflatable balloon type catheter) in the newly postoperative prostatectomy patient is to

   a.＿＿＿produce hemostasis.
   b.＿＿＿provide an irrigating system.
   c.＿＿＿keep the bladder empty of urine.
   d.＿＿＿allow for adequate drainage.

10. To secure adequate gravity drainage when a suprapubic tube is connected by rubber tubing to a drainage bottle on the floor, the nurse should check the following:

    a.＿＿＿Tubing should be long enough to allow the patient to turn on his side. Allow the tubing to reach into the drainage bottle, but not to become immersed in the drainage. Place a safety pin through the tubing and fasten it to the draw sheet to prevent the tubing from pulling out of the patient.

b._____Check all tubing for kinks and collapsed portions. Allow the tubing to have a deep U-turn before the terminal end enters the drainage bottle. To keep the tubing from slipping down over the bed, fasten a tape around the rubber tubing and pin the tape to the draw sheet.

c._____Check to see that there is no tension on the tubing. Allow the tubing to flow downward to the drainage bottle with no U-turn or loop. Be sure there are no tapering glass connecting tubes which might become clogged with mineral deposits.

11. When disinfecting a ureteral catheter in a suitable chemical solution, the following points must be observed for optimum effect:

a._____Submerge only that part of the catheter which will be introduced into a patient.

b._____Submerge the entire catheter, even though part of it need not be disinfected.

c._____Inject the solution through the catheter until all air bubbles have escaped.

d._____It is not necessary to inject the chemical solution through the catheter, because it flows into the catheter anyway.

e._____The killing of vegetative organisms can be accomplished with a suitable chemical in 30 minutes.

f._____The killing of vegetative organisms can be accomplished with a suitable chemical in 10 minutes.

12. In decompression drainage, a certain amount of urine accumulates in the bladder, creating a slight pressure which overcomes resistance presented by the "Y-tube." Physics principles involved are that

a._____fluid will flow in a system only where there is a difference of pressure at both ends of the system.

b._____when fluid flows out of a system, a drop in pressure is evidenced.

c._____the greater the diameter of the tubing, the less will be the volume of fluid flow.

d._____the flow rate of the fluid is directly proportional to the viscosity.

13. Some of the purposes of using decompression drainage, rather than straight drainage of the bladder, are that

a._____bladder surfaces are prevented from coming in contact with one another.

b._____the bladder is kept empty most of the time, which reduces the possibility of infection.

c._____gentle pressure produced by fluid in the bladder gives some hemostasis.

d._____bladder spasm, which is necessary for complete evacuation, is produced.

THE PATRIARCH—PATIENT STUDY

Samuel Epstein, an orthodox Jew of moderate means, is a patient in a semi-private room. At the age of 78, he seems very proud of his solicitous wife, 7 children, 18 grandchildren, and 6 great-grandchildren. His large family expresses its concern, respect and adoration for him by frequent visits, by many calls of inquiry and by sending food and gifts. Mr. Epstein is apparently deeply religious, evidenced by the wearing of his black skull cap and the time spent with religious books and rituals.

Mr. Epstein has been in relatively good health and only recently has shown signs associated with age, such as impaired vision and hearing, and noticeable forgetfulness. He seems dependent upon the use of a cane, and moves very slowly.

Mr. Epstein was admitted to the hospital because of urinary difficulties, which have been progressively more severe. He complains of nocturia and difficulty in starting a stream. Because of these difficulties, he has limited his fluid and food intake.

He expresses apprehension at any new procedure or treatment. He shows concern about himself by restlessness at night, inability to go to sleep, and reluctance to stay in one place.

Medical treatment was directed toward preparing Mr. Epstein for surgery since it was apparent on examination that he had a hypertrophied prostate. Because of his dehydration, malnourishment, and elevated blood non-protein nitrogen, he had a 7-day preoperative phase.

The surgical procedure of choice was a suprapubic prostatectomy done satisfactorily under general anesthesia. One hour postoperatively, Mr. Epstein went into shock, but with proper treatment he responded well. He had a suprapubic tube and a Foley 3-way catheter for drainage. The first day postoperatively, he was assisted out of the bed and ambulated. He was always reluctant to get out of bed, to move from his chair, or to walk. He seemed very sensitive about his "tube and bottle," and always tried to hide it when he had visitors.

By the time he was ready for discharge, the indwelling catheter was removed; however, he still had a suprapubic tube in place. A rubber urinal was purchased for Mr. Epstein to wear during the day. He was instructed to connect the suprapubic tube to a gallon bottle at his bedside for drainage at night. His wife was taught how to take care of Mr. Epstein's skin, the rubber urinal, and the drainage tube. She was also told how important it was to keep Mr. Epstein on an adequate fluid intake. He was to report to his own physician for follow-up care.

References

Cooper, Barber, Mitchell, Rynbergen: Nutrition in Health and Disease, 11th ed., pp. 140–143, "Jewish Dietary Habits," Philadelphia, Lippincott, 1950.

Flitter, H.: An Introduction to Physics in Nursing, pp. 75–77, "Pressure in Flowing Fluids," St. Louis, Mosby, 1948.

Hayes, B. A., and Millsop, J. G.: Retropubic prostatectomy, Am. J. Nursing 50:435, 1950.

Newton, K.: Urologic nursing, Am. J. Nursing 50:167, 1950.

Pool, T. L.: Transurethral prostatic resection on elderly patients, Geriatrics 1:121, 1946.

Van Schoick, M. R., and Higgins, C.: Carcinoma of the prostate, Am. J. Nursing 48:427, 1948.

Questions Relating to the Patient Study

1. In preparing Mr. Epstein for a cystoscopic examination, it is

    a._____necessary to encourage him to drink 1 or 2 glasses of water before going to the cystoscopic room.

    b._____necessary to be sure he has nothing by mouth for at least 4 hours before his examination.

    c._____necessary to secure his signature on an Operative Permit.

    d._____not necessary for him to sign an Operative Permit.

    e._____not necessary to give a sedative before cystoscopy because such a medication distorts the actual nature of the bladder wall.

    f._____usually necessary to give a sedative before cystoscopy, and because of this, it is often unnecessary to use a general anesthetic.

2. Mr. Epstein went into a state of shock immediately postoperatively. Shock is most commonly defined as

    a._____failure of the peripheral circulation.

    b._____failure of the cerebral circulation.

    c._____failure of the central (cardiac) circulation.

3. The surgical nurse recognized that Mr. Epstein was going into shock when the following combination of symptoms were presented:

    a. Blood pressure (normally 170/95):

     (1)_____120/80→100/75.
     (2)_____110/80→90/60.
     (3)_____100/75→120/90.
     (4)_____60/40→40/?

    b. Pulse (normally 74):

     (1)_____120→150.
     (2)_____110→80.
     (3)_____80→50.
     (4)_____150→155.

    c. Skin:

     (1)_____flushed, moist.
     (2)_____warm, dry.
     (3)_____pale, moist.

    d.

     (1)_____restless.
     (2)_____apprehensive.
     (3)_____thirsty.
     (4)_____apathetic.

4. Good psychologic understanding of the older patient who should have forced fluids can be demonstrated as follows:

   a._____Fluids are important for him; however, if he insists that he cannot or does not want to take them, do not offer him any, for it would be worse for his general condition.

   b._____A good way to get him to take fluids, if the nurse is having difficulty, is to tell him that he will "get a needle" if he does not take them by mouth.

   c._____It is not a good idea to tell him that he is doing well when he takes fluids, food, etc., for that will make him dependent in the sense that he will always look for approbation.

   d._____The nurse should learn about his favorite beverages from his family, e.g. special tea, choice soups, etc. Even though these may not be available from the floor kitchen, she should try to get them for him.

5. When Mr. Epstein goes home with a tube and bottle (constant bladder drainage), the nurse can best help him make a better adjustment by

   a._____telling his family not to let him go out in public, for he will then be conscious of his personal difficulties, and this will depress him.

   b._____telling his family to let him go out with his friends, for the sooner he accepts the fact that he must live with his incapacities, the better.

   c._____instructing him in the use of the rubber urinal for daytime use. This will make him less self-conscious with his friends.

   d._____instructing him in the use of the Pilcher or Hagnar bag for daytime use. His physical needs will be met more comfortably with this device.

6. In teaching Mrs. Epstein the best way to clean and deodorize a rubber urinal, you would recommend that she

   a._____soak it in alcohol for 30 minutes, after it has been rinsed thoroughly with water.

   b._____wash it with soap and water, and then boil it for 20 minutes.

   c._____wash it with soap and water, dry thoroughly, and then dust liberally with a deodorant powder (inside and outside).

   d._____wash it with soap and water, dry thoroughly, and allow it to air for about 12 hours near an open window, keeping walls of the bag separated.

7. Mr. Epstein's diet before surgery was high-caloric and high-protein. Because such food combinations violate Jewish dietary habits, he should not be served

   a._____broiled lamb chops, legumes, pickles, rye bread.

   b._____oyster stew, W.W. bread.

   c._____creamed vegetables (white sauce) and koshered beef.

   d._____vegetable soup.

    e._____canned fruits.

    f._____steak, buttered carrots, cucumber and tomato salad.

Questions for Discussion and Student Projects

1. What technics do you consider to be most effective in maintaining good body alignment under the following conditions:

   a. When Mr. Epstein is placed in semi-Fowler's position, the only way he can flex his knees at the proper bend of the lower Gatch is to slump down on his sacrum.

   b. When in the dorsal recumbent position, Mr. Epstein's legs have a tendency to rotate externally. The nurse's attendant has placed large sand bags on the outer side of each foot, but Mr. Epstein complains that this is most uncomfortable.

2. How can Mr. Epstein, who has urinary drainage by means of an indwelling catheter, rubber tubing and drainage bottle, have optimum function of this system while he is ambulatory? Often the rubber tubing is of ideal length when he is in bed, but when he is sitting in a chair or walking the tubing has a tendency to coil or drag, which encourages pooling of drainage.

3. How would you lessen the anxiety of Mr. Epstein and his family at the time of his discharge when you know he is still "dribbling," has suprapubic drainage, and you suspect that he is not convinced that his operation has been successful?

4. David Epstein (one of Mr. Epstein's grandchildren, who is about 24 years old and unmarried) has asked you, a young student nurse, "What is Grandpa's real problem?" What, and in how much detail, would you tell him?

5. Mrs. Epstein brought a pint jar of some kind of soup for Mr. Epstein. She asks for a bowl and a spoon but rejects your offer to heat the liquid. Obviously it has a collection of cold grease on top. What would you do in this situation?

6. Make a list of rules which would be helpful to have when caring for the dietary needs of orthodox Jewish patients.

7. What religious customs, rituals, and observations of the orthodox Jew, in addition to dietary rules, may conflict with the hospital routine? How can you handle these?

8. How do you think a student nurse reacts when she is assigned to change perineal dressings on a patient similar to Mr. Epstein? How would she react if the patient were a handsome man of 30? How can the situation be handled easily, graciously, and effectively?

9. Demonstrate an effective and comfortable way of keeping perineal dressings on a male patient. How would you teach an elderly patient to change his dressings? (List the points you would stress.)

10. What can the nurse do to help her male urology patient under the following conditions?

   a. Because of a tiny malignant tumor, a patient has had to have a bilateral orchiectomy. He misinterprets his wife's reaction to his surgery because of his own apprehension and a repressed feeling of guilt.

b. An elderly patient is worrying because he fears his wife suspects that he is disinterested in her, when actually his sexual inactivity is due to aging and illness.

11. Discuss the problem of an elderly patient who has a urethral stricture and insists on using a "hickory stick" rather than submit to surgery.

12. What part does the use of estrogens play in the treatment of cancer of the prostate? How effective are they? Why is an orchiectomy often done in conjunction with estrogenic therapy? How effective is radiation?

Section 5. Nursing Care of Patients with Disorders of the Integumentary System*

STUDY SUGGESTIONS: Before beginning the study of this Section, the student will find it helpful to

A. Review

    1. Anatomy and physiology: the integumentary system.

    2. Pathology (or introduction to medical science): neoplasms.

B. Study

    1. In surgical nursing texts: breast amputation.

C. Read the additional References listed before attempting to answer the questions relating to each patient study.

THE WIFE WHO FEARED CANCER

Background Review Questions

1. The female breast is composed mostly of

    a._____epithelial glandular and supporting connective tissue.
    b._____fatty and muscular tissue.
    c._____muscular and vascular tissue.
    d._____fatty and glandular tissue.
    e._____muscular and nervous tissue.

2. The earliest sign of cancer of the breast is

    a._____a skin attachment at the site of the mass.
    b._____pain when slight pressure is applied.
    c._____retraction of the nipple.
    d._____the presence of a mass.
    e._____slight bleeding from the nipple.

3. Cancer of the breast might be prevented if

    a._____a properly fitted and well-supporting brassière were worn.
    b._____mothers would breast-feed their babies.
    c._____the breast were guarded against any form of trauma.
    d._____a woman married before she was 20.
    e._____the cause of cancer were known.

4. The highest incidence of breast cancer is in the age group of

    a._____25–35.   c._____45–55.   e._____65 and over.
    b._____35–45.   d._____55–65.

* Skin conditions are treated in other Sections of the Guide; see patient study, pneumonia, and pediatric section.

5. Cancer of the breast can be detected best by

    a._____blood analysis.   d._____roentgenogram.
    b._____palpation.   e._____the injection of a dye fol-
    c._____biopsy of breast tissue.   lowed by roentgenogram.

6. The most accurate diagnostic aid for breast carcinoma from cell tissue is

    a._____the Papanicolaou test.   c._____gross examination.
    b._____frozen section.   d._____cytology test.

7. The surgical rate for breast carcinoma up to 5 years after diagnosis is made and treatment is instituted is

    a. with lymph-node involvement, about (1)_____25 per cent.
                                       (2)_____50 per cent.

    b. without lymph-node involvement, about (1)_____75 per cent.
                                       (2)_____100 per cent.

8. Paget's disease is a form of

    a._____benign growth.   b._____malignant disease.

    It affects

    a._____an engorged breast and may develop into an abscess.
    b._____the nipple and resembles eczema.

    It is best treated by

    a._____radical surgery.   c._____prescribed skin ointments.
    b._____hot compresses.   d._____x-ray therapy.

9. Cancer of the breast may spread

    a._____by direct extension into neighboring tissue such as the chest and the lungs.
    b._____by permeation along lymphatic channels to the brain.
    c._____by a mother to her nursing baby.
    d._____from one patient to another by a break in medical asepsis.
    e._____to the skin on the hand of the nurse if she touches the discharge from the nipple of a cancer victim.

10. The spreading cancer is referred to as

    a._____exostosis.   d._____fibrosis.
    b._____metastasis.   e._____mitosis.
    c._____malignancy.

11. A patient of yours has a benign tumor which the doctor has recommended to be removed surgically. The patient wishes to avoid surgery and tries to get you to commit yourself on the issue. Of the following courses, it probably would be best for you to

    a._____reaffirm the doctor's recommendation, because nurses should not disagree with the doctor.

    b._____support the patient's viewpoint, because a benign tumor limits its growth and is not dangerous.

    c._____reaffirm the doctor's recommendation, because some benign tumors become malignant.

    d._____reaffirm the doctor's recommendation, although you secretly agree with the patient.

12. When a biopsy is done, the procedure involved is to

    a._____take a sample of tissue from the diseased organ of a patient after he is dead and study it microscopically to confirm the doctor's diagnosis.

    b._____surgically remove an organ and study the tissue microscopically to confirm the doctor's diagnosis.

    c._____take a sample of living tissue from a patient and study it microscopically to aid the doctor to arrive at his diagnosis.

    d._____insert a tube into a closed body cavity to look at the tissue lining the tract to determine the presence of a neoplasm.

13. From the list at the right, the one which best describes the neoplasms is listed in the column on the left. Place its number in the blank space at the left.

a._____myoma.	(1) benign neoplasm of connective tissue.
b._____liposarcoma.	
c._____adenocarcinoma.	(2) malignant neoplasm of connective tissue.
d._____chondrosarcoma.	
e._____polycytosis.	(3) benign neoplasm of epithelial tissue.
f._____polyp.	
g._____leukemia.	(4) malignant neoplasm of epithelial tissue.
h._____osteoma.	
i._____fibrosarcoma.	
j._____adenoma.	

14. Listed below are certain characteristics of neoplasms. Place an "M" in the blank space at the left of those findings which occur in malignant growths. Place a "B" in the blank space at the left of those findings characteristic of benign neoplasms.

    a._____frequent mitotic cell.

    b._____a tendency to recur.

    c._____growth usually limited by a capsule.

    d._____soft, pliable consistency.

    e._____hard, firm consistency.

    f._____a tendency to remain localized.

    g._____a tendency to metastasize.

    h._____necrosis of tissue because cells increase at a more rapid rate than their blood supply.

    i._____a slow increase in size.

    j._____a rapid increase in size.

    k._____seeding into lymphatic channels.

    l._____few invasive properties.

    m._____the absence of capsules.

15. Match the following:

a. furuncle.	(1)_____run-around infection of a nail bed.
b. carbuncle.	(2)_____multiple boils.
c. paronychia.	(3)_____finger-tip infection.
d. felon.	(4)_____an open lesion with loss of substance.
e. ulcer.	(5)_____scar.
f. laceration.	(6)_____irregular tear of flesh.
g. cellulitis.	(7)_____diffuse infection.
h. cicatrix.	(8)_____boil.

THE WIFE WHO FEARED CANCER—PATIENT STUDY

As she sat in the waiting room of her doctor's office, turning the pages of *Life* magazine, the meaning of not a single picture pierced Mrs. Brennan's consciousness. In less than an hour from now, her deepest fears might be verified or relieved. Which would it be? Of course, she had made her appointment as soon as she noticed the small lump in her breast—perhaps she had come in time. But how was one to know? People had said the tumor might be widespread and yet one would not feel the slightest pain.

"The doctor will see you now, Mrs. Brennan," announced the graduate nurse from the door of the inner office.

When her examination was almost over, Mrs. Brennan became aware that the violent pounding of her heart had subsided. Dr. Stamford and his nurse always made one relax.

"So glad you came now, Mrs. Brennan. That little growth will have to come out. When we do that, it will be examined carefully. We may have to do more surgery at that time." Dr. Stamford gave her real courage when she admitted that she knew it might be cancer. Her mother had died of it because she neglected to seek medical advice until it was too late.

Mr. Brennan was quite concerned when his wife told him of her experience that day. He had been unaware that anything troubled her. "Couldn't you use salve or have massage or baking? Do you have to be admitted to the hospital? Must you have an operation?" Mrs. Brennan could answer all his questions for they were the very ones which she had asked the nurse.

The Brennans decided not to tell their two married children until the operation was over. Three days after her visit to her doctor, she was admitted as a semi-private patient, under the Blue Cross plan, to the local hospital. The nurses on the floor were amazed when she said she was 55 years old, for the years had dealt kindly with her.

The results of laboratory findings confirmed the diagnosis of adenocarcinoma. While she was still under nitrous oxide and ether, a radical mastectomy was done. Mrs. Brennan was on the operating table about 2½ hours and the estimated blood loss was 500 cc. A transfusion was given in the O.R., using a vein in her lower leg. When it came time to close the wound, it was found necessary to graft some skin from the right thigh. A Thiersch graft of approximately 5 x 12 cm. was stitched in place with interrupted black silk sutures. A stab wound accommodated a medium-size Penrose drain with gauze filler. The initial breast dressing consisted of a single layer of paraffin mesh, on top of which were placed sterile dressings and sponge rubber to act as a pressure dressing. The chest and shoulder girdle on the operated right side were snugly bandaged with 6-inch Ace bandage.

Mrs. Brennan regained complete consciousness about 2 hours after returning to her room. Her arm was supported on a pillow and she was placed in a semi-Fowler position. She thought she was thirsty. However, a few sips of water proved that she was nauseated. Within 24 hours, she was feeling much better and was allowed out of bed with her arm well protected in a sling. She received some passive exercise to this arm which showed signs of slight edema. Although her dressing was snug, she claimed it was not tight. She had some pain when she moved her arm in a shrugging manner.

Her dressings were changed down to the paraffin mesh on the second day P.O. It was only then that she fully realized some skin had been taken from her leg because the doctor dressed this wound too. She made a steady recovery and carried out prescribed arm exercises conscientiously. By the eighth day P.O. she was ready for discharge. At this time she could raise her arm upward, comb her hair and reach backward to touch the midline of her spine. She was to continue with physical therapy and under the care of Dr. Stamford.

Discharge note: a small adenocarcinomatous lesion removed intact with total resection of the right breast, pectoral muscles and a fair amount of uninvolved axillary content. Wound closing well with Thiersch skin graft from the right thigh. Close follow-up visits will reveal whether radiation therapy is necessary. Prognosis: excellent.

References

Hill, G., and Silver, A. G.: Psychodynamic and esthetic motivations for plastic surgery, Psychosomatic Med. 12:345, 1950.

Smith, G. W.: When a breast must be removed, Am. J. Nursing 50:335, 1950.

Sugarbaker, E. D., and Wilfley, L. E.: Cancer of the breast, Am. J. Nursing 50:332, 1950.

Walter, C. W.: The Aseptic Treatment of Wounds, pp. 177–185, "Disinfection of the Skin," New York, Macmillan, 1948.

Cancer Nursing, A Manual for Public Health Nurses, pp. 48–51, "Breast," Health Publications Institute, Inc., Raleigh, N.C., 1950.

A Cancer Source Book for Nurses, pp. 59–64, American Cancer Society, New York, 1950.

Questions Relating to the Patient Study

1. In reply to Mrs. Brennan's question regarding the use of ointments or massage for her breast, the nurse probably replied that

   a.____"Cocoa butter is an excellent salve for use in gentle breast massage. Use it 2 or 3 times a day for the next few days; it may work wonders in dissolving that lump."

   b.____"Although we dislike admitting it, the only salve known to be of any help is goose grease. Firm but gentle massage every morning and evening may help to shrink the mass and you will have a smaller incision."

c.____"This is one type of growth which we want to handle as little as possible because the danger of spread and injury to surrounding breast tissue is too great. Do not massage."

d.____"The use of heat often helps. Try moist compresses which are lukewarm to the touch of your wrist. Apply these 3 times a day and we may bring this infection to a head by the time of your hospital admission."

2. On the day Mrs. Brennan was admitted, it was determined that she had type AB blood. The relative incidence of individuals with this type is

a.____5 per cent.   c.____30 per cent.
b.____20 per cent.   d.____40 per cent.

3. With this type blood, Mrs. Brennan may receive blood of the following types:

a.____A only.   d.____AB only.
b.____B only.   e.____any of the above types.
c.____O only.

4. Skin preparation for surgery would include

a.____the right breast only.
b.____that quarter segment of the breast from which the biopsy would be taken.
c.____the right breast and the right axilla.
d.____an area from the nipple line of the left breast around the operative site to the back midline; from the neck to the waist.
e.____the area described in item (d) plus the right upper arm to the elbow.

5. Mrs. Brennan had nitrous oxide for her general anesthetic. This is often called

a.____"laughing gas."   c.____"sweet air."
b.____Vinethene.   d.____a volatile liquid.

6. In cases lasting longer than a few minutes, nitrous oxide is always given with

a.____ether, to intensify its effect.
b.____oxygen, to prevent cyanosis.
c.____carbon dioxide, to keep respirations stimulated.
d.____cyclopropane, to produce good relaxation as well as smooth induction.

7. The most desirable depth of anesthesia for this patient is the

a.____first stage.   d.____third phase of the third
b.____second stage.   stage.
c.____first phase of the third e.____fourth stage.
     stage.

8. In the operating room it was noted that after the knife blade was used by the surgeon to make the skin incision, it was discarded for a fresh blade. The reason for this is that

   a._____perhaps the skin was not prepared adequately.
   b._____the blade probably was dulled after going through the skin.
   c._____organisms from the skin may be transmitted to the deeper tissues.
   d._____it is considered to be good surgical technic.
   e._____it may have been a whim of this particular surgeon.

9. Principles underlying the method of chemical disinfection of the skin in the operating room are that

   a._____one should use a minimum of friction because of the danger of trauma to the underlying tissues.
   b._____friction enhances germicidal power because it aids the germicide in penetrating to the organisms.
   c._____coating the area with the germicide is sufficient inasmuch as the skin has been shaved and washed with soap and water on the ward.
   d._____no germicide is instantaneous; there must be an adequate period of exposure to the germicide.

10. An infusion or transfusion is often started in a vein in the foot of the patient in the O.R. because

    a._____fluids can be given more rapidly this way.
    b._____the leg is less likely to move and dislodge the needle than is the arm.
    c._____the uninvolved arm is then available for supplementary intravenous anesthesia.
    d._____it is more convenient for the doctor inserting the needle (during the operation).
    e._____the equipment is less likely to be disturbed by the operating team.

11. When Mrs. Brennan returned from the operating room, she had a hard rubber airway in her mouth. The nurse's responsibility for such a device is to

    a._____keep it in place until the patient has responded fully.
    b._____remove it when the patient returns to bed.
    c._____leave it in place until the patient wishes to emit it.
    d._____call the anesthetist if it appears to be coming out.

12. The most simple and effective nursing measure to prevent the aspiration of fluids (vomitus) immediately postoperatively is to

    a._____turn the patient on the operative side in Sims' lateral position.
    b._____use a small rubber catheter (No. 16) to aspirate the nose and the mouth.
    c._____keep the patients head straight (nose pointing to the ceiling) so that the airway will be patent.
    d._____turn the patient's head to the side to allow the escape of fluids.

13. Immediately postoperatively, blood pressure, pulse and respirations are taken

    a._____only as ordered by the doctor.
    b._____every 15 minutes for 2 hours and then less frequently if stable.
    c._____when the patient returns to the unit and then when she appears restless.
    d._____every half hour for the first 12 hours.

14. Copious drainage often is encountered following a radical mastectomy. For the patient's comfort, measures that may be initiated by the nurse are

    a._____to change all dressings except those directly over the wound, whenever necessary.
    b._____not to alter any dressings; to apply 2 or 3 ice bags to the bandaged area so that drainage will coagulate.
    c._____to change protecting absorbent pads and the patient's gown to prevent anything sticky or clammy contacting the skin.
    d._____to apply a snug-fitting light-weight rubber bandage over the dressings to prevent drainage coming through.

15. A Penrose drain with a gauze filler facilitates the escape of drainage from the operative area to absorbent dressings by

    a._____gravity.   c._____capillarity.
    b._____osmosis.   d._____pressure.

16. The best treatment for postoperative lymphedema is to

    a._____massage the entire arm beginning at the fingers and working toward the shoulder.
    b._____allow the arm to rest below the level of the body on a flat soft pillow.
    c._____support the arm on a pillow so that it is higher than the level of the body.
    d._____apply hot-water bottles to the sides of the arm, not allowing their weight to rest on top of the arm.
    e._____soak the arm in an arm bath containing epsom salts for 20 minutes 3 times a day.

17. The purpose of applying paraffin mesh, petrolatum gauze, etc., directly over a freshly grafted area is to

    a._____prevent dry dressings from sticking to the wound.
    b._____stimulate the process of epithelization.
    c._____prevent the newly grafted skin from being dislocated if superficial dressings are shifted.
    d._____prevent contamination of the newly grafted area.

18. The postoperative mastectomy patient has a tendency to hold her shoulder on the operated side

    a._____higher than the other shoulder.
    b._____lower than the other shoulder.

Reasons for this poor posture are that

a._____the weight of the breast has been removed; this normally creates a downward pull.

b._____the shoulder-girdle muscles are taking over the function of the absent pectorals.

c._____stitches in the axilla make the patient drop her shoulder instinctively.

d._____the instinct to protect her arm causes her to drop her shoulder as she hugs her body with this arm.

19. The final approval of the use of a suitable and safe breast prosthetic rests with the

a._____patient.

b._____nurse.

c._____surgeon.

d._____physical therapist.

e._____fitter of foundation garments.

20. The activities which will be of most help in restoring shoulder mobility in the convalescing mastectomy patient are

a._____crocheting or knitting.

b._____brushing the teeth.

c._____craftwork, such as weaving.

d._____filing the fingernails.

e._____combing the hair.

f._____writing letters.

g._____sweeping the floor.

h._____typing.

21. For inoperable breast cancer, estrogens and testosterone have provided relief. By-effects which may occur are

a._____loss of hair.

b._____serum calcium changes.

c._____development of edema.

d._____decreased libido.

22. The objectionable odor from ulcerative breast cancer may be diminished by irrigation with

a._____$KMnO_4$, 1:10,000.

b._____equal parts of hydrogen peroxide and water.

c._____isopropyl alcohol 70 per cent.

d._____Lysol 70 per cent.

e._____Zephiran chloride 1:500.

Questions for Discussion and Student Projects

1. What pamphlets or films would you recommend for the educational program of women's clubs interested in learning methods of detecting and treating breast cancer? Give the reasons for your choice. Do you think a physician should be present during the showing of the film? Why?

2. Imagine you are vacationing and a former high-school classmate calls on you. After much reminiscing she finally confides that she has a real worry. Her mother and one of her sisters had surgery for cancer of the breast. She feels that she ought to know how to examine her breasts so

that if a tumor does develop, she will be able to detect it early. Explain and/or demonstrate how you would instruct her.

3. One of the chief problems encountered with a breast prosthetic is the tendency for it to ride up and toward the midline. What effective and practical ways can you suggest to prevent this annoying problem?

4. Plan a program of rehabilitative exercises to be approved by your surgeon and physical therapist for the postoperative radical mastectomy patient in your hospital. Transcribe these exercises into useful household activities which the patient can practice while caring for her home.

5. How can a patient such as Mrs. Brennan be on intelligent guard for signs of metastases? What symptoms should prompt her to visit her physician? What effect may such constant suspicion and concern have on her? How can tendencies to be overconcerned be averted?

6. What is being done in your community to disseminate information to women regarding the early detection of breast cancer? Is this adequate? What more can be done? How can you help?

7. Collect the various types of breast prosthetics available to patients in your hospital. Compare their advantages and disadvantages, including cost and durability.

8. What are the psychodynamic and aesthetic motivations for plastic surgery, such as excessive facial wrinkles, protruding ears, pendulous breasts, etc. Discuss.

9. What problems would you expect to encounter in caring for a 22-year-old attractive college girl who has been in an automobile accident and is now having extensive facial plastic surgery? Suggest some ways of handling

   a. her concern about her future appearance.
   b. the need for repeated visits to the operating room, separated by long intervals of convalescence and healing.
   c. her resuming academic study.
   d. her resuming her social contacts.
   e. the control of odors.
   f. her mental attitude.

Section 6. Nursing Care of Patients with Disorders Due to Allergies

STUDY SUGGESTIONS: Before beginning the study of this Section, the student will find it helpful to

A. Review

    1. Physiology: body resistance, protein antibodies.

B. Study

    1. In medical nursing texts: allergic conditions.
    2. In nutrition texts: allergy diets.
    3. In pharmacology texts: drugs affecting the respiratory tract, parasympathetic drugs, antihistamine and allergenic preparations.

C. Read the additional References listed before attempting to answer the questions relating to each patient study.

THE CHOKING ASTHMATIC—PATIENT STUDY

At 8:00 P.M. Mrs. Anderson entered the admitting ward as an emergency. Hospitalization had been ordered by her physician because of irretractable asthma.

The patient, a housewife, appears older than her 52 years. She is emaciated, weighing about 100 pounds, but states that her usual weight is only 100 pounds. She appears upset, worried and acutely ill.

Mrs. Anderson's most outstanding symptom is great difficulty in breathing, which appears agonizing, even alarming. Her respirations are noisy and wheezing. She has a dry, non-productive cough. She is deeply cyanosed and her skin is dry and parched. Her pulse is rapid, thready and irregular.

Mr. Anderson, who accompanied his wife, gave the history. He stated that the patient experienced the first asthmatic attack following the removal of a nasal polyp 20 years ago. A similar operation 1 year ago seemed to aggravate the severity of the attacks.

Mrs. Anderson has been under medical care for some time and following a series of skin tests many foods have been eliminated from her diet. She feels that certain foods (for example, corn and eggs) aggravate the asthma.

Mrs. Anderson's father and two sisters also have some difficulty with "allergies." Mr. Anderson states that the family physician has suggested "neurotic tendencies" as possible contributing factors and also that Mrs. Anderson's carious teeth may be foci of chronic infection related to her condition.

With the history and physical findings the resident physician made a diagnosis of acute bronchial asthma, with emphysema. The medical ward was notified and the patient was taken to the ward at once. The following orders were written:

> Complete bed rest.
> Elevate the head of the bed.
> Helium and oxygen by mask.
> Aminophylline 0.2 Gm. in 50 per cent glucose intravenously.
> Codeine gr. 1, (h) p.r.n. for cough.
> Seconal gr. 1½ h.s.

During the night the same symptoms persisted. Mrs. Anderson alternated between periods of being quite irrational and of deep depression. She refused to take anything by mouth. By morning she was quite weak and dehydrated and appeared exhausted.

The attending physician made a diagnosis of status asthmaticus.

References

Black, J.: The treatment of asthma, J.A.M.A. **137**:453, 1948.
Criep, Leo H.: What is allergy?, Am. J. Nursing 45:721, 1945.
French, Thomas M., and Johnson, Adelaide M.: Psychotherapy in bronchial asthma, Studies in Psychomatic Medicine, New York, Ronald, 1948.
Goodall, Robert: Continuous intravenous aminophylline therapy in status asthmaticus, Ann. Allergy 5:196, 194.
Harris, M. Coleman: The present day treatment of asthma, Calif. Med. **66**:354, 1947.
Klein, Harriet: Nursing the allergic patient, Am. J. Nursing **38**:14, 1938.
London, McKinley: Bronchial asthma, Am. J. Nursing **41**:415, 1941.
Newton, Charlotte: Bronchial asthma, Am. J. Nursing **38**:413, 1938.
Rackemann, Francis: The nurse and the patient with asthma, Am. J. Nursing 47:463, 1947.
————: Other factors besides allergy in asthma, J.A.M.A. **142**:534, 1950.

Questions Relating to the Patient Study

1. Allergy is best defined as

   a.———a hypersensitivity to foreign substances.
   b.———a hypochondriac disease.
   c.———food poisoning.
   d.———irritation of the mucous membranes.

2. A tissue which has been stimulated by an amigen becomes

   a.———resistant to the amigen.
   b.———tolerant to the amigen.
   c.———more sensitive to the amigen.

3. Status asthmaticus refers to

   a.———chronic subclinical asthma.
   b.———chronic asthmatic symptoms.
   c.———an unusually severe asthmatic attack.

4. The *primary* reason for the selection of Demerol instead of morphine for Mrs. Anderson is that Demerol is

    a.____more potent as a sedative.
    b.____non-depressant of the cough reflex.
    c.____a depressant of the cough reflex.
    d.____definitely non-habit-forming.

5. Amytal is combined with ephedrine in order to

    a.____enhance the sedative effect of ephedrine.
    b.____enhance the effect of ephedrine on bronchial relaxation.
    c.____counteract the sedative effect of ephedrine.
    d.____counteract the stimulating effect of ephedrine.

6. Helium is combined with oxygen in order to

    a.____reduce the combustibility of the oxygen.
    b.____reduce the cost of continuous oxygen therapy.
    c.____decrease the respiratory effect necessary for pulmonary ventilation.
    d.____act as a mild anesthesia.

7. Aminophylline is given because of its effect of

    a.____acting as a mild sedative and analgesic.
    b.____promoting relaxation of the bronchial tubes.
    c.____acting as a depressant of the cough reflex.
    d.____acting as a stimulant to the respiratory center.

8. The desired effect of cough medications is to

    a.____depress the cough reflex.
    b.____act as an expectorant.
    c.____reduce the mucous membrane.

9. The trade name for epinephrine is

    a.____Ephedrine.   c.____Prostigmin.
    b.____Adrenalin.   d.____Ergotrate.

10. The strength of solution of epinephrine for hypodermic administration is

    a.____1:100.   b.____1:1,000.   c.____1:5,000.

11. The average dosage of this solution is

    a.____1 cc. b.____0.6 cc. c.____0.2 cc. d.____16 minims. e.____10 minims.

12. Frequent attacks of asthma may lead to

    a.____pulmonary tuberculosis.   d.____lung abscess.
    b.____pulmonary emphysema.   e.____status asthmaticus.
    c.____chronic asthmatic bronchitis. f.____no untoward effects.

Questions for Discussion and Student Projects

A. Related to Patient Study

1. What are the responsibilities of the nurse in administering helium and oxygen by mask to Mrs. Anderson? What are the therapeutic effects of the treatment? What instruction should be given to the patient? What is the daily cost of the treatment to the hospital and to the patient? How does it compare with the cost of administering oxygen by tent? What care is given to the patient's face, and how is the mask cleaned?

2. Discuss the therapeutic effects of dosage, toxic symptoms and methods of administering codeine, Seconal, Demeral, terpin hydrate elixir with codeine, as prescribed for Mrs. Anderson.

3. List the possible ways Mrs. Anderson might eat eggs without realizing it. What may be done to diagnose a food allergy? How may she be desensitized to eggs? Discuss the patient's responsibility for the treatment.

4. Discuss various types of elimination diets which might be ordered for Mrs. Anderson.

5. List the usual appointments of a bedroom which should be eliminated from Mrs. Anderson's room. What additional measures can be taken to decrease the common potent allergies from the home?

6. During a conversation with Mr. Anderson you discovered that he was "provoked" with the family physician for mentioning "neurotic tendencies" and commented that he could not believe that his wife was "imagining or deliberately producing these attacks". Explain, in detail, how you would answer him.

B. Related to Allergy in General

1. Discuss the allergy diet including the potent allergens which must be rigidly eliminated, and the less potent substances which may be tolerated in smaller quantities.

2. Investigate the current use of the antihistaminic drugs in the treatment of allergic diseases. Discuss the recent findings on the use of these drugs for the treatment of the common cold.

3. What are the nursing responsibilities for the management of a patient suffering from anaphylactic shock? What will she need to know in regard to etiology, symptoms, prevention?

4. What is meant by serum sickness? What are the symptoms, prognosis and medical and nursing care?

5. Arrange a group conference with the head nurse, dietitian and social worker to discuss all aspects of asthma in relation to one or more patients suffering with asthma. Include the etiology, signs and symptoms, treatment, prognosis, observation of causes, nursing care, teaching the patient how to live with his allergy, nutritional problems in relation to food allergy, how to help the patient with psychologic, social and economic problems such as changing environment, changing work and contacting social agencies for economic assistance.

6. What measure may the nurse take to relieve the intense pruritus of contact dermatitis?
7. Discuss the symptoms, prognosis, treatment and complication of angioneurotic edema. Relate the discussion to a patient if clinical material is available.
8. What are the nurse's responsibilities for the allergic patient in the clinic? Discuss testing, common systemic reactions, less frequent reaction, delayed reactions, and significance of testing.

Section 7. Nursing Care of Patients with Disorders of the Endocrine Glands and of Metabolism

STUDY SUGGESTIONS: Before beginning the study of this Section, the student will find it helpful to

A. Review

1. Anatomy and physiology: the endocrine glands, digestion, metabolism.
2. Chemistry: blood chemistry, urinalysis, oxidation, chemistry of carbohydrates, proteins, fats.
3. Nursing arts: the administration of fluids.

B. Study

1. In medical nursing texts: disorders of the endocrine glands and metabolism.
2. In nutrition texts: diabetic diet, high caloric diet.
3. In pharmacology texts: agents used in metabolic disorders, hormones and synthetic substitutes.
4. In surgical nursing texts: thyroidectomy.

C. Read the additional References listed before attempting to answer the questions relating to each patient study.

THE MAN IN A COMA

Background Review Questions

1. Animal carbohydrate is stored in the body in the form of

   a.____glucose.
   b.____glycogen.
   c.____amino acids.
   d.____dextrose.

2. The principal nitrogenous waste product of protein metabolism normally excreted by the kidneys is

   a.____cholesterol.
   b.____urine.
   c.____bilirubin.
   d.____amino acid.

3. The normal pH value of the human blood is approximately

   a.____6.5.
   b.____7.0.
   c.____7.4.
   d.____7.8.

4. Carbohydrate can be utilized by the cells of the human body only in the form of

   a.____fatty acids.
   b.____glycogen.
   c.____amino acids.
   d.____glucose.

5. The structural unit of proteins and also the form in which the human body utilizes protein is

a._____glucose.   c._____amino acids.
b._____fatty acids.   d._____cholesterol.

6. When more carbohydrate is taken into the body than is needed for body metabolism, the excess

a._____remains circulating in the blood stream until needed.
b._____is stored as amino acids in the liver.
c._____is converted into glycogen and stored in the spleen.
d._____is converted into fat and is stored as adipose tissue.

7. The end-product of carbohydrate digestion and the form in which carbohydrate is utilized by the body is

a._____amino acids.   c._____glycogen.
b._____glucose.   d._____fatty acids.

8. When an excessive amount of carbohydrate is taken into the body, the excess

a._____remains circulating in the blood stream until needed.
b._____is stored as amino acids in the liver.
c._____is converted into glycogen and stored in the spleen.
d._____is converted into fat and is stored as adipose tissue.

9. Normally, fats are oxidized completely in the body, releasing energy (including heat) and

a._____fatty acids and glycerol.
b._____carbon dioxide and water.
c._____ketone bodies and ammonia.
d._____glucose and glycogen.

10. The temperature-regulating center of the body is located in the

a._____medulla oblongata.   c._____cerebral cortex.
b._____thalamus.   d._____hypothalamus.

11. The CO_2 combining power of the plasma is a test used to determine

a._____acidosis.   c._____uremic poisoning.
b._____alkalosis.   d._____excessive blood sugar.

12. An increase in the pH of the blood would indicate

a._____alkalosis.   c._____uremic poisoning.
b._____acidosis.   d._____excessive blood sugar.

13. Normal fluid balance is maintained by regulation in intake and/or output. The main output is in the form of urine. The second most important output is through

a._____secretion of the sweat glands.
b._____insensible losses.
c._____the feces.
d._____expired air.

14. Acidosis results from a

    a.＿＿sudden increase in the concentration of cholesterol in the interstitial fluids.
    b.＿＿normal physiologic phenomenon following the ingestion of foods which are too highly acid in nature.
    c.＿＿decrease in the pH of the blood to a point below 7.3.
    d.＿＿rise in the pH of the blood to a point above 7.5.

15. The most important constituent of the buffer system which operates in the body to maintain the blood pH within the normal range is

    a.＿＿NaCl.
    b.＿＿$NaHCO_3$.
    c.＿＿NH_2.
    d.＿＿potassium and chloride ions.

16. When the liver utilizes the end-products of protein digestion to produce certain of the plasma proteins, which of the following substances is released (or produced) as a waste product?

    a.＿＿amino acids.
    b.＿＿carbon dioxide and water.
    c.＿＿urea.
    d.＿＿cholesterol.

17. The primary function of the parathyroid hormone is to regulate the

    a.＿＿calcium-phosphorus balance of the blood.
    b.＿＿sodium-potassium balance of the blood.
    c.＿＿rate of oxidation within the tissue cells.
    d.＿＿storage of iodine within the thyroid.

18. The accumulation of ketone bodies within the blood results from a (an)

    a.＿＿incomplete oxidation of carbohydrates.
    b.＿＿lack of insulin.
    c.＿＿incomplete oxidation of fats.
    d.＿＿increased H-ion concentration of the blood.

19. One of the most important physiologic functions of insulin is to stimulate the

    a.＿＿liver to store fat.
    b.＿＿kidney tubules to reabsorb glucose.
    c.＿＿liver and muscles to metabolize carbohydrate.
    d.＿＿muscles to convert amino acids to glycogen.

20. In the absence of insulin, the

    a.＿＿liver stores abnormally large quantities of glycogen.
    b.＿＿kidney tubules function abnormally by allowing the passage of glucose into the urine.
    c.＿＿muscles convert abnormally large quantities of glycogen to glucose.
    d.＿＿liver fails to remove sufficient quantities of glucose from the blood.

21. One of the most dangerous toxic effects of thyroxin is its stimulating action upon

a.____the respiratory center.   c.____the liver.
b.____cardiac muscle.   d.____protein metabolism.

22. The physiologic importance of thyroxin in the normal individual is its catalytic effect upon the

a.____normal oxidation of fatty acids by the tissue cells.
b.____metabolic processes of the tissue cells.
c.____calcium-phosphorus balance of the blood.
d.____storage of iodine within the thyroid gland.

23. Select from the column of hormones at the left those secreted by each of the following endocrine glands. Place the number(s) of the hormones in the blank space to the left of the glands.

a. adrenalin.   (1)____adrenal cortex.
b. adrenocorticotropic hormone.   (2)____adrenal medulla.
c. antidiuretic hormone.   (3)____pancreas.
d. corticosterone.   (4)____parathyroid.
e. cortisone.   (5)____pituitary, anterior.
f. desoxycorticosterone.   (6)____pituitary, posterior.
g. growth hormone.   (7)____thyroid.
h. insulin.
i. lactogenic hormone.
j. parathormone.
k. pitocin.
l. pituitrin.
m. pitressin.
n. thyrotropic hormone.
o. thyroxin.

24. From the hormones listed at the left, select the one responsible for each of the functions listed below; place its letter in the blank space to the left of the function.

a. adrenalin.   (1)____the hormone which stimulates the liver and muscle cells to remove glucose from the blood and store it within these organs.
b. adrenocorticotropic hormone.
c. antidiuretic hormone. (2)____the hormone which aids in normal electrolyte balance by stimulating the kidney tubules to reabsorb sodium.
d. corticosterone.
e. cortisone.
f. desoxycorticosterone.
g. growth hormone.   (3)____the hormone which stimulates only those parts of the body innervated by the sympathetic nervous system.
h. insulin.
i. lactogenic hormone.
j. parathormone.
k. pitocin.   (4)____the active ingredient of pituitrin responsible for stimulating the
l. pituitrin.
m. pitressin.

n. thyrotropic hormone.
o. thyroxin.

(5)_____the hormone which exerts its influence upon the development of the musculoskeletal system.

(6)_____the hormone responsible for controlling and regulating the normal activity of the thyroid gland.

(7)_____the hormone which stimulates the kidney tubules to reabsorb water.

(8)_____the newly recognized hormone which is released by the adrenal gland under times of stress which apparently aids the organism to adjust to the situation of stress.

(9)_____the hormone which stimulates the adrenal gland to produce the hormone released in the situation described in (8).

(10)_____the hormone which has a catalytic effect upon the oxidative process of tissue cells, stimulating the use of oxygen.

(11)_____the active principle of pituitrin which acts to stimulate the motility of the intestinal tract.

(12)_____the hormone responsible for regulating the normal calcium-phosphorus balance in the blood.

(13)_____lack of this hormone results in an improper metabolism of fats with an increase in production and accumulation of ketone bodies within the blood.

(14)_____an over-production of this hormone in an adult results in the diseased condition called acromegaly.

(15)_____marked depression in the formation of this hormone results in cretinism (if a child) or myxedema (if an adult).

(16)_____lack of this hormone leads to an increase in muscle tone and eventually to a diseased state called tetany.

smooth muscle of the body of the uterus to contract.

(17)_____the hormone responsible for hyperplasia of the mammary gland and the production of milk following childbirth.

THE MAN IN A COMA—PATIENT STUDY

Mr. Muller, a 53-year-old Jewish man of Austrian birth, was admitted to the hospital in diabetic coma.

He came to this country at the age of 22. Six years later he was married and has had a happy home life. His wife is living and well, and he has two sons, aged 22 and 23. His parents are both dead. Of his three sisters and one brother, two have diabetes. For years Mr. Muller was a storekeeper, and for the past 10 years he has been a night watchman at one of the state parks. He has always been financially independent.

Information regarding Mr. Muller's present illness was limited by several factors. Because of the type of job he holds, his family knew little of the events preceding his admission to the hospital. Secondly, the patient speaks poor English. However, he is of average intelligence and was able to give a fairly accurate history the day after admission when he was no longer comatose.

Mr. Muller had had diabetes for 12 years. His physician had placed him on a routine of insulin U. 25–0–25 daily, which he followed up to the 4 days prior to his admission. That morning he developed anorexia and constipation. He had 25 units of insulin, followed by breakfast consisting of a dish of oatmeal. From then on until admission he took no more insulin and very little food though he says he drank "a lot of water" to "clear" his urine in order to pass an insurance physical examination. He continued to work and felt good until the third day at 4 A.M. when he had a chill and vomited. Before retiring at 5 A.M. he drank some milk which he soon vomited. He felt weak and continued to vomit at irregular intervals. He was unable to drink more water, passed tarry stools and continued to vomit until admission to the hospital at 2 A.M. the next morning.

Physical examination on admission revealed Mr. Muller to be a fairly well-developed and well-nourished man in a comatose state. His respirations were deep and sighing, and there was a strong odor of acetone on his breath. Temperature was 95°F., pulse 88, respirations 38 and blood pressure 70/30. His skin was cold, dry and bluish; eyeballs were soft; lungs clear. There was slight cyanosis of the extremities and reflexes were hypoactive. The impression at that time was diabetes mellitus with severe acidosis. Blood sugar was determined and found to be 1,025 mg. per cent per 100 cc. of blood.

Mr. Muller was put on absolute bed rest, external heat applied. He was given an infusion of 500 cc. of normal saline solution containing 30 Gm. of acacia. The blood was typed, and a transfusion of citrated blood, 500 cc., was given at 4:30 A.M., two and one-half hours after admission. By 6:15 A.M. Mr. Muller's vital signs were: temperature 98.6°F., pulse 84, respirations 28 and blood pressure 118/65.

In the early stage of hospitalization Mr. Muller was under continuous medical observation. During this interval he received the following fluids and medications:

	Orally	Subcutaneously	Intravenously
Fluids	700 cc.	9,300 cc.	2,100 cc.
Salt		64 Gm.	12 Gm.
Glucose	80 Gm.	215 Gm.	225 Gm.
Insulin		275 units	20 units

The initial dose of insulin was 20 units given intravenously; thereafter, the insulin was given subcutaneously every hour in decreasing amounts from 50 units to 15 units for almost 24 hours after admission. Progress in treatment was indicated by the decreasing blood-sugar level as it slowly dropped to 460 mg. per cent per 100 cc. of blood at 11 A.M., and to 136 mg. per cent per 100 cc. of blood at 11 P.M. It was unnecessary to catheterize Mr. Muller since he voided 1,000 cc. at 6:15 A.M. and again the same amount at 7 and 9 A.M. There was a 3+ acetone reaction at 6 A.M. but in 12 hours there was none present. There was a complete reduction of sugar during the entire 24 hours.

Numerous laboratory tests were made. Albumin and acetone were cleared from the urine in 6 days. Red blood count on admission was 3.65, hemoglobin 71 per cent and white blood count 25,000. After the transfusion the red blood count was 4.24, hemoglobin 87 per cent and white blood count 5,650.

About 8 P.M. of the eighth day, Mr. Muller exhibited mild symptoms of insulin shock, and an ampul of 50 per cent glucose was given intravenously. At 10 P.M. the same evening an infusion of 10 per cent glucose was given and at 1:30 A.M. another ampul of glucose. This controlled the symptoms.

The excessive gastro-intestinal bleeding indicated several tests: gastric analysis, guaiac test of the stomach content and stools, and a gastro-intestinal series. All revealed no abnormality of the G.I. tract.

Mr. Muller remained in the hospital for 10 days. In addition to the specific treatment for the acidosis, general medical and nursing care included: regulation of diet, administration of insulin, collection and examination of urine specimens, regulation of hygienic regimen and the education of the patient regarding his responsibility toward control of the disease and prevention of its complications. He was discharged to his own physician on a diet of 80 Gm. of protein, 150 Gm. of carbohydrate, and 200 Gm. of fat, with 30 units of protamine zinc insulin daily.

References

Caso, Elizabeth K.: Revised procedure for the calculation of diabetic diets, Report of the Committee on Diabetic Diet Calculation, J. Am. Dietet. Assoc. 26:575, 1950.

Irmisch, Alice K., and Wilder, Russel M.: Diet and insulin in the care of the diabetic patient, Am. J. Nursing 46:603, 1946.

Joslin, Elliot P.: Treatment of diabetes today, J.A.M.A. 140:581, 1949.

Maureen, Sister M., and Beland, Irene: The nurse and the diabetic patient, Am. J. Nursing 46:606, 1946.

Rosenthal, Helen, Stern, Frances, and Rosenthal, Joseph: Diabetic Care in Pictures, Philadelphia, Lippincott, 1946.

Tangney, Mary E.: Diabetes and the Diabetic in the Community, Philadelphia, Saunders, 1947.
Tolstoi, Edward: Objectives of modern diabetic care, Psychosom. Med. 10:291, 1948.
Wilkerson, Hugh L. C., and Ford, Malcolm J.: Diabetes control in a local health department, Am. J. Pub. Health 39:607, 1949.
————: Public health aspects of diabetes mellitus, Am. J. Pub. Health 37:177, 1947.

Questions Relating to the Patient Study

1. Immediately upon Mr. Muller's admission the nurse should participate in or make preparation for certain therapeutic measures which will be initiated promptly:

   A. In the white space to the left of the procedures, indicate which should be carried out for Mr. Muller.

   Part A   *Procedure*   *Part B*
      1. Apply external heat.
      2. Place an ice cap to the abdomen.
      3. Prepare to administer insulin, 25 to 50 units, immediately.
      4. Prepare for the immediate administration of normal salt solution by hypodermoclysis.
      5. Prepare the patient for a blood transfusion.
      6. Assemble equipment for the administration of oxygen.
      7. Assemble equipment and prepare the patient for gastric gavage.
      8. Prepare for the administration of glucose intravenously.
      9. Give an alcohol sponge.
     10. Insert a retention catheter.
     11. Take vital signs at frequent intervals.
     12. Prepare for venipuncture for a blood specimen.

   B. From the following list of statements select those which support your choice of procedures in A. In the white space to the right of the procedure, place the number of the statement which supports your choice.

      1. Peripheral vascular collapse may be prevented by the administration of a blood transfusion, which increases the blood volume.
      2. Application of external heat stimulates the circulation of blood and assists in maintaining a normal body temperature.

    3. Alcohol applied to the body surface readily evaporates. The heat required for evaporation is drawn from the body, thus cooling the surface.

    4. When heat is removed from the tissues lying adjacent to an organ, the activity and secretion of the organ are reduced.

    5. In the presence of a sufficient quantity of insulin in the blood stream, the complete oxidation of the ketone bodies takes place.

    6. During acidosis the toxic products of fat digestion are poured into the blood stream continuously from the tissues.

    7. The administration of glucose prevents the development of hypoglycemia, which ordinarily would occur with the repeated injection of insulin.

    8. The approximate amount of insulin required for complete oxidation of ketone bodies can be estimated by the degree of hyperglycemia.

    9. An unconscious patient may be fed by placing suitable food directly into the stomach.

    10. When the patient becomes dehydrated, the sodium base in the tissues is lost through its combination with the fatty acids.

    11. Administration of sodium chloride provides the sodium necessary to re-establish the normal salt balance for the tissues.

    12. Lack of fluid in the tissues causes an increase in the concentration of sodium base in the blood.

    13. The coma is relieved by the administration of large quantities of hypertonic solution to establish a normal salt balance for the tissues.

    14. A low CO_2 combining power of the blood results in a lack of oxygen in the tissues and stimulates exaggerated breathing.

    15. Air hunger respirations are caused by the increased stimulation from excess carbon dioxide in the blood.

2. Assuming that Mr. Muller was a typical example of diabetic coma, the nurse should expect the following symptoms:

  a. Skin:

    (1)____moist, cool.
    (2)____hot, dry.

  b. Breath:

    (1)____acetone odor.
    (2)____acetic acid odor.

  c. Breathing:

    (1)____exaggerated breathing.
    (2)____quiet breathing.

  d. Urine output:

    (1)____increased amount.
    (2)____decreased amount.
    (3)____normal amount.

e. Alertness:

    (1)_____restless, irritable, rouses easily.
    (2)_____lethargic, unconscious, rouses with difficulty.

3. Mr. Muller's laboratory tests would be expected to reveal the following:

  a. Blood:

    (1)_____elevated sugar, normal acidity, high CO_2 combining power.
    (2)_____low sugar, increased acidity, high CO_2 combining power.
    (3)_____elevated sugar, increased acidity, low CO_2 combining power.
    (4)_____low sugar, decreased acidity, low CO_2 combining power.

  b. Urine:

    (1)_____glycosuria, hematuria, albuminuria.
    (2)_____glycosuria, ketonuria.
    (3)_____hematuria, albuminuria.
    (4)_____glycosuria, albuminuria.

4. The insulin used for intravenous infusion should be

  a._____protamine zinc insulin.
  b._____regular (unmodified) insulin.
  c._____either (a) or (b), dependent upon the action desired.

5. The dosage of 20 units of insulin would be administered best as

  a._____0.5 cc. of U 80 insulin.
  b._____0.5 cc. of U 40 insulin.
  c._____0.5 cc. of U 20 insulin.
  d._____1.0 cc. of U 40 insulin.
  e._____1.0 cc. of U 20 insulin.

6. In order to administer insulin 50 units subcutaneously it would be most desirable to use

  a._____2.5 cc. U 20.
  b._____1.2 cc. U 40.
  c._____10 min. U 80.
  d._____20 min. U 40.
  e._____1.2 cc. U 80.

7. During the acute period of the condition skin care for Mr. Muller is of

  a._____less importance than the patient's rest.
  b._____great importance to prevent complications.
  c._____less importance than for convalescent patients.
  d._____no more or less importance than for other patients.

8. In applying external heat to Mr. Muller the nurse should expect

  a._____increased sensitivity to heat, resulting in the patient's discomfort.

    b._____decreased sensitivity to heat, resulting in the possibility of burns without the patient's awareness.

    c._____no change in sensitivity to heat, making usual precautions adequate.

9. During the acute first few days of hospitalization each specimen of urine was tested with Benedict's solution. This should be carried out as follows:

a._____Take 2 cc. of solution,	a._____add 4 drops of urine, and
b._____Take 4 cc. of solution,	b._____add 6 drops of urine, and
c._____Take 6 cc. of solution,	c._____add 8 drops of urine, and

        a._____allow to stand 5 minutes.
        b._____allow to boil 5 minutes.
        c._____allow to stand in boiling water 5 minutes.

10. In the blank space before each resulting color change, indicate the proper interpretation of the amount of sugar present:

_____blue	_____green
_____brick red	_____yellow

11. Mr. Muller demonstrates a need of instruction in

    a._____calculation of diet.
    b._____measurement of insulin.
    c._____symptoms of insulin reaction.
    d._____precautions during illness.
    e._____hygienic care of the skin.

12. Because Mr. Muller is a night worker, the physician directed him to take protamine zinc insulin before his evening meal. With this schedule, insulin reaction would be most apt to occur

a._____during the evening.	c._____early the following morning.
b._____during the night while at work.	d._____during the following day.

Questions for Discussion and Student Projects

1. Discuss the precipitating factors of Mr. Muller's coma. Could this have been prevented? If so, how?
2. What considerations should be kept in mind in planning Mr. Muller's diet? What additional information about Mr. Muller would you need in order to plan the diet?
3. What part does the metabolism of fats play in uncontrolled diabetes? Discuss the relationship of fat metabolism to sodium ions in blood plasma. Why was Mr. Muller dehydrated? Why was there glucose in the urine after a period of vomiting?
4. Outline a desirable teaching plan for Mr. Muller, with particular emphasis on his demonstrated needs.

5. Estimate the weekly cost of Mr. Muller's insulin and of the adjustments of his diet. How much significance would these costs have for a patient in Mr. Muller's income group?
6. What resources are available in your community for a patient like Mr. Muller, if he requires assistance in planning for, or securing, the necessary diet, equipment, etc.? How would you assist Mr. Muller in contacting these resources?
7. Outline the nursing care of a patient in a diabetic coma, including participation in diagnostic procedures, observations, etc.

Questions Relating to Diabetes in General

1. Although the etiology of diabetes is not understood completely, recent studies indicate that it is

    a.____an inheritable disease.
    b.____caused by overconsumption of sweets.
    c.____caused by malignancy of the pancreas.
    d.____an infectious disease.

2. Diabetes occurs most frequently in

    a.____Jewish males.
    b.____Jewish females.
    c.____Chinese, either sex.
    d.____Teutonic males.
    e.____Teutonic females.

3. Diabetes is a disease primarily of

    a.____childhood.   d.____old age.
    b.____youth.   e.____any age.
    c.____middle age.

4. The most common symptom of diabetes is

    a.____weight loss.   d.____anorexia.
    b.____weight gain.   e.____edema.
    c.____polyuria.

5. Precipitating factors in the appearance of clinical symptoms of diabetes are

    a.____infectious diseases.   d.____overconsumption of pro-
    b.____overconsumption of   teins.
       sweets.   e.____vitamin deficiency.
    c.____emotional factors.

6. Insulin normally is produced by the

    a.____hepatic duct of the liver.
    b.____islands of Langerhans in the pancreas.
    c.____pituitary gland.
    d.____adrenal cortex.

7. Insulin is necessary for

   a._____digestion of glucose.
   b._____metabolism of carbohydrate.
   c._____pituitary function.   .
   d._____metabolism of protein.
   e._____oxidation of foods.

8. Insulin is prepared and labeled in various degrees of strength (U 20, U 40, U 80). This differential indicates varying amounts of

   a._____active ingredient per unit.   c._____inactive ingredient per
   b._____active ingredient per   unit.
         cubic centimeter.   d._____inactive ingredient per
                                             cubic centimeter.

9. A prescribed dose of insulin 30 units should be given as

   a._____0.75 cc. of U 40.   d._____1.50 cc. of U 20.
   b._____0.25 cc. of U 40.   e._____none of the above.
   c._____0.30 cc. of U 80.

10. Insulin is not administered by mouth because it

    a._____would be difficult to control the time of action.
    b._____nauseates the patient.
    c._____is inactivated by gastric juices.
    d._____acts too slowly by this route.
    e._____is not absorbed in the G.I. tract.

11. Diabetic control almost always requires insulin in

    a._____obese adults.   c._____growing children.
    b._____underweight adults.

12. Diabetes may be controlled by a low-caloric diet in

    a._____obese adults.   c._____growing children.
    b._____underweight adults.

13. The ideal diabetic diet is based on the following principles:

    a._____sufficient calories to maintain weight slightly below average, sufficient protein for tissue repair, sufficient fat to balance calories.
    b._____sufficient calories to maintain weight slightly above average, sufficient protein for tissue repair, low fat.
    c._____sufficient calories to oxidize a high-fat diet, restricted variety of foods, restricted proteins.

14. A diabetic patient, receiving insulin, should be instructed that if he has an upper respiratory infection he should

    a._____discontinue insulin, reduce caloric intake.
    b._____increase insulin, maintain caloric intake.
    c._____maintain insulin and caloric intake.
    d._____seek medical advice for the regulation of insulin.

15. Conditions frequently occurring with, or as complications of, diabetes are
    a.____arteriosclerosis, coronary occlusion, gangrene.
    b.____tuberculosis, bronchiectasis, lung abscess.
    c.____skin infections, pruritus, carbuncles.
    d.____pyelitis, cystitis, nephritis.

16. The primary use of the glucose tolerance test is to
    a.____determine the amount of insulin needed.
    b.____diagnose diabetes in patients with normal urine and high blood sugar.
    c.____diagnose diabetes in patients with normal blood sugar and glycosuria.
    d.____distinguish between hypoglycemia and hyperglycemia.

17. Preparation for the glucose tolerance test includes
    a.____restricted diet 3 days previous to the test.
    b.____unrestricted diet 3 days previous to the test.
                                and
    a.____no breakfast on the day of the test.
    b.____a normal breakfast on the day of the test.

18. Factors which may give abnormal response by normal persons in the glucose tolerance test include
    a.____infections and fever.   d.____unrestricted diet.
    b.____restricted diet.   e.____bed rest.
    c.____physical effort.

19. Compare the action of the various preparations of insulin by filling in the following table:

	Peak of Action	Duration of Action
Regular, or crystalline zinc insulin		
Protamine zinc insulin		
Neutral protamine Hagedorn insulin		

Questions for Discussion and Student Projects

1. Discuss the various preparations of insulin, and their relative value in the control of diabetes. What are some of the indications for the choice of the type of preparation to be used?
2. Discuss the significance of the recent belief that diabetes is an inheritable disease, following a mendelian recessive pattern. What percentage of cases would you expect in the children of two diabetic parents? Of one diabetic and one non-diabetic parent? What is meant by a carrier of the disease?

3. What is the primary objective of the American Diabetes Association? How is it financed? List some of the recent activities of the association. Is there an association in your community? In your state?
4. Discuss the prevalence of diabetes mellitus in this country. What special studies have been made to determine the national incidence and what factors may explain the increasing death rate? What steps may any individual take to determine if he has diabetes?
5. Discuss measures taken to stimulate, improve, and restore circulation to the extremities. Review the procedure for contrast foot baths, Pavex boot, Buerger's exercises. Why are these necessary?
6. Discuss the effect of the amputation of a leg in an elderly diabetic. How may he be assisted in adjusting to an appliance or a sedentary life? How serious is the danger of falling with subsequent fracture? What resources are available in the community for the care of such patients and the provision of necessary appliances.
7. Outline the teaching plan for a newly diagnosed diabetic patient, including testing of urine, administration of insulin, hygienic care, prevention of complications. When should this teaching begin? What are the most effective methods?
8. Prepare a list of materials suitable for reading by a patient or his family. Where may the general public secure suitable information about diabetes?

THE IRRITABLE MOTHER—PATIENT STUDY

Jennie Miller was again on the brink of tears. She had scolded Timmy, aged 4, because the little wooden train he was tugging around the kitchen linoleum made a monotonous noise. She had really not meant to reprimand him and now he was crying. Without a doubt he would waken 2-year-old Lindy from her nap.

Mrs. Miller was only 30 and she knew "these little things" ought not to upset her. The children were really wonderful, but lately she had had episodes when she felt she just could not go on any longer. Finally, her husband Jim insisted that she see their family physician.

Dr. Thomas was a kindly practitioner who immediately noted her tenseness, a nervous tapping of her foot, and a wide-eyed look filled with apprehension. Her respirations were 40, pulse 130 and forceful, and she was slightly dyspneic. When weighed, she was not too surprised to learn that she had lost 15 pounds in the past 2 months although she admitted to having a voracious appetite. Dr. Thomas tactfully suggested that she be admitted to the hospital so that she could rest and have some special tests. Mrs. Miller appeared very concerned at first but when it was explained that she had a thyroid condition which could be corrected with proper therapy, she was reconciled to the plan made for her. Dr. Thomas gave her a prescription for propylthiouracil.

Mrs. Miller's concerns which she expressed to her husband on their way home were, "Whom can we get to take care of the children?" "Maybe I have cancer; my sister died of cancer of the breast." "I can't bear to be left alone in the hospital. Will someone be near me?"

Mr. Miller did his best to reassure her. His mother lived in the same community and would be happy to help with the children. He would be on hand to make a request that she be placed near some pleasant patient in the hospital. As for the possibility of cancer, he had never heard of anyone having cancer of the thyroid. She seemed to be satisfied with his solutions.

Several days later, Mrs. Miller arrived on the surgical ward in a wheel chair. She was restless and over-active, but when directed to a pleasant semi-private room was a little less upset. The house officer was expecting her and knew that her diagnosis was exophthalmic goiter. He left the following orders:

> Bed rest.
> High-vitamin 4,000-calorie diet.
> Fluids ad lib.
> Chloral hydrate gr. xv q.n. p.r.n.
> Lugol's sol. gtts. v t.i.d.
> Basal metabolism test q. 2 day.

After 10 days in the hospital, her B.M.R. came down from plus 65 to plus 13 and surgery was planned. Mrs. Miller was started on procaine penicillin and vitamin K. Mentally and emotionally, she appeared ready for her operation and had a successful subtotal thyroidectomy.

On the second postoperative day she was allowed out of bed and on the sixth day she was discharged to the care of Dr. Thomas.

Reference

Lidz, Theodore: Emotional factors in the etiology of hyperthyroidism, Psychosomatic Med. 11:2, 1949.

Questions Relating to the Patient Study

1. To prepare Mrs. Miller for a B.M.R. the nurse should tell her that

   a. the purpose of the test is to determine

      (1)＿＿bodily utilization of oxygen and nitrogen.
      (2)＿＿bodily utilization of oxygen and nitrogen excretion of CO_2.
      (3)＿＿the rate of circulation and heat production.
      (4)＿＿the rate of heat production and CO_2 excretion.
      (5)＿＿all of the above.

   b. the test will be made

      (1)＿＿in the morning, after a normal breakfast.
      (2)＿＿in the morning, after no breakfast.
      (3)＿＿in the late afternoon, after fasting all day.
      (4)＿＿in the late afternoon, after normal meals.

   c. she will be asked to co-operate by

      (1)＿＿alternately holding her breath and then breathing forcefully.

(2)＿＿＿breathing naturally and relaxing.

(3)＿＿＿alternately holding her breath and then taking deep breaths.

(4)＿＿＿talking and exercising as instructed.

d. the test will involve

(1)＿＿＿no pain.

(2)＿＿＿very little pain.

(3)＿＿＿anesthetic to prevent pain.

2. The test probably will be omitted if Mrs. Miller

a.＿＿＿eats a small breakfast.

b.＿＿＿fails to eat breakfast.

c.＿＿＿drinks a glass of water.

d.＿＿＿failed to sleep the previous night.

e.＿＿＿seems emotionally upset.

3. Mrs. Miller's over-activity was due to

a.＿＿＿an inability to face reality and her family problems.

b.＿＿＿an inadequate intake of iodine.

c.＿＿＿an excessive amount of thyroxin.

d.＿＿＿worry about the possibility of having cancer.

4. When giving Mrs. Miller her admission bath, the nurse would be likely to find

a.＿＿＿swollen ankles.　　　　f.＿＿＿palpitation.

b.＿＿＿fatigue on exertion.　　g.＿＿＿depression.

c.＿＿＿a fine tremor of the hands.　h.＿＿＿constipation.

d.＿＿＿a flushed skin.　　　　i.＿＿＿nystagmus.

e.＿＿＿ascites.　　　　　　　j.＿＿＿apathy.

5. The nurse should expect that Mrs. Miller will be

a.＿＿＿sensitive to cold, requiring extra blankets, etc.

b.＿＿＿intolerant of heat, requiring little covering and a cool room.

c.＿＿＿normally responsive to heat and cold, requiring the usual covering and room temperature.

6. Lugol's solution is the name for

a.＿＿＿potassium iodide.

b.＿＿＿potassium iodide with aqueous iodine solution.

c.＿＿＿a tinted aqueous iodine solution.

7. Lugol's solution was ordered for Mrs. Miller to

a.＿＿＿increase glandular hyperplasia, decrease basal metabolism.

b.＿＿＿decrease glandular hyperplasia, decrease basal metabolism.

c.＿＿＿reduce exophthalmus, induce weight gain.

d.＿＿＿increase basal metabolism, induce weight gain.

8. The nurse should administer Lugol's solution in fruit juice or in milk in order to

    a._____prevent the reaction of iodine on tooth enamel.
    b._____prevent irritation of the gastric mucosa.
    c._____insure adequate fluid intake.
    d._____provide additional calories.
    e._____disguise its bitter taste.

9. The purpose of the propylthiouracil for Mrs. Miller is to

    a._____interfere with the utilization of iodine by gland and to block the formation of thyroxin.
    b._____promote the utilization of iodine by gland and to block the formation of thyroxin.
    c._____interfere with the utilization of iodine by gland and to stimulate the formation of thyroxin.
    d._____produce atrophy of gland.
    e._____produce hyperplasia of gland.

10. Thiamine hydrochloride was ordered for Mrs. Miller because of a (an)

    a._____increased amount of fat in the diet.
    b._____increased protein destruction.
    c._____greatly augmented metabolism.
    d._____depletion of glycogen store in the liver.

11. a. Because of Mrs. Miller's need for a high-caloric and high-protein intake, the following groups of foods would be indicated:

    (1)_____50 Gm. of cottage cheese and 1 serving of Junket with 1 tbsp. of whipped cream.
    (2)_____an egg, 200 cc. of whole milk and 1 serving of Jello.
    (3)_____a toasted American cheese (20 Gm.) sandwich and 1 cup of cocoa.
    (4)_____60 Gm. of chicken and 1 baked custard.

    b. From the groups of foods above, the highest in calories would be

    (1)_____. (2)_____. (3)_____. (4)_____.

    c. From the groups of foods above, the richest in protein would be

    (1)_____. (2)_____. (3)_____. (4)_____.

12. Of the following measures the most effective in assisting Mrs. Miller to consume extra food would be

    a._____large servings of food at regular meal hours.
    b._____small servings of food frequently.
    c._____increased fat content of the diet.
    d._____large amounts of concentrated carbohydrates.
    e._____placement near another patient on a similar diet.

13. The purpose of vitamin K for Mrs. Miller was to

    a.____decrease emotional tension before surgery.
    b.____shrink the thyroid tissue.
    c.____decrease the blood clotting time.
    d.____prevent postoperative infection.

14. After responding from the anesthetic, the most desirable position for Mrs. Miller would be

    a.____high Fowler.
    b.____semi-Fowler.
    c.____flat.
    d.____with the head of the bed on 6-inch blocks.
    e.____with the foot of the bed elevated.
    f.____any way she finds comfortable.

15. Emergency equipment which should be at Mrs. Miller's bedside postoperatively includes

    a.____aspiration needle and syringe, sterile dressings, sterile drainage tubing and bottle.
    b.____tourniquet, packing set, aspiration needle and syringe, vitamin K.
    c.____intratracheal aspiration set, suction tubing and bottle.
    d.____tracheotomy set, packing set, sterile gloves.
    e.____nasal oxygen set-up, electric fan, ice bags.

16. A sudden temperature elevation to 106° accompanied by restlessness and delirium would lead you to suspect

    a.____pneumonitis.
    b.____thyroid crisis.
    c.____hemorrhage.
    d.____atelectasis.
    e.____emphysema.

17. Since the situation described in question 16 is an emergency, the nurse would

    a.____immediately cover Mrs. Miller with blankets to prevent chilling.
    b.____administer whatever sedative has been ordered.
    c.____stop the intravenous infusion if one is running.
    d.____place her in an oxygen tent.
    e.____reduce the number of covers, add ice bags and ice packs.
    f.____have calcium gluconate ready for the surgeon to give intravenously.

18. Dyspnea or aphonia would lead you to suspect

    a.____hemorrhage.
    b.____excessive tightness of dressings.
    c.____hysteria.
    d.____injury to the larynx.
    e.____injury to the recurrent laryngeal nerve.

19. Tetany may occur as a postoperative complication and must be watched for by the nurse. Symptoms suggestive of this complication are

    a._____sardonic grin, trismus, generalized convulsion resulting from the least stimulus.

    b._____hyperirritability of the nerves, spasms of the hands and feet, muscular twitching.

    c._____stimulation of nervous tissue of the spine, opisthotonus, excessive fatigue.

20. Tetany postoperatively may occur as a result of

    a._____an increased amount of calcium in the blood.

    b._____a decrease in the amount of calcium in the blood.

    c._____the invasion of *Bacillus tetani.*

    d._____an increase of phosphorus in the blood serum.

    e._____a decrease of phosphorus in the blood serum.

    f._____the removal of one or more parathyroid glands.

21. Treatment for tetany is

    a._____thorough cleansing of the wound.

    b._____injection of tetanus toxoid.

    c._____intravenous administration of soluble calcium salts.

    d._____immediate administration of phosphorus compounds.

22. Six weeks after her discharge from the hospital, Mrs. Miller returned to the Endocrine Clinic for a basal metabolism test. The results showed it to be —18. Symptoms which would be expected to accompany this drop are

    a._____a 20-pound weight loss.

    b._____difficulty in concentrating on the Woman's Club treasury report which she had to prepare.

    c._____perspiring profusely upon the least exertion.

    d._____extreme tiredness.

    e._____unusual sensitiveness to cold.

23. After being started on thyroid therapy because of her low B.M.R., within 2 weeks she would be expected to notice that

    a._____she was gaining weight.   c._____she was less alert mentally.

    b._____her skin seemed less dry.   d._____she had more energy.

Questions for Discussion and Student Projects

1. Could Mrs. Miller, or any patient who develops an exophthalmic goiter, have prevented this condition? Discuss this from the point of view of hereditary influences, environmental factors and preventive aspects. Substantiate your point of view.

2. What means would you employ to lessen the anxiety when preparing a patient such as Mrs. Miller for her operation?

3. What instruction or information will Mr. Miller require to insure an

optimum environment for his wife when she goes home? What precautions, if any, will she need to follow in her convalescent care? Will she be able to resume care of the children? What are the possibilities of a malignancy developing?

4. Congress has rejected a law requiring all table salt in interstate commerce to be iodized. Many housewives in iodine-poor areas suspect iodized salt of being "medicated." People living near the coasts used to get ample iodine in seafood and in vegetables grown in iodine-bearing soils, but nowadays much produce is shipped to the coasts from iodine-poor areas. Old-fashioned refining methods left the iodine in, but modern, high-temperature processes have been taking it out. What are the implications of this problem? What can nurses do about it?

5. When a patient has a total thyroidectomy for carcinoma, what adjustment in his future life will he have to make? Discuss the following aspects:

   a._____activity.   d._____medications.
   b._____type of occupation.   e._____prognosis.
   c._____dietary modifications.

6. What may be the relations between pathologic fractures, renal, calculi and Von Recklinghausen's disease? What is the surgical treatment?

7. It has been suggested that the repeated use of radioactive iodine for thyroid pathology carries with it the possibility of causing a malignant growth of the thyroid in later years. Canvas the literature for the current thinking about this form of treatment and its results.

Nursing Care of Patients with Other Disorders of the Endocrine Glands

Reference

Quimby, E. H.: Safety in the use of radioactive isotopes, Am. J. Nursing **51:** 240, 1951.

1. Hypofunctioning of the thyroid gland in a very young child results in the diseased condition known as

   a._____cretinism.   d._____micromegaly.
   b._____myxedema.   e._____diabetes insipidus.
   c._____acromegaly.

2. A cretin may be described as one with

   a._____a relatively small head, broad shoulders, wide hips, short legs.
   b._____a moonlike face, winged scapulae, cervical kyphosis, lumbar lordosis.
   c._____small ears, a big head, long legs, pawlike hands, mental slowness.

    d._____shortness of stature, a pot-belly, a narrow pelvis, the mouth open, a dry, cold skin.

3. In the adult, if the entire thyroid gland is removed, and the patient fails to take the prescribed doses of thyroid extract, myxedema results. Symptoms of this condition are

    a._____increased mental and physical vigor.
    b._____an increased sensitivity to heat.
    c._____subnormal temperature and pulse rate.
    d._____weight gain.
    e._____the hair grows more thickly.

4. A condition which often develops rapidly in a patient with myxedema is

    a._____hypertension.   d._____intestinal obstruction.
    b._____arteriosclerosis.   e._____hyperparathyroidism.
    c._____tetany.

5. A radioactive isotope is

    a._____the name of a ray emanating from the element radium.
    b._____a synthetic substance charged with penetrating activity.
    c._____an element which, when treated by a cyclotron, "can become radioactive."
    d._____an element which is in a high state of ionization.

6. Necessary precautions in handling radioactive isotopes are

    a._____if active material gets on the hands or other skin surfaces, to scrub thoroughly for 1 full minute.
    b._____to place radioactive material in a thick-walled copper box if it must be transferred from one place to another.
    c._____to check the radioactive substance on clothing or skin by means of a monitoring device.
    d._____to have the patient drink the material through a drinking tube while it is still in the shielded carrying case.
    e._____if he is ambulatory, to have the patient under treatment urinate in the toilet (providing it is not necessary to save the urine). This will not endanger other persons.

7. The effect of radioactive iodine (I_{131}) is to

    a._____bombard radiosensitive tissues of the body.
    b._____irradiate the thyroid gland without jeopardy to other tissues.
    c._____supply the necessary vehicle for stimulating the growth of healthy thyroid cells.
    d._____immediately replace the element iodine, which was lacking for a long period of time in the diet.
    e._____destroy the glandular cells of the hyperactive thyroid gland.

8. Gout is essentially a disease of

   a._____young adult males.
   b._____young adult females.
   c._____middle-aged males.
   d._____middle-aged females.
   e._____either sex, age not significant.

9. Gout is best described as

   a._____a hereditary disease of purine metabolism.
   b._____the result of over-indulgence in alcohol.
   c._____the result of over-indulgence in high-protein foods.
   d._____an acute infection of the joints.

10. Hyperinsulinism is a

   a._____term synonymous with diabetes mellitus.
   b._____rare disease just the opposite of diabetes mellitus.
   c._____term synonymous with Addison's disease.
   d._____complication of diabetes mellitus.

11. The most effective treatment of hyperinsulinism is

   a._____control with insulin.
   b._____control with diet.
   c._____surgery of the pancreas.
   d._____liver and iron.

12. Addison's disease (chronic renal insufficiency) in most cases is due to

   a._____an over-intake of vitamin D.
   b._____tuberculosis of the adrenal glands.
   c._____carcinoma of the adrenal glands.
   d._____overstimulation of the sympathetic nerve.

13. The patient in acute Addison's disease should be

   a._____encouraged to exercise and to keep alert.
   b._____protected from exertion.
   c._____treated by psychotherapy.

14. The major factor in obesity is

   a._____glandular dysfunction.
   b._____a caloric intake in excess of caloric needs.
   c._____heredity.
   d._____lack of exercise.

Section 8. Nursing Care of Patients with Disorders of the Musculoskeletal System*

STUDY SUGGESTIONS: Before beginning the study of this Section, the student
will find it helpful to

A. Review

   1. Anatomy and physiology: the musculoskeletal system.

B. Study

   1. In medical nursing texts: diseases of the musculoskeletal system.
   2. In surgical nursing texts: conditions of the musculoskeletal system,
      antisepsis, asepsis.
   3. In pharmacology texts: hormones and synthetic substitutes, vitamins.

C. Read the additional References listed before attempting to answer the
   questions relating to each patient study.

"WILL I BE A CRIPPLE?"
Background Review Questions

1. Match the following:

   a. genu.
   b. manus.
   c. hallux.
   d. osteo-.
   e. chondr-.
   f. myo-.
   g. spondyl.
   h. cubitus.
   i. syno-.
   j. coxa.
   k. valgus genu.
   l. varus genu.

   (1)_____joint.
   (2)_____hip.
   (3)_____foot.
   (4)_____elbow.
   (5)_____bow-legged deformity.
   (6)_____spine.
   (7)_____bone.
   (8)_____cartilage.
   (9)_____hand.
   (10)_____muscle.
   (11)_____knock-knee deformity.
   (12)_____knee.
   (13)_____large toe.
   (14)_____joint lining.

2. Match the following:

   Fracture

   a. Colles'.
   b. pathologic.
   c. comminuted.

   Description

   (1)_____ankle involvement.
   (2)_____skin intact but bone is broken.
   (3)_____broken bone pierces the skin.

---

* Additional material on orthopedic nursing is included in Section 2, on amputation.
Other musculoskeletal conditions are considered in the pediatric section.

d. simple.
e. greenstick.
f. compound.

(4)_____the result of disease process.
(5)_____contains 3 or more fragments.
(6)_____wrist involvement.
(7)_____incomplete break in bone.

3. Match the following:

Pathologic Manifestation

a. caseation of bone.
b. elevated scapulae.
c. sequestrum.
d. cold abscess.
e. involucrum.
f. aseptic necrosis.
g. low back pain.
h. displaced L_4 or L_5 vertebrae.

Specific Orthopedic Disease or Condition of Which It Is Characteristic

(1)_____osteomyelitis.
(2)_____spondylolisthesis.
(3)_____Legg-Perthe's disease.
(4)_____osteoarthritis.
(5)_____Sprengel's disease.
(6)_____tuberculosis of bone.
(7)_____tuberculosis of bone and joint.
(8)_____ruptured intervertebral disc.

4. In the blank space to the left of each descriptive phrase, place the name of the type of movement described:

a._____movement of the forearm which turns the palm of the hand downward.
b._____movement of the forearm which occurs when the triceps brachii contract.
c._____movement of the leg which occurs when the gastrocnemius contracts.
d._____movement of the leg which occurs when the sartorius contracts.
e._____movement which brings the arms out from the side of the body to a horizontal position.
f._____movement by which the palms of the hands are brought to face upward.
g._____movement which moves the leg away from the midline of the body.
h._____movement of the arm which would occur after placing a parcel under the arm in order to carry the object in that position.
i._____backward movement of the arm and forearm taken before the ball is brought forward when bowling.
j._____forward movement of the arm which occurs when rolling a bowling ball.

5. Joint motion can be measured by a

a.___tonometer.
b.___goniometer.
c.___osteometer.

d.___angulometer.
e.___manometer.

6. Of the following types of joints, the elbow joint is an example of a (an)

a._____diarthrotic joint.   c._____amphiarthrotic joint.
b._____synarthrotic joint.   d._____ball-and-socket joint.

7. The typical cervical vertebra may be differentiated from other types of vertebra because of the

a._____absence of the structure known as a body.
b._____unusually long length of the spinous processes.
c._____presence of small foramina in the transverse processes.
d._____unusually small size of the vertebral foramina.

8. The area of bone where longitudinal bone growth occurs is the

a._____endosteum.   c._____epiphyseal line.
b._____epiphysis.   d._____medullary canal.

9. Sensations of fatigue and cramping within active skeletal muscles are due to a (an)

a._____lack of oxygen for the conversion of adenosinetriphosphate from organic phosphates.
b._____increased flow of blood through the active muscle.
c._____accumulation of carbon dioxide within the muscle.
d._____accumulation of lactic acid within the muscle.

10. During muscular exercise, if the active muscles do not receive sufficient quantities of oxygen, this leads to a (an)

a._____cessation of muscular contraction.
b._____accumulation of lactic acid within the muscle.
c._____retarded conversion of creatine and phosphoric acid to phosphocreatine.
d._____accumulation of carbon dioxide within the muscle.

11. Skeletal muscles work with greater efficiency

a._____if the fibers pull against a load.
b._____if there is an accumulation of lactic acid within the muscle.
c._____in a cool rather than a warm environment.
d._____in an environment rich in nitrogen.

12. The increase in production of heat occurring within active muscles is physiologically significant because it

a._____increases the temperature of the blood, which stimulates the respiratory center.
b._____tends to reduce the irritability of muscle fibers and to hasten fatigue.
c._____increases the rate at which oxygen will dissociate from the hemoglobin of the blood.
d._____increases the rate at which resynthesis of glycogen can take place.

13. The chemical constituent of skeletal muscle fibers which is the first to become depleted with prolonged muscular activity is

a.____glycogen.   c.____phosphocreatine.
b.____adenosinetriphosphate.   d.____adenosinediphosphate.

14. A chemical which, when present in large amounts around muscle cells, causes fatigue is

a.____lactic acid.   d.____creatinine.
b.____uric acid.   e.____carbon dioxide.
c.____glycogen.

15. Fatigue in muscle is due to depletion of

a.____organic phosphates.   d.____glycogen.
b.____lactic acid.   e.____creatin.
c.____oxygen.

16. The chemical process which is necessary to provide energy for prolonged muscular work is

a.____ionization.   c.____oxidation.
b.____hydrolysis.   d.____reduction.

17. Match the following:

   Type of Joint   *Description*
   a. synarthroses.   (1)____freely movable joints.
   b. diarthroses.   (2)____immovable joints.
   c. amphiarthroses.   (3)____slightly movable joints.

18. Check the correct statement regarding muscle action:

a.____Muscles which move a part usually lie directly over that part.
b.____As a muscle contracts, one of the bones must remain stationary to act as an anchorage for the muscle to pull against as it draws the other bone toward it.
c.____A muscle acts singly; when one contracts, a pull is exerted on the adjoining muscle which in turn contracts.
d.____Skeletal muscles contract in response to stimulation; the natural stimulus is a nerve impulse brought to the muscle by sensory nerves.

19. Skeletal changes which take place as one progresses from infancy to young adulthood are that

a.____the vertebral column develops two curves not present at birth —the cervical and the lumbar.
b.____the legs become proportionately shorter and the trunk proportionately longer.
c.____the thorax changes its shape, from elliptical to round.
d.____the head becomes proportionately smaller.

"WILL I BE A CRIPPLE?"—PATIENT STUDY

Mrs. Carter, a 35-year-old housewife, was referred from the orthopedic clinic to the medical clinic because of swelling and pain in the joints of her hands and feet. About 6 months ago, at Christmas time, she had had a severe sore throat and swelling and stiffness of her fingers, toes and right ankle. The sore throat disappeared, leaving the swelling in the extremities. It has been painful for her to walk so that she gets around poorly and is also unable to do any fine work requiring finger movements.

The positive findings on physical examination were marked fusiform swelling of the proximal phalangeal joints of the hands and feet; tenderness in the right ankle, with swelling at the proximal end of the metatarsal bone; and a small telengectasis present on the lateral surface. On standing the right foot was slightly pronated; there was no redness or heat about the infected area. A diagnosis of rheumatoid arthritis was made.

The treatment prescribed was use of hot wet soaks and massage of the feet and hands. She was also referred to the orthopedic clinic where pads were fitted into her shoes. These gave her much relief and aided her in walking. She developed pain in her knees and was advised to apply hot magnesium sulfate soaks to her knees, and to take aspirin gr. x for pain.

On a subsequent visit to the Medical Clinic, Mrs. Carter complained of severe heart palpitation when anxious or excited. No pathologic reason was discovered for this complaint.

Mrs. Carter seems fairly intelligent and able to carry out the instructions for treatment herself. Her family consists of her husband and 3 children, aged 11, 7 and 2 years. The care of the children is difficult as they demand considerable attention. She feels that she is very nervous and becomes upset easily, particularly at the present time when she finds she is unable to do the things she wishes to do. She has not been going out, and, with the exception of visits from some friends, has had few outside contacts. Friends wanted her to go to the seashore for a month and others want her to go with them to a health resort for "natural water baths." The clinic physician advised her to go away for 3 or 4 weeks and assured her that the baths should be beneficial for her condition.

Mrs. Carter needs help in adjusting, and considerable encouragement. She is not underweight but requires instruction regarding a proper diet. If she does go away for a rest, this vacation away from the family will be beneficial only if her mind is at ease. Arrangements will have to be made for the care of the family so she will not worry about them. The economic status of the family is such that they do not require financial aid of agencies, although they are appreciative of guidance. Mrs. Carter has confidence in the physicians and the clinic, and her co-operation with them has obtained relief of her symptoms.

References

Blodgett, Margaret L.: The place of occupational therapy in the treatment of arthritis, Occupational Therapy and Rehabilitation 21:277, 1942.

Boland, Edward W., and Headley, Nathan E.: Effects of cortisone therapy on rheumatoid arthritis, J.A.M.A. **141**:301, 1949.

Editorial: Rheumatic fever control program, J.A.M.A. **134**:1094, 1947.

Hench, Philip, et al.: Effects of cortisone acetate and pituitary ACTH on rheumatoid arthritis, rheumatic fever and certain other conditions: a study in clinical physiology, Arch. Int. Med. **85**:545, 1950.

Holmquist, Emily W.: The patient with atrophic arthritis, Am. J. Nursing **49**:302, 1949.

Ludwig, Alfred O.: Emotional factors in rheumatoid arthritis: their bearing on the care and rehabilitation of the patient, Physiol. Rev. **29**:344, 1949.

Margolis, H. M.: Rheumatoid arthritis, Am. J. Nursing **47**:787, 1947.

Marsh, Edith L.: Nursing Care in Chronic Diseases, pp. 88–103, Rheumatoid Arthritis, Philadelphia, Lippincott, 1946.

Norcross, Bernard M., and Lockie, Maxwell: Help for the arthritic, Pub. Health Nursing **40**:90, 1948.

Scheele, Leonard A.: Arthritis as a public health problem, Pub. Health Rep. **65**:1351, 1950.

Questions Relating to the Patient Study

1. In order to prevent deformities due to muscular contraction it is important that the patient have

   a._____complete rest, with immobilization of the inflamed joints.
   b._____exercise of non-infected joints, but rest for the inflamed joints.
   c._____frequent change of position of the infected joints, regular exercises and avoidance of muscle and joint strain.

2. Mrs. Carter should be encouraged to

   a._____continue to assume all of the care of her home and children.
   b._____avoid over-exertion but continue some normal activities.
   c._____plan for long-term complete relief from all activities.

3. Pads were fitted into Mrs. Carter's shoes because of

   a._____changes in the bony structure of her feet.
   b._____the need for cushioning the inflamed joints.
   c._____improperly fitted shoes.
   d._____the need of all adults for this type of support.

4. If Mrs. Carter complains of pain in her knees at night she should be advised to take aspirin, apply heat and

   a._____flex the knees and support them with pillows.
   b._____immobilize the knees with elastic bandage.
   c._____change the position of the knees frequently.

5. When Mrs. Carter complains of palpitation she should

   a._____be assured it is of no significance.
   b._____be told it is to be expected with this disease.
   c,_____have complete cardiac examination.
   d._____be placed on digitalis therapy.

6. Aspirin gr. x was selected for relief of pain for Mrs. Carter because

    a._____only a mild analgesic is needed as the pain in this condition is not severe.

    b._____her symptoms are primarily imaginary and any drug would satisfy her.

    c._____more effective habit-forming drugs must be avoided because of the chronicity of the disease.

7. Mrs. Carter complains that the aspirin ordered for relief of pain makes her feel nauseated. You should advise her

    a._____that she must choose between the nausea and the pain.

    b._____that taking a glass of milk with the aspirin may prevent nausea.

    c._____to crush the aspirin and take it in solution.

    d._____to ask the physician for an order for hypodermic medications.

8. Mrs. Carter asks you about the value of vitamin D. She has heard of an article reporting cures of arthritis from massive dosages of vitamin D. You should tell her that

    a._____this information is correct and she should take vitamin D.

    b._____increased amounts of vitamins are essential to her improvement.

    c._____her doctor would have ordered vitamin D if it were indicated.

    d._____not only is there no evidence that this vitamin cures, but also there is a real danger from overdosages.

    e._____all vitamins are good and the more she takes of them the better.

9. The diet for Mrs. Carter should be

    a._____low-purine.   d._____normal well-balanced.

    b._____low-salt.   e._____reinforced with vitamin D.

    c._____low-carbohydrate.

The following questions relate to arthritis in general:

1. The onset of rheumatoid arthritis usually is

    a._____insidious, with slight pain and stiffness in one joint, followed by migratory joint symptoms.

    b._____acute, with pain and swelling of many joints, fever.

    c._____acute, with pain and swelling of one joint, followed by migratory joint symptoms.

2. Rheumatoid arthritis occurs most frequently

    a._____in men.   c._____during childhood.

    b._____in women.   d._____between 20 and 40 years of age.

                      e._____during old age.

3. The drug considered as the best single therapeutic measure in the treatment of arthritis is

    a._____vitamin D, in massive doses.   c._____antibiotics.

    b._____gold salts.   d._____sulfonamides.

4. Cortisone and ACTH administered to patients with rheumatoid arthritis
   a._____produce prompt remission of symptoms.
   b._____provide a permanent cure of the condition.
   c._____have been shown to have no value.
   d._____prevent deformities.

5. From the following items select those which describe the toxic effects of the drugs listed below

   a. dermatitis, agranulocytosis, gastroenteritis, nephritis, bleeding gums.
   b. urticaria, marked fatigue, ataxia, upset carbohydrate metabolism, jaundice.
   c. acne, hirsutism, edema, glycosuria, retention of sodium.
   d. acne, leukopenia, rounding of the face, stomatitis, disturbing mental changes.
   e. cyanosis, vertigo, nystagmus, tremors, thick speech.

   (1)_____barbital.
   (2)_____gold salts.
   (3)_____ACTH and cortisone.

Questions for Discussion and Student Projects

A. Related to Patient Study
  1. What practical suggestions should the nurse give Mrs. Carter which would assist her in securing needed rest? In maintenance of good posture?
  2. What explanation would the nurse give Mrs. Carter in relation to using hot magnesium sulfate soaks to her knees, and hot soaks and massage to her feet and hands? Discuss various ways dry or moist heat may be applied to arthritic joints.
  3. What arrangements could be made with Mr. Carter to relieve his wife of family responsibilities? How would you help them both to accept and to understand her physical condition?
  4. What type of suggestions might be given to Mrs. Carter by the Social Service Department where psychotherapy and diversional therapy are more significant than financial aid?

B. Related to Arthritis in General
  1. Distinguish between
    a. traumatic arthritis,
    b. infectious or suppurative arthritis,
    c. rheumatoid arthritis,

giving consideration to the

  (1) etiology or precipitating factors.
  (2) symptoms and diagnosis.
  (3) treatment.
  (4) prognosis (including the probability of deformity).

  2. Discuss the incidence of arthritic conditions in the United States and the social and economic significance of the protracted illness and disabling conditions.

3. What types of diversions and occupations are suitable for patients crippled with arthritis? How may they be rehabilitated? What community agencies are available for the chronic patient for re-education and rehabilitation?

4. What suggestions may be made to a patient for developing a healthy mental attitude toward physical limitations of arthritis?

5. Discuss the purpose and activities of the Arthritis and Rheumatism Foundation.

6. Discuss the care of patients suffering with atrophic arthritis, including

a. supervised rest.
b. adequate diet.
c. improvement of posture and prevention of de-formity.
d. heat.
e. massage.
f. exercises.
g. good body alignment.
h. breathing exercises.
i. occupational therapy and psychotherapy.

7. What measures may combat the serious results of continued muscle spasm, such as flexion and adduction of the joints and ankylosis?

8. If you were a public health nurse calling on an elderly patient with hypertrophic arthritis, what suggestion would you make to the family for proper care? What responsibilities would you assign to the patient? How would your advice differ if the patient were obese and had a chronic heart condition?

9. Discuss the importance of providing adequate care for patients having hypertrophic arthritis, giving particular consideration to the emotional factors resulting from incapacity.

10. How would you tell a young patient with rheumatoid arthritis that she must keep her mind free of worry and anxiety as part of treatment? Could you use this as a reason for discharge to a nursing home? How would you persuade an older person with hypertrophic arthritis that more adequate care might be given in a nursing home than in his own home?

11. Discuss the use of ACTH and cortisone. What is the purpose of these drugs? Dosage, therapeutic effect and untoward action? May they be given for an indefinite period?

12. What steps have been taken nationally to provide added research on ACTH, cortisone and other drugs helpful in the treatment of arthritic conditions? What local resources are available to provide these necessary drugs in needy cases?

"I DIDN'T MEAN TO BOTHER YOU"—PATIENT STUDY

Early one May morning, Grandma Holland fell while walking in the dark to the bathroom in her home. She was unable to get up and noted severe pain in her left hip. By calling, she was able to waken her daughter and son-in-law, who helped her back to bed. She remained there all morning but her pain was unrelieved by aspirin. By noon she was suffering so acutely that the family physican was called. He ordered her immediate transfer to the hospital where she was x-rayed before admission to the ward. The diagnosis was trochanteric fracture of the left femur.

Mrs. Holland is an 87-year-old widow, of medium size, with loose false teeth and slight hearing and sight defects. Her complexion was somewhat sallow but her skin was clear. She was immaculately clean from her white long braided hair to her feet, which were well cared for though calloused along the outer edge of the great toes. At first she seemed somewhat confused by the hustle of the open ward but later appeared resigned to her status and was neither irritated nor consoled by the amount of attention she received.

The day after admission she was taken to the operating room and given a general anesthesia. After reduction of the fracture on a Hawley table, an incision was made over the trochanter and down the side of the thigh. A hole was drilled about 3 cm. below the trochanter and a guide wire inserted. Under roentgen-ray control, a blade plate was inserted and screwed in place. Mrs. Holland received 800 cc. of normal saline during the procedure. Her condition was satisfactory when she came back to her bed and Buck's traction was applied.

The following day, Mrs. Holland was given infusions. A continuous bladder irrigation was started and gantrisin 2 Gm. daily was ordered. Her progress appeared to be satisfactory until 3 days later when she developed slight swelling with tenderness in the left leg and hip. It was thought that this symptom might indicate incipient thrombophlebitis. Because her prothrombin time was 43 per cent, she was given Dicumerol 150 mg. Buck's extension was removed and the bladder irrigation was discontinued. Ten days postoperative the stitches were removed; the calf tenderness had disappeared. She was now able to begin physical therapy exercises. She tired easily but persisted with her push-ups and other activities.

During this time, her daughter had tried to have Mrs. Holland transferred to a nursing home in order to save expenses. The surgeon might have given his permission but Mrs. Holland returned one day from physical therapy and mentioned "feeling poorly," but had no specific complaints. The next day there was a marked change in her condition and it was thought that she had a slight cerebral hemorrhage. She improved slowly and within a week was taking fluids and speaking coherently again. Her exercises were resumed. With this improvement, her daughter again pursued the possibility of having her mother moved to a nursing home. The daughter "felt she had put up with her mother long enough."

When Mrs. Holland was transferred, there were tears in her eyes. She had had hopes of going back to the home she had lived in for the past 20 years. Physically, she was very well for her age. Her skin condition was excellent and she was just beginning to adapt herself to her new crutches.

References

Benton, M.: Buck's extension, Am. J. Nursing 34:539, 1934.

Flitter, H.: An Introduction to Physics in Nursing, pp. 22–27, "Scalar versus Vector Quantities—Equilibrium," St. Louis, Mosby, 1948.

Funsten and Calderwood: Orthopedic Nursing, 2d ed., St. Louis, Mosby, 1949.
Knocke and Knocke: Orthopaedic Nursing, Philadelphia, Davis, 1951.
Newton, Kathleen: Geriatric Nursing, pp. 17–127, 361–370, St. Louis, Mosby, 1950.

Questions Relating to the Patient Study

1. Satisfactory methods which might be employed in the home to immobilize a fracture such as Mrs. Holland sustained are

   a._____first to straighten the limb by grasping the foot and heel and moving it gently into a normal position; while someone holds the foot with moderate traction, another can tie the trunk and involved leg to a long wooden lateral splint; another long splint can be slipped under the patient.

   b._____with sufficient help, to move her to a bed so that she lies in exactly the same position as she was found; when transferred to the stretcher prior to her trip to the hospital, the same technic will be followed.

   c._____to straighten the involved limb gently; while one person is maintaining traction, another may tie the legs together; the patient must be moved carefully in one piece; the good leg acts as a splint for the injured one.

2. The purpose of emergency traction is to

   a._____reduce the fracture.

   b._____prevent further injury to the soft parts.

   c._____reduce pain and shock to the patient.

   d._____prevent the patient from moving an injured part.

   e._____maintain muscle tonus by keeping it contracted.

3. Forgetting that he was using a term which Mrs. Holland did not know, Dr. Silver asked her to "pronate" her arm. The nurse's explanation would be:

   a._____"Move your arm straight out to the side."

   b._____"Bring your arm back to your side."

   c._____"Turn your forearm so as to bring the palm forward."

   d._____"Turn your forearm so as to bring the back of the hand forward."

4. Compound benzoin tincture is often used before applying skin traction to

   a._____lessen the incidence of skin irritation.

   b._____present a more adhesive surface.

   c._____act as a depilatory.

   d._____prevent the growth of hair.

   e._____serve as a disinfectant for the skin.

5. During the time Mrs. Holland had Buck's extension, she frequently slid down toward the foot end of the bed. Possible causes which should be investigated are that

    a._____skin in the older aged person is more sensitive; hence there is a danger of necrosis owing to pressure of skin traction tapes. Mrs. Holland may have been trying to relieve such pressure and altered her position.

    b._____the weights might be too heavy for her size; the nurse has the right in such a situation to remove some of the weights.

    c._____countertraction may not have been adequate; the use of 6-inch blocks under the head of the bed should be tried.

    d._____the knee may not have been flexed sufficiently; a stiff pillow or several rolled towels placed under the knees and kept there may alleviate the problem.

6. Bed sideboards are often used for older patients. Are they desirable? (Check the best answer or answers).

    a._____No, because an older patient tends to resent being inhibited. He feels he is being treated like a child.

    b._____No, because a patient who is in traction already has a reminder that he must remain in bed.

    c._____Yes, because in many hospitals they are required legally. The nurse would be violating a law if she eliminated them.

    d._____Yes, because they offer a means of support in shifting from one position to another.

    e._____Yes, because they serve as a reminder to an elderly patient that he is to remain in bed. This is especially true at night when he may be half asleep.

7. One of the chief responsibilities of the nurse in her care of bed patients is to prevent contractures. A contracture is

    a._____an exostosis of a joint.

    b._____the formation of callus between two bones.

    c._____the foreshortening of a group of muscles.

    d._____the stretching of a tendon beyond its capability.

8. Some nursing measures which are helpful in preventing contractures are

    a._____place the patient in proper body alignment and encourage him to stay in this position without moving.

    b._____put all unaffected joints through a full range of motion at least once daily.

    c._____since the knees are most comfortable in a slightly flexed position, maintain this position regardless of what general position the patient assumes.

    d._____the foot need not be maintained at a 90° angle to the leg because ordinarily, when one sleeps, a dorsiflexion occurs; overcorrection is often more hazardous than under-correction.

9. In caring for a patient with a fractured femur in traction, the nurse should

a._____turn the patient frequently to avoid chest and vascular complications.

b._____move the patient in the line of traction.

c._____supply counter-traction by raising the head of the bed.

d._____remove weights only when changing sheets.

e._____see that the spreader is in contact with the foot of the bed.

10. In caring for Mrs. Holland's skin the nurse must consider the patient's age. This would mean that in Mrs. Holland's case

a. she should be bathed with soap and water

(1)_____more frequently than average patients.

(2)_____less frequently than average patients.

b. massage of pressure areas should be

(1)_____frequent and vigorous.

(2)_____frequent and gentle.

(3)_____infrequent and gentle.

(4)_____infrequent and vigorous.

c. the best preparation for a backrub would be

(1)_____oil or cream.

(2)_____alcohol.

(3)_____talcum powder.

11. If Mrs. Holland is typical of her age group you would expect that she

a. recalls distant events in time

(1)_____more readily than recent events.

(2)_____less readily than recent events.

b. welcomes changes in her routine, regular diet, etc.

(1)_____less readily than younger patients.

(2)_____more readily than younger patients.

Questions Relating to Fractures in General

1. Skeletal traction can be brought about by

a._____Buck's traction.

b._____Steinmann pin.

c._____Crutchfield tongs.

d._____Bryant's extension.

e._____Russell's extension.

f._____Kirschner wire.

2. Russell traction is an example of the use of two traction forces to secure a desired resultant. Characteristic features of this type of traction are as follows:

a._____there are 3 pulleys operating in this system and all are freely movable.

b._____the traction force exerted on the sling under the knee is double the original weight applied.

    c._____traction is exerted in the long axis of the tibia by two parallel ropes which double the original amount of weight applied.

    d._____the resultant of the two forces is in the long axis of the femur and is more than three times the original weight.

3. Important nursing points to follow in caring for a patient in Russell's traction are

    a._____the thigh and the calf of the involved leg should be freely suspended; supporting pillows must not be used because of interference with traction.

    b._____the heel of the foot in traction should just clear the bed; provision should be made to prevent dorsiflexion.

    c._____it is very important that the patient does not shift his position for the various angles of this system must be maintained.

    d._____sponge rubber or other soft padding should be placed in the knee sling for comfort and to prevent skin damage.

4. When an individual has a fracture or injury of an extremity, his clothes are removed, first from the

    a._____uninjured side of his body, and then from the injured side.

    b._____injured side of his body, and then from the uninjured side.

5. Pott's fracture involves the

    a._____wrist.   c._____hip.

    b._____ankle.   d._____spine.

6. A complication which should be watched for within 24 hours in a patient who has a diagnosis of fractured ribs is

    a._____empyema.   d._____atelectasis.

    b._____bronchopleural fistula.   e._____emphysema.

    c._____esophagospasm.

7. In an elderly person, the most common fracture is

    a._____Colles'.   c._____of the neck of the femur.

    b._____Pott's.   d._____supracondylar fracture of femur.

8. When several pieces of broken bone protrude through the skin the fracture is a

    a._____compound greenstick.   c._____incomplete comminuted.

    b._____compound comminuted.   d._____simple greenstick.

9. Which of the following are correctly stated as principles of pulley systems?

    a._____Effort equals resistance multiplied by the number of ropes supporting the resistance.

    b._____A single pulley transmits the exact force of the weight applied, the pulley merely changing the direction of the force.

    c._____By using pulleys to double the number of ropes pulling on the limb, the traction force can be halved.

    d._____By doubling the number of ropes supporting the weight, the traction force can be doubled.

10. The Pott's and Colles' fractures usually are treated by the application of

    a._____Russell's traction.   d._____skeletal traction.

    b._____a Smith-Petersen nail.   e._____a cast.

    c._____a blade plate.

Questions for Discussion and Student Projects

A. Related to Patient Study

1. How could you help Mrs. Holland solve the following problems:
   a. She regarded the indwelling catheter for constant bladder irrigation as a source of irritation because it seemed to create a continual urge to void.
   b. With Buck's extension she often slid down in bed and the soles of her feet would then rest against the spreader, which in turn rested against the pulley wheel.
   c. She was told that she must drink 10 glasses of fluid a day. To her, this seemed like an enormous quantity of water.
   d. Because of her loose teeth, she found it difficult to chew many of the foods.
   e. She was sensitive about cleaning her own false teeth; consequently it was not done so frequently as it should have been.

2. When Mrs. Holland was allowed out of bed in a wheelchair, the physician asked that her involved leg be kept extended at the knee. Demonstrate, using a classmate as a patient, how you would get such a patient out of bed and into a wheelchair.

3. Mrs. Holland showed a tendency toward vascular problems. For what signs and symptoms should one be on the alert in view of this tendency, her age and her orthopedic problem? What emergency measures could be administered to minimize long-range effects in the event of such attacks?

4. Discuss the use of Dicumerol. What precautions are indicated in its use?

5. Discuss the relative advantages of homes for the aged versus keeping old people in their own homes. What is the cost of maintaining older people who do not live with their families?

6. Discuss the social-psychologic needs of older people. To what extent were Mrs. Holland's needs being met? How could her last years be made more satisfying?

7. Describe the nursing responsibility for a patient with a retention catheter and continuous drainage. What was the purpose of this treatment for Mrs. Holland? What was the purpose of gantrisin?

8. What other complications might have retarded Mrs. Holland's recovery? How could they be prevented?

B. Related to Fractures in General

1. Make a study of home accidents as follows:

    a. Of all fractures, what percentage occurs in the home?
    b. What is the incidence of fractures in those over 65 which occur at home?
    c. What are the three most common types of fractures which occur at home?
    d. What are the causative factors for fractures occurring in the home?
    e. Make a list of recommendations which would be applicable in most homes to prevent the high incidence of fractures?

2. Prepare a study of the histories of 10 to 20 patients in your hospital who have had fractures of the femur and are in the age group over 65.

    a. What types of repair were done?
    b. How long were they hospitalized?
    c. What complications resulted from their hospitalization?
    d. What was their condition upon discharge?
    e. What was the attitude of their immediate family toward post-hospital care?
    f. How was the cost of medical care met?

3. If a patient with a fractured femur is in a state of balanced traction, what effect would sliding down toward the foot of the bed have on the traction? Differentiate between vector and resultant forces using this situation.

4. Describe the advantages and disadvantages of the following types of fixation devices used in fracture of the femur:

    a. Smith-Petersen nail.   c. blade plate.
    b. Moore pins.   d. Neufeld nail.

Nursing Care of Patients with Other Orthopedic Disorders

References

Baily, J.: Care of the patient with a Taylor spine brace, Am. J. Nursing 44: 665, 1944.

Flitter, H.: An Introduction to Physics in Nursing, pp. 34–38, "Gravity— Center of Gravity," St. Louis, Mosby, 1948.

Grice, Williams and MacDonald: Talipes equinovarus, Am. J. Nursing 51: 707, 1951.

Miller, B. L.: Well-leg and well-hip splints, Am. J. Nursing 48:572, 1948.

Morrissey, A. B.: The nursing techniques in rehabilitation, Am. J. Nursing 49:545, 1949.

O'Brien, R. M.: Osteomyelitis, Am. J. Nursing 50:17, 1950.

Schaar, C. M.: The Stader-splint, Am. J. Nursing 44:215, 1944.

Westcott, F. H.: Oral chlorophyll fractions for body and breath deodorization, N.Y. State J. Med. **50**:698, 1950.

A. Bunion

Janet Tabor was admitted to the Orthopedic Ward with complaints of pain over the medial aspect of the right great toe, inability to find shoes that fit comfortably and tenderness and swelling over the localized area. She was scheduled for an excision of a hallux valgus.

1. Hallux valgus is

   a.____a plantar wart.   c.____a corn.
   b.____a bunion, (affecting   d.____a bone deformity.
       the soft tissues).

2. The most common cause of hallux valgus is

   a.____ill-fitting shoes.   c.____congenital deformity.
   b.____sudden trauma.   d.____osteomyelitis.

3. Complications postoperatively for which the nurse will have to be on guard are

   a.____footdrop.   c.____shock.
   b.____constriction of tissues   d.____hemorrhage.
       because of tight dress-
       ings.

B. Legg-Perthes' Disease

A 10-year-old Polish boy, Joe, was seen in the out-patient department. He had been well until a month ago when he began to limp; his limp tended to disappear and reappear. He complained of pain in the right hip and knee and it was noticed that he was unable to abduct or externally rotate his left leg. Roentgenograms show fragmentation of the femur. The diagnosis of Legg-Perthes' disease was made and Joe was placed in traction for 2 months. After that he was allowed up in a Thomas non-weight-bearing walking caliper. His mother was told how he could reduce his weight by proper dieting. After being instructed in the use of crutches, he was allowed to go home.

1. Legg-Perthes' disease is also known as

   a.____"coxa plana."   d.____Scheuermann's disease.
   b.____Osgood-Schlatter's dis-   e.____osteochondrosis.
       ease.
   c.____osteochondritis.

2. The age and sex group most commonly affected is

   a.____males, 5–10 years.   c.____females, 5–10 years.
   b.____males, 10–15 years.   d.____females, 10–15 years.

3. Legg-Perthes' disease is

a._____a progressive disease.
b._____a self-limiting disease (heals automatically).
c._____communicable.
d._____caused by tubercle bacilli.
e._____a condition thought to be caused by trauma.

4. Dietary adjustment for Joe should be to

a._____increase calcium intake.
b._____increase protein intake.
c._____increase carbohydrate intake.
d._____increase vitamin D concentrate intake.
e._____limit calcium intake.
f._____limit protein intake.
g._____limit carbohydrate intake.
h._____limit vitamin D concentrate intake.

C. Osteomalacia

1. Osteomalacia is a metabolic disease of adults related to the childhood disease of

a._____scurvy.
b._____cretinism.
c._____beriberi.
d._____rickets.

2. The most common deformities resulting from osteomalacia are

a._____kyphosis of the spine.
b._____outward protrusion of the acetabula of the pelvis.
c._____bowing of the tibiae and femora.
d._____scoliosis of the spine.

3. Foods which are most valuable in the treatment and prevention of osteomalacia are

a._____green, leafy vegetables.
b._____fish-liver oils.
c._____carrots and "yellow-colored" vegetables.
d._____cereals and wheat germ.
e._____eggs and cheese.

D. Postoperative Spinal Fusion

1. For a patient who has had a spinal fusion, the activity of the patient, insofar as his spine is concerned, is

a._____encouraged to prevent contractures of the muscles of the back.
b._____encouraged to prevent pulmonary and vascular complications.
c._____restricted to allow for the deposition of new bone cells in the fusion site.
d._____encouraged to stimulate the adequate functioning of the circulatory, nervous and muscular structures.
e._____restricted to prevent the development of infection in cases of tuberculosis of the spine.

2. When a spinal fusion patient is in a body cast and in a regular bed, which of the following methods should be followed to place him on a regulation bedpan?

    a._____With the patient in a side-lying position, place supporting pillows to the back, head, shoulders and thigh before he is turned carefully on to the pan.

    b._____Instruct the patient to bend his knees while he is lying on his back; with your left hand, depress the mattress before sliding the bedpan under with your right hand.

    c._____Ask your patient to bend his knees and place his feet so that they are flat on the mattress; ask him to elevate his body using the overhead trapeze; he can then gently lower himself onto the pan.

E. Osteomyelitis

1. Osteomyelitis is caused primarily by

    a._____staphylococcus.   c._____tubercle bacilli.
    b._____streptococcus.   d._____pneumococcus.

2. Patients who have osteomyelitis frequently have a history of

    a._____upper respiratory in-   c._____boils and abscesses.
           fections.   d._____impetigo.
    b._____dental caries.   e._____vascular disorders.

3. The necrotic bone found as a result of an osteomyelitis is known as

    a._____gangrene.   d._____involucrum.
    b._____slough.   e._____sequestrum.
    c._____gibbus.

4. Specific treatment for osteomyelitis is the

    a._____aspiration of any abscess which may form.
    b._____injection of saline into the cavity.
    c._____skin traction to prevent infection from spreading to adjoining bone.
    d._____prescribed activity to encourage good blood circulation.
    e._____administration of large doses of penicillin.

5. During the acute phase of osteomyelitis, the nurse may make her patient more comfortable by

    a._____giving him a complete admission bath since it is likely that he has been too ill at home for such care.

    b._____passive exercise to the involved joint; in this way an adequate blood supply to the site of infection can be assured.

    c._____supporting the joints nearest the involved area in slight flexion; this can be accomplished with pillows and pads.

    d._____bandaging the involved joint snugly with an Ace bandage or immobilizing the part with a splint.

F. Tuberculosis of the Bone

    1. Tuberculosis of bone is found most frequently in the

        a._____knee.   c._____ankle.
        b._____spine.   d._____hip.

    2. Positive diagnosis of tuberculosis of the bone in adults is made by

        a._____tuberculin test.   d._____roentgenogram.
        b._____sputum test.   e._____biopsy.
        c._____aspiration.

    3. Tuberculosis of the bone first involves the

        a._____diaphysis.
        b._____shaft side of the epiphyseal line.
        c._____joint side of the epiphyseal line.
        d._____shaft of the bone.

    4. Tuberculosis of the bone is characterized by

        a._____a rapid onset.   c._____an insidious onset.
        b._____no pathognomonic   d._____moderately rapid onset.
             signs.

    5. Greatest deformities occur when tuberculosis of the spine is in the

        a._____sacral spine.   c._____dorsal spine.
        b._____lumbar spine.   d._____cervical spine.

    6. Braces perform an essential part of rehabilitation in many orthopedic patients. Fundamentals of good care of patients with back braces and corsets are as follows:

        a._____supports or straps should be adjusted from the highest tapes downward.
        b._____supports or straps should be adjusted from the lowest tapes upward.
        c._____when a patient is ambulatory, a back brace or corset should be put on while the patient is standing as erect as possible.
        d._____when a patient wears a brace, he can turn from side to side with no potential danger since the brace will provide completely rigid support.

G. Patients in Casts

    1. Plaster of paris is

        a._____calcium sulfide.   d._____hydrated calcium gluco-
        b._____calcium oxide.   nate.
        c._____hydrated calcium sul- c._____calcium lactate.
            fate.

    2. A plaster cast which has been applied too tightly to an extremity will produce the following signs of arterial circulatory impairment:

        a._____pain, numbness, tingling, redness, swelling.

b.____cold, pallid-numbness, swelling.
c.____blotchiness, petechiae, tingling, itchiness.
d.____swelling, tiny water blisters, pallor, pain.

3. Pressure exerted on the peroneal nerve by a long-leg cast may result in

a.____dorsiflexion of the foot.   c.____adduction of the foot.
b.____abduction of the foot.   d.____inversion of the foot.

4. A spica is a cast which includes

a.____the foot and leg including the upper thigh.
b.____a leg cast with an extension for weight bearing.
c.____the trunk and no extremities.
d.____the trunk and one or more extremities.

5. When a plaster cast has been removed, the skin often appears to be caked with dry, scaly exudate. The most effective way to care for such skin is

a.____first, to gently scrape as much exudate away as is possible, using coarse gauze. Then scrub the part thoroughly with a soft brush, soap and water.
b.____to peel off the exudate as well as possible; follow this with a sponging of alcohol. Use a heat lamp to help in the drying and healing process.
c.____to apply mild soap or warm olive oil poultices; follow by gentle cleansing, exposure to air and moderate heat.

6. Turning a patient in a hip spica is done best by

a.____moving the patient to the side of the bed toward the uninvolved leg; turning him as one piece on the leg encased in plaster; giving adequate support to the uppermost leg which is encased.
b.____moving the patient to the side of the bed toward the leg encased in plaster, turning him as one piece on the leg not involved, giving adequate support to the uppermost leg which is encased.

7. A mild chemical which aids in softening a plaster cast when used along the proposed cutting line prior to cast removal is

a.____acetic acid.   d.____hydrogen peroxide.
b.____alcohol.   e.____zinc oxide.
c.____phenol.

8. In drying a plaster cast, points to remember are

a.____a radiant heat lamp used close to a cast is a quick and inexpensive method for drying a cast.
b.____a stream of moving air should be guarded against while a cast is drying for the patient is susceptible to chilling.

  c.____large body casts and spicas may take several days to dry thoroughly.

  d.____it is better not to turn a large cast until the uppermost side is thoroughly dry, otherwise cracking or breaking may occur.

9. When the motion at a joint is eliminated by fusing the articular surfaces of the bones which form the joint, the operation is called an

  a.____arthrodesis.   c.____arthroplasty.

  b.____ankylosis.   d.____arthrotomy.

10. The purpose(s) of the operation (question 9) is (are) to

  a.____stabilize an unstable flail joint, as in poliomyelitis.

  b.____eliminate painful motion, as in an osteoarthritic hip.

  c.____hasten the process of joint immobilization, as in arthritis.

  d.____provide good body alignment, as in congenital hip dislocation.

  e.____aid in the healing of disease, as in joint tuberculosis.

H. Congenital Hip Dislocation

1. A congenital dislocation of the hip

  a.____cannot be recognized at birth.

  b.____cannot be recognized until the child begins to walk.

  c.____can be recognized at birth by the presence of a broadened perineum.

  d.____can be recognized by an additional gluteal fold on the affected side.

2. Secondary changes in unreduced, congenital hips are

  a.____retroversion of the neck of the femur.

  b.____filling of the true acetabulum with bony tissue.

  c.____lengthening of the soft tissues connecting the pelvis and the thigh.

  d.____stretching of the hip-joint capsule.

  e.____flattening, irregularity, and delayed ossification of the femoral head.

3. When a dislocation is incomplete, the condition is referred to as a

  a.____sprain.   c.____internal derangement of
  b.____strain.   the joint.
              d.____subluxation.

4. Treatment for a congenital dislocation of the hip may be

  a.____a closed reduction by manipulation under anesthesia.

  b.____an adduction splint to maintain the reduction.

  c.____the construction of a shelf of bone at its superior margin.

  d.____a reconstruction of the femoral head by means of an inert plastic.

I. Clubfoot

1. A clubfoot is characterized by

   a.____adduction of the forefoot; versus position of the heel; equinus position of both the ankle and the forefoot.

   b.____abduction of the forefoot; versus position of the heel; equinus position of both the ankle and the forefoot.

   c.____adduction of the forefoot; valgus position of the heel; equinus position of both the ankle and the forefoot.

2. The cause of clubfoot is

   a.____still debatable.

   b.____a primary defect in the germ plasm.

   c.____an abnormal position *in utero.*

   d.____an insufficiency of calcium and phosphorus in fetal life.

3. The Denis-Browne splint used to correct congenital clubfoot can be described as a (an)

   a.____plaster cast which is wedged at intervals as the correction progresses.

   b.____pair of specially constructed shoes which are constructed to meet the problem of the individual patient.

   c.____apparatus in which the feet are strapped to footplates attached to a crossbar.

   d.____brace which is applied to the deformed foot only; a specially constructed shoe completes the splint.

4. The nurse may help the mother of a child with a clubfoot by giving the following advice:

   a.____Exercises which may be prescribed are best done after rather than before the child is fed.

   b.____If the foot is in a cast and circulation of the foot is impaired and she cannot contact the clinic or physician the mother should remove the cast.

   c.____When a Denis-Browne splint is used, it is imperative that the child's feet remain in the apparatus continuously.

   d.____The child should be restrained as much as possible in his activities so that full concentration of effort be made on the correction of the deformity.

J. Body Mechanics and Posture

1. In lifting an object from the floor, such as a suitcase, the best posture to maintain is to

   a.____separate the feet; stand close to the object; flex the hip, knee and ankle as the object is grasped.

   b.____stand away from the object; keep the feet close together; bend from the hips; keep the knees straight.

c._____stand facing the object; separate the feet; flex the hip, knee and ankle; grasp the object with both hands; lift, using the forearm muscles.

2. When seated, the weight of the body should be borne on the

a._____thighs.   c._____dorsal spine.
b._____ilium and thighs.   d._____ischia and thighs.

3. In moving or turning a patient, the following principles of good body mechanics should be observed by the nurse:

a._____The feet should be close together to give a better base of support.
b._____Bending from the hips with the knees straight is the most effective method.
c._____Knees and hips should be flexed sufficiently to bring the arms on a level with the part of the patient being moved.
d._____Lifting upward is more conservative of time and energy than moving an object horizontally.

4. A worn pair of shoes may serve as real evidence of the proper or improper bearing of weight. Normally, the following characteristics are true:

a._____Usually the heel is worn down slightly more on the outer side than in the direct mid-center.
b._____Usually the heel is worn down in the direct mid-center.
c._____The heel wears more rapidly than the sole.
d._____The heel and sole wear down fairly evenly.

5. Which of the following comments are true of "modern" shoes:

a._____Heelless or counterless shoes with a strap may be harmful because they do not furnish stability.
b._____"Loafers" and "ballets" without heels are recommended as an adolescent girl's shoe because the foot is placed in the most natural position.
c._____Wedge soles and platform heels have more eye appeal than sensible construction.
d._____Young girls can wear high heels all day without getting into difficulty because their muscular and bony structure is pliable.

6. In moving a paralyzed lower leg, the most acceptable method is to

a._____grasp the toes gently but firmly and move the leg to the desired position; in this way, footdrop is also prevented.
b._____cradle the heel in the palm of the hand while the other hand supports the leg beneath the knee.
c._____cradle the area of the tendon of Achilles in one hand while the other hand supports the leg beneath the thigh.
d._____grasp the anterior surface of the foot with one hand and the anterior aspect of the lower leg with the other.

Questions for Discussion and Student Projects

1. Every Easter contributions are sought for the National Society for Crippled Children and Adults by the sale of Easter seals.

   a. Describe the program of this society under the following headings: (1) health.   (2) welfare.   (3) education.   (4) recreation.
   b. Does this society have the support of any medical authority?
   c. Under what conditions, and how, could you secure assistance for one of your patients from this society?

2. Briefly trace the development of national legislation which has helped the orthopedically handicapped. Include

   a. state services.
   b. U.S. Children's Bureau.
   c. state registers of crippled children.
   d. surveys of crippled persons.
   e. rehabilitation.

3. What is being done in your community to employ the handicapped? Do you think that undesirable attitudes toward the physically handicapped still exists? What can be (is being) done about this?

4. What educational facilities should be provided for the orthopedically handicapped child who cannot attend regular classes? Are these facilities available in your community?

5. Demonstrate the various methods which can be used at home to keep a plaster cast clean.

6. Describe how you would teach a mother to protect a body cast on her child from developing odors and soiling, especially around the perineal area.

7. Discuss nursing measures which might be employed for the comfort of the patient on a Whitman frame, considering the following:

   a. maintaining warmth.
   b. maintaining comfort during eating.
   c. preventing eyestrain.
   d. maintaining comfort of the extremities.

8. Imagine that you have as a patient a little old lady of about 4'10" who continually slides down in bed from a Fowler's position. Demonstrate with a classmate how such a position can be maintained with adequate and comfortable support.

9. Meeting the psychologic needs of the handicapped is often a real problem. Discuss possible implications and solutions of the following problems:

   a. Johnny is over-protected by his parents; this manifestation may be due to genuine sympathy or to feelings of guilt or anxiety.
   b. Marilyn's parents have threatened to institutionalize her because of the excessive care, financial burden and social stigma attached to keeping her at home.
   c. The Martins, who are uninformed, ignorant and poorly educated, unwittingly are depriving young Jim of having the necessary medi-

cal care and attention. They look upon his physical impairment as punishment for evil and are determined to bear their burden without help from anyone.

10. Give 5 examples of situations in which you encouraged your patients to "help themselves" this past week. Analyze these examples as follows:

    a. Should you have helped them more?
    b. Was each able to accomplish the prescribed activity to the limit of his ability? Could he have done more?
    c. What was the attitude of the patient toward your suggestion? Could it have been improved? How?

11. Assume that you have a patient in a body cast and that he is to remain in his cast for several more weeks. The cast lining has become soiled and greasy. Describe how you would replace such a stockinet cast lining with the least discomfort to the patient.

12. Review the literature for the latest effective means of deodorizing drainage in osteomyelitis, considering

    a. deodorizing agents in plaster.
    b. charcoal and charcoal dust.
    c. systemic approach.

13. What instructions should be given to those who will take care of the cast patient at home?

    a.____verbal.   b.____demonstration.   c.____printed.

14. Describe how you would turn a patient from a hyperextension (Whitman) frame to a face-lying position in the bed. What precautions must be observed? Why?

15. Prepare a list of instructions which can be given to patients as a guide when they are discharged from the hospital with a brace. Include

    a. care of locks and joints.
    b. care of shoes.
    c. care of leather parts.
    d. care of screws.
    e. pressure areas.
    f. care of the brace when not worn.

16. The Stader splint allows for ambulatory convalescence with maximum use of the afflicted part. What is the current attitude toward this device?

17. Secure a Roger Anderson well-leg splint from your orthopedic department and describe the principles involved in reducing a fracture of the femur. What are the nursing problems involved? How can such a patient be turned safely in bed?

18. How may a knowledge of the center of gravity of the human body aid in conserving the energy of the nurse? Illustrate with several examples and give the principles of physics involved.

Section 9. Nursing Care of Patients with Neurologic Disorders*

STUDY SUGGESTIONS: Before beginning the study of this Section, the student will find it helpful to

A. Review
   1. Anatomy and physiology: the central nervous system, blood pressure.
   2. Nursing arts: care of the unconscious patient, lumbar puncture.
B. Study
   1. In medical nursing texts: diseases of the arteries, disorders of the nervous system.
   2. In pharmacology texts: drugs affecting the central nervous system, anticoagulants, drugs used in the treatment of epilepsy.
   3. In surgical nursing texts: surgery of the brain and spinal cord.
C. Read the additional References listed before attempting to answer the questions relating to each patient study.

THE ACCIDENT VICTIM

Background Review Questions

1. The motor area of the cerebrum which controls the muscles of the lower extremities can be identified as the

   a._____pre-Rolandic convolution, lower part.
   b._____pre-Rolandic convolution, upper part.
   c._____pre-Rolandic convolution, middle part.
   d._____post-Rolandic convolution, lower part.
   e._____post-Rolandic convolution, upper part.
   f._____post-Rolandic convolution, middle part.

2. The medulla oblongata is the

   a._____most vital part of the whole brain.
   b._____second most important part of the brain.
   c._____third most important part of the brain.

3. The function(s) of the medulla oblongata is (are) to

   a._____act as the nerve center for the control of respiration, blood pressure and the heart.
   b._____act as a bridge between the pons varolii and the midbrain.
   c._____harbor the centers for vomiting, sneezing and coughing.
   d._____control the function of co-ordinating muscles.

4. The formation and circulation of the cerebrospinal fluid may be traced

   a._____from blood plasma in the capillaries of the choroid plexuses → lateral ventricles → third and fourth ventricles → spinal canal → capillaries to the azygos vein and into the portal circulation.

* Other disorders of the nervous system are considered in the pediatric section.

211

b.____from blood plasma in the capillaries of the choroid plexuses →
lateral, third and fourth ventricles → subarachnoid space of
the cord and the brain → gradually absorbed by the venous
blood of the brain.

c.____from the choroid plexuses → lateral, third and fourth ventricles → subarachnoid space of the cord and the brain → gradually absorbed by the meninges.

5. The amount of cerebrospinal fluid in the average person is normally
about

a.____10–20 cc.   c.____50–80 cc.   e.____120–160 cc.
b.____20–50 cc.   d.____80–120 cc.

6. A neuron is made up of a cell body, a dendrite and an axon. There are
afferent, efferent and central neurons. Match the following:

a. afferent.   (1)____motor.
b. efferent.   (2)____sensory.
c. central.   (3)____connecting.
                            (4)____dendrites are short and multiple.
                            (5)____axons are single and long.
                            (6)____dendrites are long.

7. Check the statements which are true of neurons:

a.____An adult has the same number of neurons as he had at birth.
b.____Nerve cells can be replaced if they are destroyed.
c.____The passage of messages from an axon to a dendrite is possible;
passage in the opposite direction is impossible.
d.____Afferent neurons may be subdivided on a functional basis into
motor, secretory, accelerator or inhibitory.
e.____Accelerator neurons carry impulses which increase or speed
up activity in an organ which is already active; they do not
necessarily initiate activity.

8. Match the following areas of the brain with the correct function:

a. parietal lobe.   (1)____concerned with vision and the end station
b. temporal lobe.   for visual perception.
c. occipital lobe.   (2)____the principal region for the initiation of
d. frontal lobe.   motor function.
                      (3)____receives impressions of taste and smell.
                      (4)____concerned principally with personality
                           and behavior.
                      (5)____receives sensations from the opposite side
                           of body.

9. Match the following names of diagnostic roentgen-ray tests with the
correct description:

a. myelogram.   (1)____recording of the electrical activity of
b. arteriogram.   the brain on a graphic chart.
c. angiogram.   (2)____introduction of air or O_2 directly into
d. pneumo-encephal-   the lateral ventricles.
   ogram.   (3)____introduction of air or O_2 into the

e. ventriculogram.
f. electro-encephal-
   ogram.

subarachnoid space by lumbar or cisternal puncture.

(4)_____introduction of a radiopaque liquid into the blood vessels and/or the lymphatics.

(5)_____injection of a radiopaque substance into the internal carotid artery.

(6)_____introduction of a gas or radiopaque liquid into the subarachnoid space, lumbar or cysternal.

10. Match the following neurologic terms with the correct description:

a. aphasia.
b. agnosia.
c. apraxia.
d. ataxia.
e. aphonia.
f. agraphia.
g. dysphonia.
h. diplopia.
i. tonic.
j. clonic.
k. flaccid.

(1)_____loss of voice.
(2)_____inability to perform co-ordinated movements.
(3)_____double vision.
(4)_____inability to express ideas in writing.
(5)_____without tone.
(6)_____a persistent involuntary muscular contraction.
(7)_____difficulty in speech.
(8)_____inability to use an object properly in spite of knowing its name and function.
(9)_____rapidly alternating involuntary contraction and relaxation of a muscle in response to a sudden stretch.
(10)_____hoarseness.
(11)_____inability to recognize an object.

11. A common early symptom suggestive of an intracranial space-occupying lesion is papilledema.

a. This is

(1)_____a swelling of the optic nerve head.
(2)_____a dilatation of the pupil.
(3)_____increased intra-ocular fluid pressure.
(4)_____an edema of the oculomotor nerve.

b. It can be observed

(1)_____during a gross examination of the eye.
(2)_____by measuring eye pressure with a tonometer.
(3)_____with the aid of an ophthalmoscope.
(4)_____when the pupil is refracted.

12. When a tumor compresses the optic chiasm at its midpoint, an impaired type of vision results in

a._____bitemporal hemianopsia.
b._____homonymous hemianopsia.
c._____diplopia.
d._____Argyll Robertson pupil.

13. The impairment of vision which results (in question 12) can be described as follows:

    a._____light reflex is absent.
    b._____the individual sees "double."
    c._____blindness results in the two outer (lateral) halves of vision.
    d._____blindness results in the same lateral halves of vision.

14. Match the following types of brain tumors with the correct description:

    a. astrocytoma.
    b. glioblastoma multiforme.
    c. medulloblastoma.
    d. acoustic neuroma.
    e. pituitary.

    (1)_____malignant, occurs in the cerebellum (children); sensitive to roentgen-ray but the prognosis is poor; has a tendency to seed and spread.
    (2)_____benign, occurs in the cerebellum (children); can be completely removed; prognosis is good.
    (3)_____affects abnormal growth, menstrual flow; located near the optic nerve, hence may impair vision.
    (4)_____malignant; prognosis 6 months to 1 year.
    (5)_____benign; occurs in the cerebrum of adults; prognosis not good (2–5 years).

15. What percentage of all tumors of the body are brain tumors?

    a._____1 per cent.   d._____20 per cent.
    b._____5 per cent.   e._____35 per cent.
    c._____10 per cent.

16. Of all brain tumors, what is the incidence of cancerous (malignant) growths?

    a._____1 per cent.   c._____10 per cent.
    b._____5 per cent.   d._____20 per cent.

17. Heightened sensitivity of tissue without an objective cause is referred to as

    a._____hypesthesia.   c._____hyperesthesia.
    b._____analgesia.   d._____paresthesia.

18. In preparing a patient for a ventriculogram, the usual procedure is

    a._____the same as for any major surgery; that is, obtain operative permit, nothing P.O. after midnight if study is done in morning, evacuate rectum and bladder, shave the back of the head, administer preoperative medication.
    b._____much like any other roentgen-ray procedure; explain to the patient that he will have an injection of local anesthesia and a radiopaque dye in the roentgen-ray rooms; he should not eat or drink for 2 hours prior to his visit to the roentgen-ray rooms;

it is not necessary to have an enema but a sedative taken before the study is desirable.

19. Following a ventriculogram, the nurse's responsibility is to help the physician in preventing the development in her patient of

a.____respiratory collapse.   d.____decreased intracranial pres-
b.____opisthotonus.   sure.
c.____hydrocephalus.   e.____hemorrhage.

20. After an air-injection study (encephalogram, ventriculogram), it is important to encourage the patient to take fluids because

a.____blood volume is replaced in this way.
b.____absorption of air is hastened.
c.____production of spinal fluid is increased.
d.____increased intracranial pressure is prevented.
e.____the condition of shock is prevented.

21. Postoperatively, comfort of the ear can be maintained and pressure sores can be prevented by

a.____including the ear in the snug-fitting head dressing.
b.____placing a tightly made cotton doughnut over the ear.
c.____placing a small pad of cotton behind the pinna before a head-dressing bandage is applied.
d.____not turning the head of the patient on its side.

22. If a patient has had a large lateral brain tumor removed, lying on the operated side is

a.____recommended to facilitate drainage.
b.____desirable so that infection will not be allowed to spread to the unaffected side.
c.____contraindicated because of the possible shift of the brain to the resulting cavity.
d.____discouraged because drainage may seep through the dressings and infection may be introduced.

23. Match the following:

a. Bell's palsy.   (1)____upper arm type of brachial birth
b. Ménière's syndrome.   palsy.
c. bulbar palsy.   (2)____loss of ability to move the muscles
d. Erb's palsy.   of one side of the face.
e. tic douloureaux.   (3)____a condition affecting one or more
                                     branches of the trigeminal nerve.
                        (4)____disturbance of the peripheral ele-
                                     ments of the eighth nerve within
                                     the internal ear.
                        (5)____involvement of the ninth and the
                                     tenth cranial nerves.

24. When a person has had all branches of the trigeminal nerve severed, he needs the following instruction:

a.____Always wear dark glasses to protect the eye on the operated side since the corneal reflex is lost.

b.____Shave the involved side of the face carefully to avoid cutting the skin without your knowledge.

c.____Chew food on the uninvolved side of the mouth since otherwise you will not be able to taste it.

d.____Visit your dentist regularly for a cavity may develop on the operated side without toothache.

25. Aneurysms of the cerebral carotid arteries are a vital neurosurgical problem because the mortality rate is about 50 per cent with the first spontaneous subarachnoid hemorrhage. Those who survive have a high chance of succumbing during the next hemorrhage. Surgical treatment(s) which has (have) been done with some degree of success is (are)

a.____ligation of the common carotid artery in the neck.

b.____ligation of the innominate and the left common carotid arteries.

c.____clipping the vessel leading to and away from the aneurysm with metal clips.

d.____ligation of the jugular vessels in the neck.

26. Important principles of care for a patient with an aneurysm which should be practiced by the nurse are

a.____if his blood pressure is stable, to elevate the head of the bed 30 to 40° to facilitate venous drainage.

b.____if his blood pressure is low, 100 mm. systolic or less, to lower the head of the bed (Trendelenburg position) to prevent shock.

c.____if he develops a sudden sharp headache, to apply a hot-water bottle; meanwhile, to call the surgeon and describe the nature of the headache.

d.____to prevent the patient from straining himself on defecation; this is best accomplished by giving him a cleansing enema daily.

27. Inasmuch as angiography is an important diagnostic procedure for the patient with a possible aneurysm, the nurse must be acquainted with the following reactions which may be expected following the roentgenogram:

a.____petechiae occasionally develop on the face and neck.

b.____sore throat and some swallowing difficulties may occur.

c.____temporary hemiparesis may develop.

d.____nausea and vomiting often occur.

e.____not any of the above symptoms is expected.

THE ACCIDENT VICTIM—PATIENT STUDY

Imagine that, as you are walking toward the business section of your community, you suddenly become aware that an accident has occurred in the next block. Curiosity impels you to hurry toward the stopped trolley car, the traffic jam and the growing collection of people. It soon becomes apparent that a man is lying unconscious in the street. By the time you get near enough to evaluate the situation, the victim is being moved carefully to an ambulance.

Two hours later you are back in uniform and by coincidence a Mr. Boling, aged 45, has just been admitted to your ward with a diagnosis of fractured skull and minor injuries. He is unconscious and placed in a unit near the nurses' station.

In the admission room it was verified that he had multiple scalp lacerations, a simple linear fracture, and possible trauma to the brain (extent undetermined). He had skull roentgenograms and a transfusion of whole blood, which was still running on arrival to the ward.

The nurse was told to be on the alert for any evidence of returning consciousness, convulsions, pupillary changes and bleeding. She was to keep an accurate record of vital signs and to report immediately any signs of shock, respiratory difficulty or intracranial pressure.

For 24 hours, Mr. Boling had stable vital signs but remained unconscious. Then he began to show signs of restlessness and within an hour responded completely. He could not remember what had happened and was much surprised to discover that he was a patient in a hospital. His passing complaints were a headache, blurry vision and some nausea. He then lapsed into a state of drowsiness and had to be aroused periodically. The nurse noticed a Jacksonian convulsion of the right leg persisted for about a minute. She carefully described it in her notes and notified the surgeon.

On the second day, and for 3 days thereafter, Mr. Boling appeared symptomless except for a slight headache. He was allowed out of bed on the fourth day but was kept under close observation. He had had a neurologic examination and a lumbar-puncture test. Reflexes appeared normal, spinal pressure was 150 mm. and only a slight trace of blood was noted in the spinal fluid. On the fifth day, he complained of feeling dizzy. He showed an unsteadiness in his gait and seemed to have some speech difficulty. He asked the nurse, "Where am I?" and "Who are you?"

As the nurse was getting him back into bed, she noticed twitching movements of the muscles of his lower right leg which was followed by a generalized convulsion. This lasted only 30 seconds and following the attack Mr. Boling appeared conscious but somewhat dazed. The nurse noticed a dropping in the rate of pulse and respirations and dilatation of one pupil. She reported this to the surgeon who examined Mr. Boling and wrote orders for the patient to be prepared for surgery. Tentative diagnosis was hemorrhage plus a subdural hematoma. This was confirmed on the operating table where a blood cyst was evacuated and minor bleeding was controlled. He was returned to the division in good condition.

Postoperatively Mr. Boling progressed rather slowly at first. During the first 24 hours, he had two generalized convulsions and remained unconscious, except in response to painful stimuli. The third day postoperatively he responded and tried to speak. But the fifth day he could speak more clearly and in sentences. He insisted on holding his drinking glass and tube himself. Soon he was taking his own bath, climbing out of bed and settling himself into his chair.

Before his discharge, he was given a list of instructions which would acquaint him with untoward symptoms suggesting the need for further medical supervision and advice. These were reviewed with him by the nurse and the surgeon. He also received an appointment for his first follow-up visit in the out-patient department.

References

Carini, E., and Robinson, F.: Acute craniocerebral injuries, Am. J. Nursing 50:423, 1950.
DeGutierrex-Mahoney, C. G., and Carini Esta: Neurological and Neurosurgical Nursing, St. Louis, Mosby, 1949.
Norcross, MacDonald, and Sinclair: The nursing care of patients with brain injuries, Am. J. Nursing 45:259, 1945.

Questions Relating to the Patient Study

1. In a head injury the first concern of the neurosurgeon is to
   - a._____prevent hemorrhage from scalp lacerations.
   - b._____repair the fracture in the skull.
   - c.___determine the extent of brain damage.
   - d._____note whether speech is coherent.
   - e._____do a neurologic examination.

2. When Mr. Boling was brought into the admitting room, for which of the following conditions should he be treated first?
   - a.___oozing scalp lacerations.
   - b._____fractured skull.
   - c.___shock.
   - d._____fractured right leg.
   - e._____watery drainage from the ear.

3. The reason that the condition selected in question 2 should be treated first is that this condition would lead to
   - a._____hemorrhage.
   - b._____embolus formation.
   - c._____brain injury.
   - d._____infection.
   - e.___anoxia.

4. The length of time a patient remains unconscious is usually directly proportional to the extent of injury. Match the following:

Types of Injury	Description
a. concussion.	(1)_____rupture of the middle meningeal artery; within a course of hours, there may be lucid intervals and a state of drowsiness; surgery is imperative immediately.
b. contusion.	
c. subdural hematoma.	(2)_____unconscious for a considerable period; feeble pulse, shallow respirations; may be aroused but slips back to unconsciousness.
d. epidural hematoma.	(3)_____lesion produced is microscopic; mild symptoms; perhaps dizziness, spots before the eyes.

5. Head injuries may affect the function of certain cranial nerves. Match the following symptoms with the nerve which may be affected:

   a. the turning inward of an eye.   (1)_____first nerve.
   b. the drooping of a corner of   (2)_____third nerve.
      the mouth.   (3)_____sixth nerve.
   c. deafness.   (4)_____seventh nerve.
   d. inability to differentiate pro-   (5)_____eighth nerve.
      nounced odors.
   e. the losing of pupillary reflex.

6. A contrecoup injury of the head can be compared to a

   a._____rubber ball which hits a surface but bounces back to its original shape.
   b._____fresh egg which, when hit, cracks, and a part of the contents protrudes.
   c._____soft orange which, when dropped, shows injury produced on the side opposite the original impact.

Mr. Boling was unconscious for several days. The following are important aspects of care for which the nurse must plan:

A. Care of the Eyes

7. Periocular edema may be relieved most effectively and safely by applying

   a._____hot compresses.
   b._____cold compresses.
   c._____a pressure dressing.
   d._____compresses moistened with supersaturated magnesium sulfate.

8. A thin coating of petrolatum applied to the skin prior to treating with hot compresses is done to

   a._____hasten the process of conduction.
   b._____decrease the process of conduction.
   c._____hasten the process of evaporation.
   d._____prevent the process of evaporation.

9. When unconsciousness is due to an organic cause, the corneal reflex is often absent. To prevent the development of corneal ulcers, keratitis, etc., the nurse should

   a._____irrigate the eyes with a germicidal solution such as 1 per cent zephiran chloride.
   b._____swab the eyelashes carefully with sterile mineral oil to prevent the collection of dried secretions.
   c._____lift up the upper eyelid and gently pass a sterile cotton ball across the cornea to test for reflex action.
   d._____depress the lower eyelid and instill 2 gtts. of 5 per cent silver proteinate daily.
   e._____irrigate the eye until the exudate is removed and then insert 1 or 2 drops of sterile mineral oil.

B. Care of the Nose

10. Following a head injury, if bleeding is present or there is watery fluid drainage from the nose, the nurse's responsibility is to

a._____insert cotton tamponades snugly to act as compression dressings.
b._____place sterile cotton loosely in the nares and change when soiled.
c._____swab the nostril gently with an applicator which has been dipped in mineral oil.
d._____swab the nostril and apply gentle pressure with an applicator which has been dipped in adrenalin.

C. Care of the skin

11. Because the blood supply to the skin may be poor, tissue repair may be inadequate. Measures which may be initiated by the nurse are to

a._____apply lanolin daily to the hands and the feet to prevent a deficiency of cutaneous oils.
b._____apply hot-water bottles to the extremities to insure an adequate peripheral blood supply.
c._____refrain from changing linen slightly moist with perspiration to aid in the maintenance of normal body temperature.
d._____place the patient in the sun or to secure permission for the use of an ultraviolet lamp.

D. Care of the Mouth

12. Frequently the unconscious patient is a mouth breather. When this is true the nurse should

a._____allow dentures to remain in the mouth in order to retain normal contour.
b._____swab the lips with alcohol several times a day to prevent fever blisters and subsequent infection.
c._____aspirate secretions in the oro-/and nasopharynx with suction (not exceeding 5 lb./sq. in.), using a soft rubber catheter.
d._____swab the mouth with full-strength hydrogen peroxide to remove thick mucus.

E. Position and Posture

13. The patient should spend most of his time

a._____on his back, for it is in this position that the organs of the body function best.
b._____lying on the side, for this facilitates the circulation of oxygen through the lungs and lessens the danger of obstruction of the airway.

14. For proper placement of the patient on his side, place a small firm pillow under his head, support the upper extremity on a doubled pillow;

a._____the upper leg, flexed at the knee at a right angle to the hip, is supported from knee to foot on a large pillow; the foot is kept in dorsiflexion; the back is straight and the lower leg is hyper-extended.

    b._____the upper leg is hyperextended with the foot supported at a right angle to the leg; the lower leg is flexed at the knee at a right angle to the hip; from knee to foot this leg is supported on a large firm rubber-covered pillow; the back is straight.

15. In caring for a patient during a convulsion, the nurse should

    a._____try to keep the head of the patient elevated to prevent asphyxiation.

    b._____insert a padded tongue depressor between his front teeth.

    c._____insert a padded tongue depressor between his side and back teeth.

    d._____do nothing for the patient since a seizure must run its normal course.

    e._____prevent his injuring himself by getting him into a recumbent position, loosening tight clothing, etc.

    f._____slap his face since this sudden stimulus usually brings the victim to consciousness.

    g._____note the march of symptoms, such as where the movements start, stop, etc.

16. Match the following descriptions of state of consciousness with the correct term:

    a._____stupor.   (1)_____can be aroused by simple address.
    b._____coma.   (2)_____can be aroused only with unpleasant stim-
    c._____drowsy.   uli, loud speech, shaking, etc.
                         (3)_____cannot be aroused.

17. The sense of awareness of environment which leaves the patient last is

    a._____seeing.   b._____touching.   c._____smelling.   d._____hearing.

18. Early symptoms indicating an I.I.P. (increasing intracranial pressure) which the nurse should report immediately are

    a._____marked irregularity in the pulse, respirations and/or blood pressure.

    b._____dilatation of both pupils simultaneously.

    c._____apathy which then changes to restlessness and marked irritability.

    d._____increasing pulse pressure.

    e._____cold and clammy skin noted in the extremities only.

19. Often, indisputable evidence of increasing intracranial pressure is a lowering of pulse and respiration and a rise of blood pressure.

    a. The reason for the lowered pulse and respiration is

        (1)_____pressure in the medulla from edema, hemorrhage.

        (2)_____constriction of the peripheral vascular system due to shock.

(3)____pressure on the medulla from its herniation.

(4)____inadequate oxygen-carbon dioxide exchange in the lung alveoli due to limited air intake.

b. Increase in blood pressure is due probably to

(1)____collapse of the peripheral vascular system.

(2)____a compensatory rise in an effort to re-establish normal medullary circulation.

(3)____an emotional strain brought on by the accident and other related conditions.

(4)____a re-stimulation of nerves which parallel the circulatory system and which were "stunned" during the accident.

20. Increased intracranial pressure due to edema following a fracture of the skull can be relieved by

a.____drilling occipital burr holes and inserting ventricular needles for tapping the ventricles.

b.____injecting 50 per cent glucose intravenously.

c.____injecting supersaturated magnesium sulfate.

d.____placing the patient in Trendelenburg position.

21. The pulse pressure important to observe during an increase of intracranial pressure is the

a.____difference between the systolic and diastolic pressure.

b.____perceptible intensity of pressure one feels when counting the pulse at the wrist.

c.____systolic reading as recorded by the sphygmomanometer.

d.____difference between the usual pulse of the patient under normal conditions and the present pulse rate.

22. The sedative which should never be given to a patient showing signs of increased intracranial pressure is

a.____codeine sulfate.   d.____morphine sulfate.

b.____Demerol.   e.____hyoscine hydrobromide.

c.____barbiturates.

23. The reasons for not giving this particular sedative in I.I.P. (see question 22) is that

a.____pressure will be increased rather than decreased.

b.____the rate at which pressure is decreased is rapid, therefore it is hazardous.

c.____the function of the medulla oblongata is stimulated.

d.____it often establishes a state of euphoria which is not easily given up later.

e.____pupillary changes needed for diagnosis are disguised.

24. The action of caffeine sodium benzoate which assists in the reduction of I.I.P. is

a.____stimulation of the respiratory center in the medulla.

b.____increased strength of cardiac contraction.

    c._____stimulation of the kidneys to produce diuresis.
    d._____stimulation of the central nervous system.

25. In attempts to relieve I.I.P., a lumbar puncture is

    a._____recommended, because it is easy to do and effective in withdrawing excess fluid.
    b._____preferred, because this equipment is usually always available.
    c._____contraindicated, for the medulla may be embarrassed as it is drawn downward into the foramen magnum.
    d._____not desirable, for the amount of fluid thus obtained does not affect appreciably the increased fluid in the ventricles.

26. Mr. Boling's symptoms suggest that he is going into shock at any time. The nurse should call the physician and immediately

    a._____place the patient in Trendelenburg position.
    b._____place hot-water bottles next to his body.
    c._____prepare for transfusion or infusion.
    d._____add one or two cotton blankets to his bed clothing.

27. A brain cannula (ventricular tap needle) which should be sterile and at the bedside of every patient who has a head injury or lesion has the following characteristics:

    a._____blunt tip.   d._____multiholed.
    b._____sharp bevel edge.   e._____equipped with stylet.
    c._____single opening.   f._____no stylet.

28. For hyperthermia in the patient who has had cerebral surgery or injury, often the nurse is requested to give alcohol sponges. Acceptable procedure is to

    a._____concentrate on those areas where most blood vessels come near the surface, such as the axilla, groin, etc.
    b._____concentrate only on those portions of the body which are warm.
    c._____sponge the entire body in a routine manner including those portions which are warm or cold.

29. The reason(s) why body temperature may be reduced following an alcohol sponge is (are) that

    a._____small areas of the body are wet at one time; the effect is more concentrated.
    b._____alcohol has a much lower freezing temperature than water.
    c._____by rapid evaporation from the skin, the effect is cooling.
    d._____by its astringent action, alcohol causes a contraction of tissue.

30. When a rectal-tap of ice water is used in patients whose temperature is over 102.5°F., the following technic is employed:

    a._____add a glass of cracked ice to half a glass of cold water, using a number 22–24 F. catheter and funnel; administer the fluid rectally and allow it to be retained for about 15 minutes; siphon.

b._____fill a liter enema can with cracked ice and add water until the ice is melted; administer the solution slowly via a No. 30 rectal tube (taking about 30 minutes for 1,000 cc. of fluid).

c._____take a rectal temperature 30 minutes after treatment.

d._____rectal temperature may not be taken for 2 hours after treatment.

31. Occasionally an aspirin enema is ordered to reduce an elevated temperature. This is administered as follows:

a._____crush the tablets, add to 1000 cc. of tap water and administer the same as a cleansing enema.

b._____crush the tablets, dissolve in 75 cc. of hot water; add about 75 cc. of cold water; check temperature of the solution and administer as a retention enema.

c._____deposit the aspirin tablets in the rectum just as one inserts rectal suppositories; follow in 10 minutes with a regular tap-water enema.

d._____instruct the patient to take the aspirin by mouth; within a half hour, give him a 1,000 cc. tap-water enema.

32. In comparing an axillary temperature with a mouth or rectal temperature, we find that the axillary temperature is

a. one degree higher than   (1)_____mouth temperature.
b. one degree lower than   (2)_____rectal temperature.
c. the same as
d. two degrees higher than
e. two degrees lower than

33. Severe headache following brain surgery may be treated with most sedatives except morphine because morphine

a._____is a respiratory depressant.
b._____masks pupillary changes.
c._____is habit-forming.
d._____may provoke nausea and vomiting.
e._____may increase intracranial pressure.

34. The bandage turn most satisfactory for head bandaging is

a._____spiral.   d._____recurrent.
b._____figure-of-8.   e._____circular.
c._____spica.

Questions for Discussion and Student Projects

1. Discuss the medico-legal implications facing the nurse who witnesses an accident such as Mr. Boling's. Should she have a right to administer first aid to such a victim at the place of the accident before the police arrive? When is it advisable to move such a patient from the point of view of

    a. his safety.
    b. fulfilling legal requirements.
    c. eliminating traffic congestion.

2. What is the practice in your hospital with regard to the use of restraints on senile patients, neurosurgical patients, etc.? Is this a wise policy? Substantiate.

3. Is the basal metabolism requirement of 1,700 calories sufficient to meet the daily needs of an unconscious patient? If this figure should be modified, what factors have influenced the change?

4. Make a study of two unconscious patients in your division as follows: Record the daily nutritional intake of your patients for 4 days, showing the daily caloric intake as well as the daily intake of the various food elements (CHO, vitamins, etc.). Are your patients receiving their basic requirements? Comment. If not, what can be done about it?

5. Devise a plan of care for an unconscious patient that is time-saving and effective in preventing skin irritation and decubiti of the sacrum under the following conditions: The patient is incontinent of feces and urine. The surgeon is undesirous of having the patient catheterized or equipped with an indwelling catheter because of a known cystitis. The patient is allergic to the antibiotic drugs.

6. Prepare a 12-hour-day schedule of the convalescent care of a 16-year-old boy with a head injury. He may be ambulatory but has asphasia, loss of memory, and personality changes. His attitude varies from that of co-operation to that of belligerency. He is very willing to help with ward activities but must be supervised constantly. He has aroused antagonism in most of the other patients as he constantly takes articles from their bedside stands.

7. What is the incidence of epilepsy following head injury? How can this be anticipated and prevented?

8. To what extent has the incidence of head injuries increased in the past 20 years (approximately) as a result of increased hazards in industry, war and travel (automobile and airplane)? What is being done to decrease this incidence? What group or groups have programs for this purpose?

THE OLD GENTLEMAN WITH THE STROKE

Background Review Questions

1. Arteriosclerosis is described best as
    a._____a degenerative process producing loss of elasticity and thickening and hardening of the arteries.
    b._____a chronic increase in blood pressure of unknown origin.
    c._____essential hypertension.
    d._____hypertension due to renal insufficiency.

2. Recent research indicates that a possible factor in arteriosclerosis is
    a._____excessive protein intake.
    b._____disturbance of cholesterol metabolism.
    c._____vitamin deficiency.
    d._____disturbance of calcium metabolism.

3. In arteriosclerosis it is thought that arterial lesions are produced by

a._____excessive blood sugar.   d._____excessive blood urea.
b._____excessive blood nitrogen.   e._____excess blood lipids.
c._____excessive blood calcium.

4. Arteriosclerosis of the senile type is primarily

a._____necrosis of the muscular coat.
b._____necrosis of the media.
c._____calcificaction of the muscular coat.
d._____calcification of the media.
e._____calcification of the intima.

5. In arteriosclerosis the inner coat thickens and muscular media may atrophy. This results in

a._____narrowing of the lumen.   d._____phlebitis.
b._____dilation of the lumen.   e._____rupture of the smaller ar-
c._____closure of thrombosis.   teries.

6. Cerebral accident is the result of

a._____disease of the cranial nerves.
b._____disease of the cerebral artery.
c._____disease of the motor areas.
d._____erosion of the venous sinus.
e._____erosion of the choroid plexus.

7. Hemorrhage most often occurs in the

a._____internal carotid artery.
b._____middle vertebral artery.
c._____middle cerebral artery.
d._____fourth ventricle.
e._____lateral ventricles.

8. The effect of hemorrhage on body temperature is to produce

a._____an increase.   b._____a decrease.   c._____no change.

9. If a patient suffers from damage to the right internal capsule, he probably will exhibit inability to

a._____perceive light touch or discriminate between warmth and coolness on the left side of the body.
b._____perceive light touch or discriminate between warmth and coolness on the right side of the body.
c._____identify the position of his head in space, with his eyes closed.
d._____locate and identify sounds coming from the right side of his body.

10. The patient with a damaged corpus striatum will exhibit symptoms of

a._____true flaccid paralysis.
b._____marked rigidity of his muscles.

    c._____nystagmus.

    d._____loss of equilibrium.

11. If, during the course of a physical examination, the doctor determines that the patient has a positive Romberg, this means that the patient

    a._____exhibits fanning dorsiflexion of the toes when the sole of the foot is slightly stroked.

    b._____"overshoots" when trying to touch his nose with his finger when his eyes are closed.

    c._____exhibits no abnormal reflexes.

    d._____sways and cannot keep his balance when standing with his eyes closed.

12. The Babinski reflex is positive when there is damage to the

    a._____primary neuron of the vestibulospinal tract.

    b._____ventral horn cells.

    c._____cells of the spinothalamic tract.

    d._____first neuron of the pyramidal tract.

13. If a patient has a positive Babinski reflex, he will

    a._____be unable to stand erect with his eyes closed.

    b._____exhibit fanning and dorsiflexion of the toes following stroking of the sole of the foot.

    c._____exhibit plantar flexion of the toes following stroking of the sole of the foot.

    d._____"over-shoot" when attempting to touch the heel of one foot to the knee of the other leg.

14. Conscious recognition of the location and the position of one's extremities, head, etc., in space is interpreted by the

    a._____somesthetic area of the cerebral cortex.

    b._____motor area of the cerebral cortex.

    c._____pre-motor area of the cerebral cortex.

    d._____temporal lobe of the cerebral cortex.

15. If a patient had a tumor growing within the occipital lobe of the cerebrum, you could expect that he might have

    a._____impairment of his hearing.

    b._____loss of temperature discrimination.

    c._____impairment of his vision.

    d._____muscular rigidity.

16. The primary symptom of damage to any part of the extrapyramidal system is

    a._____extensive flaccid paralysis of the affected muscles.

    b._____loss of ability to discriminate between fine degrees of difference in tactile sensations.

    c._____true paralysis and inability to initiate voluntary muscular acts.

    d._____some degree of muscular rigidity and in-co-ordination.

17. The cranial contents are encased within the rigid inelastic cranium. Because of this, a rise in cerebral venous blood pressure will result in

   a._____a fall in cerebrospinal-fluid pressure.
   b._____a rise in cerebrospinal-fluid pressure.
   c._____no change in cerebrospinal-fluid pressure.

18. The normal lumbar cerebrospinal-fluid pressure in a healthy adult lying in a horizontal position is from

   a._____80–110 mm. of water.   c._____140–160 mm. of water.
   b._____110–130 mm. of water.   d._____180–200 mm. of water.

19. Damage to the left internal capsule, such as frequently occurs in cerebrovascular accidents, may leave the patient with a

   a._____flaccid type of paralysis on the left side of his body.
   b._____spastic type of paralysis on the left side of his body.
   c._____spastic type of paralysis on the right side of his body.
   d._____flaccid type of paralysis on the right side of his body.

20. The symptoms of damage to the internal capsule described in question 19 involves the

   a._____cerebrospinal tract.   c._____rubrospinal tract.
   b._____spinothalamic tract.   d._____pyramidal tract.

21. If a patient, following a cerebrovascular accident, exhibited marked facial paralysis, difficulty in tasting food, and partial loss of sensation in the face on the affected side, the doctor would suspect damage to which cranial nerve?

   a._____trigeminal nerve.   c._____hypoglossal nerve.
   b._____oculomotor nerve.   d._____facial nerve.

22. An increased intracranial pressure, as in brain tumor or hemorrhage, frequently is accompanied by a projectile type of vomiting. This vomiting is due to

   a._____toxic substances produced by the nervous tissue in response to the pressure.
   b._____the creation of impulses in psychic centers which stimulate the vomiting center.
   c._____depletion of the body's glycogen store with resulting ketosis.
   d._____anoxia of the vomiting center due to compression of the cranial blood vessels.

23. If a patient has a cerebrovascular accident involving the internal capsule, which of the following symptoms would he most likely exhibit when he regains consciousness?

   a._____a positive Romberg with inability to determine the location of his hands or his fingers with his eyes closed.
   b._____a positive Babinski on the opposite side of the body and difficulty in discriminating between fine degrees of temperature.

    c._____a flaccid type of paralysis on the opposite side of the body, but no impairment of sensation of temperature or pain.

    d._____symptoms of "over-shooting" and a positive Romberg.

THE OLD GENTLEMAN WITH THE STROKE—PATIENT STUDY

Mr. Harris, a 64-year-old man, was brought to the hospital shortly after his wife found him having a convulsion at his home. On arrival at the hospital he was unconscious; his respirations were slow, deep and stertorous. The left side of his body was flaccid, and his mouth drooped on the left. Shortly after admission he had two more convulsions. His eyes showed conjugate deviation to the right.

Mrs. Harris told the physician that her husband had lived a busy life managing his small upholstering business. Lately he had been inclined to worry over business and she noticed that he had been confused, uncertain and forgetful, tiring readily. He seemed to lose interest in Christmas preparations and became over-emotional, crying easily and showing unusual fondness for her. On the morning of the accident he remarked that he felt tired and stayed in bed. Later he decided to take a bath and Mrs. Harris found him on the bathroom floor.

The admitting physician made a diagnosis of generalized arteriosclerosis with cerebrovascular accident. Mr. Harris was taken to the medical unit, with the following orders:

> Place on the danger list.
> Bed rest, crib sides.
> Nothing by mouth.
> Blood pressure, pulse and respirations every 2 hours for 2 days.
> Lumbar puncture.
> Hypodermoclysis, 750 cc. of normal saline.
>   750 cc. of 5 per cent glucose.

Mr. Harris was comatose for 2 days. When he began to respond he was given sips of water, and gradually the diet was increased from liquids to a soft diet.

After 2 weeks, he was able to move about the ward with a cane, although some paralysis remained in the left arm and leg.

At times he appeared delightfully euphoric and disoriented. At other times he would seem aware of his condition and attempt to conceal his difficulty and restlessness. At these times he would be worried and apprehensive, and chloral hydrate was ordered for restlessness. Mr. Harris was very weak and tired easily.

After 3 weeks the patient was discharged to a nursing home. Mrs. Harris is attempting to sell the upholstery shop to provide an income for his future care.

References

Dade, Lucy S.: Diversional activities for patients, Am. J. Nursing 47:384, 1947.

Flick, Stephan: Emotional effects of a long term illness on the family, Pub. Health Nursing 41:495, 1949.

Knocke, Lazelle: Role of the nurse in rehabilitation, Am. J. Nursing 47:238, 1947.

Lowman, Edward W.: Rehabilitation of the hemiplegic patient, J.A.M.A. **137**:431, 1948.

Manwell, Elizabeth: Three basic needs, Am. J. Nursing **40**:403, 1940.

Morissey, Alice B.: Psychosocial and spiritual factors in rehabilitation, Am. J. Nursing **50**:763, 1950.

Prochazka, Anne: Nursing care in hemiplegia, Am. J. Nursing **46**:118, 1946.

Rusk, Howard: Rehabilitation, J.A.M.A. **141**:282, 1949.

Questions Relating to the Patient Study

1. In Mr. Harris, the probable cause of the hemorrhage was

   a._____transitory epileptiform attack.

   b._____brain tumor.

   c._____rupture of a cerebral artery.

   d._____thrombosis of a small vessel.

   e._____extended aortic aneurysm.

2. The immediate cause of the convulsion was a rise in the blood pressure due to

   a._____acute apprehension.

   b._____sentimentality toward his wife.

   c._____unusual fatigue.

   d._____mental confusion, forgetfulness.

   e._____muscular exertion.

3. Increase in intracranial pressure usually is indicated by

   a._____slowing of the pulse and respirations and increase of the blood pressure.

   b._____increase of the pulse and respirations and decrease of the blood pressure.

   c._____slowing of the pulse and respirations and decrease of the blood pressure.

   d._____increase of the pulse, respirations and blood pressure.

4. During the period when convulsions are to be expected, the equipment at the bedside must include

   a._____an ampule of magnesium sulfate.

   b._____a can of ether.

   c._____a mouth gag.

   d._____restraints.

5. The optimum position for Mr. Harris would be with his head

   a._____lowered.   b._____level.   c._____elevated.

6. During the period of bed rest, it is important that the patient

   a._____be disturbed as little as possible.

   b._____have his position changed frequently.

   c._____have his position changed only if he seems uncomfortable.

7. Three specimens of Mr. Harris' spinal fluid are necessary in order to

   a.____determine the color.
   b.____determine the cell count.
   c.____determine the spinal pressure.

   d.____determine the presence of R.B.C.
   e.____determine the colloidal gold curve.

8. If Mr. Harris complained of headache immediately following the lumbar puncture, it would probably be due to

   a.____sudden rise in cerebrospinal-fluid pressure in the cranial subarachnoid space.
   b.____gradual fall in cerebrospinal-fluid pressure within the fourth ventricle.
   c.____gradual rise in cerebrospinal-fluid pressure within the lateral ventricles.
   d.____sudden fall in cerebrospinal-fluid pressure within the third ventricle.

9. When preparing a stomach tube for gavage, it should be brought to the bedside

   a.____dry.
   b.____well lubricated.
   c.____in a basin of warm water.

   d.____in a bowl of cracked ice.
   e.____in a basin of 2 per cent Lysol.

10. Mr. Harris' flaccid paralysis signifies

    a.____loss of reflexes and muscle tonus of the paralyzed part.
    b.____combined motor and sensory paralysis.
    c.____paralysis due to pressure during convulsions.
    d.____paralysis due to lesions of the spinal cord.
    e.____hyperactive reflexes and muscle tonus.

11. Mr. Harris' coma probably is caused by

    a.____compression of the brain from edema.
    b.____escaping lymph from the ventricles.
    c.____blocking of the venous return.
    d.____paralysis of the vital centers.
    e.____compression of the pons by posture.

12. Mr. Harris' paralysis affected

    a.____the same side as the brain lesion.
    b.____the side opposite that of the brain lesion.
    c.____both sides, irrespective of lesion.
    d.____alternate parts, irrespective of lesion.
    e.____the upper parts nearest the lesion.

13. In coma, Mr. Harris' respirations would be expected to be

    a.____orthopneic.
    b.____air hunger in type.
    c.____Cheyne-Stokes in type.

    d.____slow, deep, silent.
    e.____slow, deep, sonorous.

14. After several hours Mr. Harris' subnormal temperature changed with the onset of fever due to

    a._____the return of conscious-   d._____the onset of infection.
    ness.   e._____the onset of bronchopneu-
    b._____the development of hemi-   monia.
    plegia.
    c._____inflammatory reaction.

15. The usual dosage of chloral hydrate is

    a._____0.5–1 gr.   c._____2–5 gr.
    b._____1–2 gr.   d._____15–30 gr.

16. The desired action of chloral hydrate is

    a._____stimulant.   c._____analgesic.
    b._____hypnotic.   d._____tonic.

17. Toxic effects of over-dosage of chloral hydrate are

    a._____destruction of kidney tissue.
    b._____depression of vasomotor center and the heart.
    c._____delirium.
    d._____spasticity of the respiratory muscles.

Questions for Discussion and Student Projects

1. Of what specific significance are the changes in the temperature, pulse and blood pressure in cerebral accident?
2. Describe the supportive care of Mr. Harris, including the prevention of contractures and other complications. What special care of back and mouth is indicated?
3. List the foods to be included in a liquid diet during the period of semi-consciousness. What specific precautions are necessary when feeding Mr. Harris?
4. What considerations are necessary in making a daily nursing care plan for Mr. Harris on the second day of illness? On the fourth day? During convalescence?
5. Discuss the probability of the comatose or unconscious patient's awareness of activities around him? Can you tell if the patient hears voices? How should the workers speak in the patient's room?
6. List the equipment you would assemble for the physician to perform a neurologic examination.
7. List the equipment you would assemble for a lumbar puncture. Indicate which items should be sterile.
8. List the factors which might cause a second cerebrovascular accident. What activities should Mr. Harris avoid?
9. Where may Mrs. Harris secure help in meeting financial problems? In helping Mr. Harris regain function?
10. What is the cost of hospital care for Mr. Harris? What financial pro-

visions will be necessary for continued care? Whose responsibility
is this?

11. What resources are available in the community for the care of
chronically ill patients such as Mr. Harris?

12. What is the usual cost of care in nursing homes? Try to secure information about nursing homes in your community. How are the
standards of care regulated in your state? What facilities are available for chronically ill patients who are unable to afford private
nursing homes?

THE ALERT BOY SCOUTS

Background Review Questions

1. With reference to the spinal cord, the meninges terminate

  a.____at the same level.   d.____just below the first lumbar vertebra.
  b.____above the cord.   e.____just below the first thoracic vertebra.
  c.____below the cord.

2. The spinal cord usually ends in the spinal column

  a.____between the first and second lumbar vertebrae.
  b.____between the first and second thoracic vertebrae.
  c.____at the first sacral vertebrae.
  d.____between the third and fourth lumbar vertebrae.

3. The main function of the spinal cord is to act as a great conduction
pathway between the peripheral nerves and the

  a.____cranial nerves.   c.____autonomic nervous system.
  b.____cerebrum.   d.____portal system.

4. A lumbar-puncture needle is inserted in the

  a.____subdural space between the third and the fourth lumbar verte-
    brae.
  b.____subarachnoid space between the third and the fourth lumbar
    vertebrae.
  c.____spinal cord between the third and the fourth lumbar vertebrae.
  d.____subdural space between the first and the second lumbar verte-
    brae.
  e.____subarachnoid space between the first and the second lumbar
    vertebrae.

5. The sympathetic nervous system is the

  a.____craniosacral division of the autonomic nervous system.
  b.____thoracolumbar division of the autonomic nervous system.

6. The sympathetic nervous system controls

  a.____automatic activities in times of emotional stress.
  b.____the activities of the viscera.
  c.____the size of the blood vessels.
  d.____glandular secretion at ordinary times.
  e.____autonomic activities in times of great energy expenditure.

7. The primary purpose of a reflex is an action to bring about

   a._____conditioning.   d._____protection.
   b._____integration.   e._____oxidation.
   c._____interpretation.

8. The proper functioning of the diaphragm is dependent on the

   a._____vagus nerve.   d._____thoracodorsal nerve.
   b._____thoracic nerve.   e._____phrenic nerve.
   c._____supraclavicular nerve.

9. The nerve referred to in question 8 comes from the

   a._____first and second cervical spinal nerves.
   b._____third and fourth cervical spinal nerves.
   c._____seventh and eighth cervical spinal nerves.
   d._____first and second thoracic spinal nerves.
   e._____third and fourth thoracic spinal nerves.

10. Injury to the spinal cord above the level of the nerve in question 9 would result in

    a._____respiratory paralysis.
    b._____facial paralysis.
    c._____loss of sight and hearing.
    d._____loss of bladder control.

11. Reflexes such as the abdominal reflex, knee jerk, ankle jerk, etc., are tested by the neurosurgeon because they indicate

    a._____whether muscle has the proper tonus.
    b._____the adequacy of function of the different levels of the cord.
    c._____whether the thalamus is relaying efferent impulses adequately.
    d._____whether the hypothalamus is effective in integrating responses.

12. The significance of the brachial plexus is that

    a._____it is often used as a site for the injection of a local anesthetic when surgery on the hand or arm is indicated.
    b._____the nurse may accidentally injure this collection of nerves during an intramuscular injection into the deltoid.
    c._____it may be injured while the patient is lying in Trendelenburg position on the O.R. table if shoulder braces are not padded adequately.
    d._____if it is injured at birth or later, the condition of torticollis or wryneck results.

13. Below are listed 10 body activities controlled by the autonomic nervous system. If the activity is controlled primarily by the parasympathetic system, place a check mark in the column under that heading. If the activity is brought about through dominance of the sympathetic system, place a check mark in the column under that heading.

Parasympathetic Sympathetic

a. dilatation of the coronary arterioles.   _____   _____

b. increased secretion of the gastric digestive juice.   _____   _____

c. constriction of the pupil.   _____   _____

d. vasoconstriction of the splanchnic blood vessels.   _____   _____

e. increased intestinal motility.   _____   _____

f. vasoconstriction of the cutaneous blood vessels.   _____   _____

g. secretion of the sweat glands.   _____   _____

h. vasodilatation of the skeletal blood vessels.   _____   _____

i. dilatation of the bronchioles.   _____   _____

j. contraction of the bladder wall with relaxation of the trigonal sphincter.   _____   _____

THE ALERT BOY SCOUTS—PATIENT STUDY

Jimmie Dougherty, a 16-year-old well-developed and healthy boy, was delighted that senior exams were now over and that he could look forward to the Memorial Day weekend with no worries. He and several of the fellows planned to try a new swimming-hole which had developed out of an abandoned and caved-in mine.

The party reached their destination and the uninhibited spirits of the six lads remained high until Jimmie, who dove eagerly into the water, failed to "come up" as fast as he should. Sensing that something was wrong, his closest friend, Pete, swam out and soon was grasping for what appeared to be Jimmie's head. He dragged the boy to shore by his hair and wisely called the other fellows to help him get Jim out of the water as carefully as they could.

Fortunately, the boys were Scouts and had had some training in first aid. Jim, who recovered his breath, winced as he muttered, "My neck." He lapsed into unconsciousness before answering Pete's question, "Can you move your feet?"

Assured that he was breathing all right, Pete informed the frightened boys that they had better find something on which to place Jim so they could move him "in one piece." A plank about 18 inches wide and 6 feet long answered their purpose and Jim was placed on the board. They then placed the makeshift stretcher on the window frames of the old convertible sedan ready for a slow drive to the hospital 6 miles away.

The physician in the admitting room was impressed by the first aid measures practiced by the boys. It was apparent that Jim had sustained an injury of the lower cervical vertebrae when he dove into a shallow part of the pond. He was now conscious but could not move his legs or arms.

Jim was treated for shock, given a sedative and sent to the x-ray department while still immobilized on the wooden plank. Then he was moved to the operating room where, under local anesthesia, Crutchfield tongs were inserted. When he finally arrived on the ward, the Stryker frame was in readiness for him.

He was kept in traction for a week. During the early part of the week he had no motion in his upper or lower extremities. As hemorrhage and edema subsided, some motion began to return. It was thought that skeletal traction alone would reduce the possible fracture. However, as time went on, it became evident that a laminectomy had to be performed to remove the fragments of bone compressing the spinal cord. Following this operation, he was again placed on the Stryker frame. Jim's postoperative treatment was similar to that following the insertion of the tongs. An indwelling catheter was kept in place but it was removed within a week in an attempt to evaluate his bladder function. This began to return, as did increasing muscular activity of his extremities.

The prognosis was favorable, inasmuch as he had only mild cord and surrounding tissue damage. Skin care and psychotherapy were the chief problems. As function returned, his pessimism gradually began to turn to optimism. After 3 weeks he was moved to a regular bed and continued with active exercises under the direction of the physical therapist. Antibiotics reduced the probability of infection so that his recovery was not marred by untoward complications. Jim is a grateful lad who will need a tremendous amount of patience when he goes home so that he will not exceed his physical limitations.

References

Chandler, F. A.: Laminectomy, Am. J. Nursing 51:156, 1951.
Collins, E. M., and Solowinski, H.: Bedsores—their prevention and treatment, Am. J. Nursing 45:370, 1945.
Mella, M. R.: The mental rehabilitation of patients with spinal cord injuries, Am. J. Nursing 45:370, 1945.
Skinner, Geraldine: Head traction and the Stryker frame, Am. J. Nursing 52: 694, 1952.

Questions Relating to the Patient Study

1. Symptoms of spinal-cord injury for which one should watch at the place of the accident are

   a.____pain in the region of the neck; respiratory difficulty; muscle weakness; numbness of the extremities.

   b.____increasing intracranial pressure; headache; dilated pupils; clear, colorless discharge from the ears and the nose.

   c.____acute sensitivity of the extremities to slight stimulation; dizziness; blurry vision; nystagmus.

   d.____drop in pulse rate; warm, flushed skin; restlessness; apprehension; pain at the site of injury.

2. Symptoms suggesting a cervical vertebral injury are

   a.____inability to move the feet or the toes.

   b.____headache.

  c._____inability to open and close the fingers readily.
  d._____painful abdominal cramps.
  e._____shooting pains down one or both legs.
  f._____severe pain at the level of injury.

3. Emergency first-aid treatment for cervical injury includes:

  a._____If conscious, gently lift the patient's head and give him a stimulant to drink in order to prevent shock.
  b._____If the injured person is found in a twisted position, he must be moved to a stretcher by a sufficient number of persons so that he continues to maintain the position in which he was found.
  c._____A patient with a back or neck injury needs immediate medical attention; therefore, every effort should be made to rush him to a physician.
  d._____The most desirable position for a potential neck injury is the prone position with no pressure exerted on the straight back.
  e._____When sufficient help is available, the victim should be carefully placed on a flat surface in the supine position with no pillow but with a padded object placed on either side of the head for immobilization.

4. Morphine is not given to Jimmie because

  a._____the severity of the pain does not warrant such a strong sedative.
  b._____the action of the diaphragm and intercostals may be decreased.
  c._____pupillary changes may mask other significant symptoms.
  d._____the reflex center controlling vomiting may be stimulated; this would be undesirable.

5. Match the following: Fractures and dislocations at

Site	Result
a. C_1 and C_2	(1)_____phrenic nerve may be involved, causing death by respiratory paralysis.
b. C_3, 4 and 5	(2)_____almost always fatal.
c. C_6 and C_7	(3)_____some arm movement can be elicited.
	(4)_____motion in both arms is lost.

6. The Queckenstedt test is often done to determine the presence of an obstruction between

  a._____any two points along the vertebral column.
  b._____the medulla and the coccyx in the spinal cord.
  c._____the cranial cavity and the lumbar puncture needle in the subarachnoid space.
  d._____the highest cervical and the lowest lumbar vertebra.
  e._____the cerebral hemispheres.

7. In the Queckenstedt test

  a._____a radiopaque dye is injected into the cerebrospinal system via a cisternal puncture.

b._____air is injected into the spinal canal after a specific amount of spinal fluid has been tapped at the lumbar site.

c._____pressure is exerted against the jugular veins of the neck and manometric-pressure readings are taken at 10-second intervals until it is stabilized.

d._____dye is injected into the spinal canal through the third and fourth lumbar vertebral interspaces; the patient is then x-rayed.

8. A myelogram is often done to determine the extent of spinal-cord compression. This is a study in which

a._____a gas or radiopaque liquid is introduced into the subarachnoid, lumbar or cisternal space, for x-ray study.

b._____various measurements are taken of the thickness of the myelin sheath as it surrounds the spinal cord.

c._____a dye is introduced into the internal carotid artery in conjunction with special roentgenologic studies.

d._____several planes of roentgenograms are taken which serve to illustrate the progression or diminution of damage to the spinal cord.

9. Failure to keep the buttocks supported while the patient is lying on the posterior shell of the Stryker frame may result in

a._____lordosis.	c._____ankylosis.

b._____scoliosis.	d._____amblyopia.

10. The advantages of the Stryker frame over a regulation bed for a patient with a spinal injury are

a._____the patient may turn himself from prone to supine position and vice versa.

b._____pulmonary emboli, pneumonia and decubitus ulcers can be largely eradicated by proper use of the frame.

c._____Crutchfield-tong traction may be applied continuously before, during and after turning.

d._____the frame may be adjusted to assume the Trendelenburg, Fowler and semi-Fowler position.

11. Proper positioning of the knees and feet while the patient is on a Stryker frame is important for good body alignment. This can be accomplished by

a._____allowing the legs to be hyperextended; the placement of a roll under the knees is to be discouraged because of possible nerve pressure and injury.

b._____flexing the knees slightly; place a small towel roll under them; this position is much more relaxing and comfortable.

c._____keeping the feet at about a 30° angle to the leg; this is the natural position when one sleeps.

d._____keeping the feet at right angles to the legs; this is the correct alignment in the standing position.

12. Counter-traction during the use of Crutchfield tongs (or similar treatment) can be accomplished by
   a.____raising the foot of the bed.
   b.____raising the head of the bed.
   c.____instructing the patient to keep his chin as far from his neck as is possible.
   d.____applying skin traction and counter-weights to his legs.

13. The most important consideration in moving Jim is to prevent
   a.____jarring of the bed.
   b.____excoriation of the skin.
   c.____disturbing the dressing.
   d.____extension or flexion of the head.

14. As a postoperative complication Jim is most likely to experience
   a.____aphasia.
   b.____nausea and vomiting.
   c.____difficulty in voiding.
   d.____difficulty in swallowing.
   e.____dyspnea.

15. An approved method of applying external heat to Jim would be by means of
   a.____an electric pad.
   b.____a hot-water bottle.
   c.____a light cradle.
   d.____warm bath blankets.

16. When an air mattress is used to reduce pressure areas, the safest measure is to fill the mattress
   a.____to its capacity and check the air valve to insure "air tightness."
   b.____to less than its capacity to allow for resiliency.
   c.____minimally so that the sides are barely separated.

17. Advantages of a sawdust bed used to prevent body decubiti are
   a.____it is comfortable and economical because it saves linen and dressings.
   b.____it is porous and has deodorizing properties, especially if the wood is of beech or some similar wood.
   c.____the resins of the wood are germicidal in their action; hence a sawdust bed of pine is ideal.

18. Cotton doughnuts as an aid to preventing decubiti are
   a.____excellent, because they eliminate pressure to a localized area.
   b.____taboo, because they restrict blood supply to an area which needs it most.
   c.____economical, because they can be made easily and used over and over again.
   d.____desirable, because they have been tried and tested for years.
   e.____undesirable, because they are difficult to keep in position.

Questions for Discussion and Student Projects

1. What can be done to prevent neuroses or traumatic hysteria in a situation such as Jim's? What can the nurse do in her daily contacts with such a patient?

2. Suppose Jim had severed his cervical cord. What additional problems would have been presented?

3. Two problems which confront patients who have to wear Sayre chin halters (a leather fitted head-traction device) are that the male patient notices (1) irritation from the friction of a growing beard against the chin strap and (2) soreness of the muscles of mastication because of the interference of the strap during eating. What can be done to alleviate these problems?

4. What are the available resources in your community for the convalescent and chronic care of paraplegics? How are they financed? Are the facilities adequate for the needs?

5. How are paraplegic and quadriplegic patients rehabilitated in your hospital? What community resources are available to further their instruction and to place them in suitable forms of occupation?

6. Imagine that you are the wife or mother of a paraplegic who is about to return home from the hospital. List the conveniences you would try to have available for him. Try to improvise with equipment ordinarily found in a home.

7. Investigate the teaching program in schools in your community for the purpose of finding out what instruction is given to students in the prevention of accidents. Is it adequate? What more can be done?

8. Imagine that a member of your family has been injured in an automobile accident and has sustained a back injury. Demonstrate on a classmate how you would direct the lifting and moving of such a victim from a twisted position to one satisfactory for transportation.

9. What types of anesthesia are used for a patient who has a cervical injury? What factors must be taken into consideration? What restrictions or precautions in preoperative medications, if any, should the nurse be aware of?

10. What variations in the following would you expect as normal symptoms in a patient with spinal-cord injury? What deviations would you consider significant? Why?

a.____vital signs.

b.____motor and sensory functions of the extremities.

c.____color.

d.____state of consciousness.

e.____pain.

f.____bladder and bowel function.

g.____dressings.

h.____mental attitude.

11. What is meant by a "cord bladder"? An "automatic bladder"? Describe the Munro apparatus, including the way it operates and the nursing care involved in its use.

Background Review Questions—(*Continued*)

1. A rupture of an intervertebral disc is

a.____a punctured cartilage which exists between the vertebra and is the result of a fracture of one of the vertebra.

b.____the pinching of a segment of spinal cord between the bodies of two vertebrae due to trauma.

c._____a simple fracture of the spinous or transverse process of one of the vertebrae.

d._____a herniation of a part of the nucleus pulposus which may push against the dural sac or spinal nerve.

2. The causative factor(s) for a rupture of an intervertebral disc is (are)

a._____congenital weakness.

b._____secondary involvement following a history of primary infection.

c._____trauma which may or may not be recalled (remembered).

d._____tumor or bizarre tissue growth.

3. Ruptured intervertebral disc occurs most commonly in the

a._____cervical region.　　　　c._____high lumbar region.

b._____thoracic region.　　　　d._____lower lumbar region.

4. Symptoms of a ruptured intervertebral disc are

a._____pain in the lower back with radiation down the back of one leg to the foot.

b._____knifelike pain in the back with a moderate amount of respiratory embarrassment.

c._____pain in the subcostal region radiating around the back to the region of the scapula.

d._____pain in the back followed by nausea, vomiting and headache.

5. Often the treatment for a ruptured intervertebral disc is a neurosurgical operation. The following surgery is done:

a._____A small wedge of damaged spinal cord is removed; the remaining bundles are anastomosed for continuity.

b._____The damaged disc is removed through a small opening between the laminae of the vertebrae.

c._____Usually a fusion of the spine is done at the site of the greatest difficulty.

d._____Segments of spinal processes are removed; in this procedure the nerves are free from potential injury.

Questions for Discussion and Student Projects

1. What factors from the anatomy and physiology point of view are involved in the development of the following:

a. hydrocephalus. b. microcephalus. c. meningocele. d. encephalocele.

2. What observations and applications of nursing care must be made in caring for patients with the above problems in regard to

a. bowel and bladder control.

b. meeting nutritional needs.

c. motor and sensory function of the extremities.

d. maintaining optimal body posture.

e. care of the fontanelles.

f. general behavior and development.

g. special therapies for this problem.

3. What provisions are made in your hospital and/or community for the rehabilitation of postoperative neurosurgical patients who have some motor impairment and who, upon discharge from the hospital, are not prepared to be financially independent?
4. Why is the nearest relative usually asked to sign the operative permit of a neurosurgical patient?
5. What provisions are made in your hospital for the comfort of the patient's family during his long operative procedure?
6. List the principles involved in determining the proper position of the following types of postoperative neurosurgical patients:

   a. cerebellar craniectomy.   d. surgery for cerebral aneurysm.
   b. craniotomy.   e. laminectomy.
   c. surgery for tic douloureux.

7. List the many complications to which a patient with trigeminal neuralgia is susceptible. How can these be prevented?
8. Imagine that you are attending a popular theatrical production. You are seated in the middle of the playhouse. Soon after the curtain rises in the second act, a girl who is sitting next to you mutters something incoherently, slips forward in her seat and goes into a generalized convulsive seizure. Describe how you would direct the handling of this situation so that the safety of the victim is respected and a minimum number of persons in the audience are disturbed.
9. Occasionally a nurse has a patient with a diagnosis of brain tumor or head injury who demonstrates over-activity. This is manifested by his being seemingly tireless, physically over-active, mentally over-productive. emotionally unstable and demonstrating extreme self-confidence. Outline

   a. a "plan of approach" to this patient.
   b. aspects of nursing care.
      (1) insurance of adequate rest and sleep.
      (2) diversional therapy.
      (3) control of external environment.
      (4) keeping records.
      (5) protective therapy.
      (6) maintenance of bodily necessities, such as nutrition, elimination, etc.

10. Repeat the project of question 9 using the under-active patient as your subject. This patient, let us imagine, has offered assurance to you that he would never harm himself.
11. Suppose you have a patient who is recovering from brain surgery and is struggling with speech disturbances. Make a list of suggestions which would be helpful in caring for this person who has impairment of the comprehension, elaboration and expression of ideas.
12. "Death Be Not Proud"* is the story of a boy who died at the age of 17 following a 14-month illness. His diagnosis was a malignant brain

* By John Gunther, Harper & Brothers, 1949.

tumor for which he received every available treatment. After reading this book, discuss

  a. the manner in which the parents were prepared for the dismal prognosis.
  a. the morale and the accomplishments of the patient throughout.
  c. the reaction of the writer to the neurosurgeons and neurosurgery.
  d. the nature of the symptoms in the progression and regression of the tumor.
  e. whether the role of a nurse could have been more effective throughout? How?
  f. your reaction to the book as a whole.

THE YOUNG EPILEPTIC—PATIENT STUDY

Miss Evans, a 29-year-old nurse's aide, was admitted to the hospital from the medical clinic for observation and treatment. Her diagnosis was idiopathic epilepsy. Although she was admitted in a wheel chair, she did not seem acutely ill. Her adjustment to the enivronment was made easily and her responses were friendly and cheerful.

She related that at the age of 13 she had had measles; following this she had had a number of seizures which were diagnosed as idiopathic epilepsy. Phenobarbital gr. 2 daily was prescribed to control the attacks. This was quite effective and she had had no further difficulty until the past few months when she began to have recurring attacks.

Four months ago, in October, the attacks recurred following a series of unfortunate happenings. In March she was in an automobile accident and suffered fractures of the third and fourth lumbar vertebrae, necessitating a long hospitalization. Then, the mother had pneumonia and was ill for a long time. Finally, Miss Evans broke off with a man whom she had been dating for several years.

She said that her attacks last from 6 to 7 minutes and are preceded by nervousness, tightness in the muscles and faintness. This is followed by a loss of consciousness in which she writhes, kicks, and has facial contortions. There is complete amnesia of the seizure.

She complained of frequent afternoon headaches and poor appetite and has been troubled by constipation.

The medical program included:

  Regular diet.
  Fluid as desired.
  Luminal gr. ¼ 4 times a day.
  Sodium bromide gr. x 3 times a day.
  Aspirin gr. x every 2 hours p.r.n.
  Mineral oil ounces 1 and cascara drams 1, each night as necessary.
  Lumbar puncture.
  Roentgenogram of skull.
  Pneumo-encephalogram.
  Electro-encephalogram.

Miss Evans had 2 convulsions during hospitalization. They were both on the same evening one week after admission. Each lasted one minute. They were generalized, starting with a sharp outcry and spastic contractions of the arms and legs, the head was then thrown back, the hands clenched and the trunk twitched. At the end of the convulsion, the patient lapsed into a deep sleep from which she could not be aroused for two minutes. She finally responded and fell asleep again.

Miss Evans withstood the special diagnostic treatments well and seemed anxious to know the truth about her condition. She was given specific suggestions in relation to diet, medications, rest and activities. It was felt that if she engaged in an occupation that was not too taxing on her emotional and nervous disposition and followed a well-regulated health program, she might continue to live an independent and moderately useful life as long as there is no further mental deterioration. She was discharged after 3 weeks with orders for Dilantin gr. 1½ twice a day, limited fluids, well-balanced diet. She is to return to clinic if she has further attacks.

References

Caveness, W. A.: A survey of public attitudes toward epilepsy, Epilepsia 4:19, 1949.

Eley, R. Cannon: Encephalography, Am. J. Nursing 32:1013, 1932.

Kalkman, Marion E.: What the nurse should know about a neurological examination, Am. J. Nursing 36:1085, 1936.

Knocke, Lazelle: Role of the nurse in rehabilitation, Am. J. Nursing 47:238, 1947.

Lennox, W. G.: Marriage and children for epileptics, Human Fertil. 10:97, 1945.

————: Social therapy of epilepsy, Canad. Med. Assoc. J. 56:638, 1947.

————: The epileptic patient and the nurse, Am. J. Nursing 46:219, 1946.

Roseman, Ephraim, and Taylor, Anne: Progress in the treatment of epilepsy, Am. J. Nursing 52:437, 1952.

U.S. Congress, House Committee on Labor, Aid to physically handicapped, Part II, Epilepsy. Washington, D.C., U.S. Government Printing Office, 1945.

Questions Relating to the Patient Study

1. In column 1 (labeled Part I) check the items pertinent to the management and nursing care of Miss Evans during an epileptic convulsion.

Part I   *Part II*
                                                                         Reason

   a._____notify the physician.

   b._____elevate the foot of the bed.   _____

   c._____loosen any tight clothing.   _____

   d._____keep the patient warm and dry.   _____

   e._____induce vomiting.   _____

   f._____insert a mouth gag between the teeth.   _____

   g._____with a flashlight test the reaction of the pupils to light.   _____

   h._____prepare to administer oxygen.   _____

   i._____prepare a tray to secure a blood specimen.   _____

j.____note the course of the convulsion. ____
k.____note the duration of the convulsion. ____
l.____restrain the patient. ____
m.____initiate necessary precautions to prevent the patient
from injuring herself during seizure. ____
n.____observe any derangement or overt behavior during
unconsciousness. ____
o.____prepare a tray for giving hypodermoclysis. ____

Part II: Reasons. Below are statements, some true and some false, some pertinent and some not pertinent to the principles involved in the patient's management. By placing the number of the reason below in the column above which is marked *"Reason,"* indicate those statements which support the answers you gave in Part I.

1. Various toxic substances circulating in the blood irritate vital centers and produce convulsions.
2. Vomiting may eliminate toxic substances in the stomach.
3. Removing gastric contents by aspiration and lavage reduces irritation to the walls of the stomach, eliminating toxic products.
4. Applications of external heat increase circulation, thus increasing body temperature.
5. Elevating the feet above the head promotes the flow of blood to the head through the action of gravity.
6. Placing the patient in shock position decreases cerebral irritation.
7. Injecting fluids into the blood stream dilutes the toxic substances which produce cerebral irritation.
8. During a convulsion there is involuntary spasmodic contraction of the muscles of the body.
9. Involuntary spasmodic contraction of skeletal muscles results in random movements.
10. During a convulsion there is a temporary contraction of the diaphragm which immobilizes it.
11. During a convulsion the strong flexor muscles dominate the extensors.
12. Spasmodic contraction of body muscles impairs circulation and results in cerebral anemia.
13. Anti-social behavior may take place during the period of unconsciousness, which the patient does not remember after recovery from the seizure.
14. The order in which twitching progresses may indicate the cerebral areas involved.
15. The duration of the convulsion is an indication of the extent of cerebral involvement.
16. Constricting garments impair circulation.
17. Pupillary reaction to light is not lost in a hysterical convulsion.
18. Assistance may be necessary if complications arise.
19. Medical reporting has priority over immediate nursing care.

2. If Miss Evans does not tolerate drugs well, she may be given a ketogenic diet which maintains a state of ketosis. This is thought to be effective in

   a._____reducing weight.
   b._____reducing convulsions.
   c._____reducing sensitivity.
   d._____relieving insomnia.
   e._____relieving tension.

3. A ketogenic diet is

   a._____low-fat, high-carbohy-
   drate.
   b._____high-fat, high-carbohy-
   drate.
   c._____high-fat, low-carbohy-
   drate.
   d._____high-fat, high-protein.
   e._____low-fat, high-protein.

4. Disadvantages of the ketogenic diet are the

   a._____monotony, expense and length of the program.
   b._____inadequacy of vitamin and minerals.
   c._____inadequacy of laxative foods.
   d._____inadequacy of calories.

5. The ketogenic diet is usually

   a._____calculated for each individual and weighed.
   b._____calculated for each individual and estimated.
   c._____given in amounts to satisfy the patient.
   d._____given in amounts slightly above those desired by the patient.

6. From the following lists of foods, check with a + those to be included in the ketogenic diet; indicate by O, those to be avoided.

   a._____cream, butter, salad oils.
   b._____meat, poultry, fish.
   c._____cereals and bread.
   d._____sweets.
   e._____eggs and cheese.

7. The aura of epileptic seizures is

   a._____a strange light seen by the patient during attack.
   b._____the tissue damage following an attack.
   c._____a peculiar sensation preceding an attack.

8. During her menstrual period, Miss Evans may need to

   a._____increase her medications.
   b._____decrease her medications.
   c._____omit her medications.

9. In order to determine the *area of the cortex* involved in Jacksonian epilepsy, the nurse should note the

   a._____type of aura.
   b._____area in which convulsive movements start.
   c._____area in which convulsive movements terminate.
   d._____duration of convulsion.

10. Luminal, which was ordered for Miss Evans, is a barbital compound given for the following effects:

    a.____narcotic.
    b.____anticonvulsant.
    c.____hypnotic.
    d.____stimulating.
    e.____stomachic.

11. The daily dose of Luminal required in adults varies from

    a.____0.001 Gm. to 0.005 Gm.
    b.____0.004 Gm. to 0.008 Gm.
    c.____0.01 Gm. to 0.05 Gm.
    d.____0.06 Gm. to 0.6 Gm.
    e.____1 Gm. to 6.0 Gm.

12. Untoward effects of Luminal may be

    a.____nausea.
    b.____headache and dizziness on awakening.
    c.____vivid dreams during sleep.
    d.____scarletiniform rash.
    e.____ulcerous lesions.
    f.____prolonged sleep.
    g.____rapid pulse, stertorous breathing.
    h.____slow pulse, shallow breathing.

13. The average daily dose of sodium or potassium bromide is

    a.____0.5 Gm. to 1.5 Gm. b.____2 Gm. to 6 Gm. c.____8 Gm. to 10 Gm.

14. Toxic effects due to slow excretions result in

    a.____somnolence.
    b.____headache.
    c.____acnelike eruptions.
    d.____constipation.
    e.____bone-marrow changes.

Questions for Discussion and Student Projects

A. Related to Patient Study

1. Discuss the relationship of Miss Evans' emotional trauma or tension to her convulsive seizures.
2. What suggestions might be helpful to Miss Evans in regard to warding off a seizure?
3. Discuss the use of codeine sulfate, aspirin, mineral oil and cascara for Miss Evans. Discuss the theory that constipation aggravates the frequency of seizures. What would you teach Miss Evans to help her correct constipation?
4. Prepare a discussion for a ward class in which several students participate in teaching Miss Evans about diet, medication, rest, activities and acceptance of her condition in preparation for discharge. One student might act as Miss Evans and ask pertinent questions.

5. List the equipment for the following procedures:
   Lumbar puncture.
   Pneumo-encephalogram.
   Ventriculogram.
   Skull roentgenogram.
   Neurologic examination.
   Electro-encephalogram.

Discuss the nurse's responsibility in preparing Miss Evans for these procedures.

6. Why are the vital signs, temperature, pulse and blood pressure watched closely in Miss Evans?
7. How would you answer Miss Evans if she told you she was hoping to (a) enter a school of nursing and (b) marry and have a family.

B. Related to Epilepsy in General
   1. What is the purpose of the American Epilepsy League? How does it serve patients and their families? Is there any group in your community interested in helping epileptics? What resources are available for treatment, guidance, training or other assistance?
   2. In what conditions other than epilepsy may convulsions occur? What are the nurse's responsibilities when she observes a person having a generalized convulsion?
   3. What are the responsibilities of the nurse in the administration of sedatives? Illustrate the discussion with a description of your specific responsibilities in the administration of 3 separate medications.
   4. What should a nurse record in the symptom record of a patient who has convulsions?
   5. What observations should be made and charted for a person admitted for neurologic observation?
   6. Discuss the responsibilities you should assume for a person who had a seizure on the street; in a hospital ward.
   7. What measures are used to protect the skin of incontinent patients?
   8. What observations would you make when admitting an unconscious patient for whom no diagnosis has been made?

THE EMOTIONALLY UPSET FIANCÉE—PATIENT STUDY

Miss Mary Salvatori, an 18-year-old girl of Italian parentage, was brought to the hospital by her parents and fiancé. The fiancé stated that he had insisted, over the protests of the parents and of Mary, that she come in to find out what was causing a "weakness" in the extremities.

Miss Salvatori seemed unconcerned about her condition. The parents were excited and volatile, but because of language difficulties a good bit of interpretation by Tony, the fiancé, was necessary before the history was complete.

The Salvatoris live on a small chicken farm in a remote section of the city. They have mingled little with their American neighbors, and, because of inaccessibility of the farm, have not seen many of their countrymen.

Mary was graduated from high school and, in spite of the protests of her family (who felt that woman's only rôle in life is marriage), has almost completed business college. Her family have noticed that she has become nervous lately, with frequent crying spells and temper tantrums, but have blamed it on her "abnormal" life.

The first pertinent episode occurred 9 months ago when Mary, while attending a cousin's funeral, became hysterical, fainted and fell. Following this, she experienced numbness of the left side of her body, which finally disappeared.

Two weeks ago she had a severe cold, following which she had slight numbness of the left foot which progressed until the foot failed to support her weight. Two days before admission she developed numbness and weakness of the left hand and arm.

Neurologic test results were:

> Slightly positive Babinski on the left foot.
> Sustained left ankle clonus.
> Abdominal reflexes less responsive on the left side.
> Some decrease in position sense of the left foot and the left hand; relatively little leg sensory defect; heat and cold less well perceived on the sole of the left foot.
> Hoffman's test (fingers) positive on the left.
> Left shoulder cannot be hunched, though the head can be rotated to the left (eleventh nerve).
> Visual fields grossly intact, fine nystagmus on lateral gaze.

Laboratory tests showed:

> White blood cells 13.650 on admission, 8.450 later.
> Lumbar puncture, monocytes 8
> > colloidal gold 00000
> > proteins 65. slight elevation

A diagnosis of multiple sclerosis was made.
The orders included:

> High-vitamin diet.
> Light treatments and massage by a physiotherapist.
> Intravenous injection, vitamin B_1.
> Histamine gr. $\frac{1}{60}$ intramuscularly q.d.

There were no changes in her condition during hospitalization, and after 10 days Miss Salvatori was discharged to her home, with a clinic appointment in 2 weeks.

References

Fritz, Edna L., and Wolf, George A. Jr.: Multiple sclerosis, Am. J. Nursing 47:519, 1947.

Horton, Bayard T., et al.: Treatment of multiple sclerosis by intravenous administration of histamine, J.A.M.A. 124:800, 1944.

National Multiple Sclerosis Society: Multiple sclerosis; diagnosis and treatment, J.A.M.A. 135:569, 1947.

Schermerhorn, Richard, These Our People, Boston, Heath, 1948.

Questions Relating to the Patient Study

1. Multiple sclerosis is described best as
   a.____✓a diffuse disseminated disease of the central nervous system.
   b.____a malignancy of the central nervous system.
   c.____a diffuse infection of muscular tissue.
   d.____a functional disease.

2. Miss Salvatori's symptoms probably were caused by
   a.____emotional tension and anxiety.
   b.____syphilis of the central nervous system.
   c.____trauma to the central nervous system from a fall.
   d.____✓factors as yet unknown.
   e.____generalized infection, following U.R.I.

3. The progress of the disease is apt to be
   a.____excellent, with proper treatment.
   b.____terminal, within a few months.
   c.____✓chronic, with remissions and exacerbations.

4. Miss Salvatori should be encouraged to
   a.____learn to accept personal and economic dependence; rest constantly; avoid outside contacts.
   b.____secure absolute bed rest; restrict diversional activities to reading, listening to radio, etc.
   c.____✓assume as much responsibility as possible; seek part-time employment when feeling well; participate in new activities and hobbies.

5. If Miss Salvatori becomes completely bedridden, hypostatic pneumonia may be avoided by
   a.____early ambulation.
   b.____✓frequent changes of position.
   c.____✓suction removal of mucus.
   d.____inhalations of carbon dioxide.
   e.____inhalations of oxygen.

6. Massage would be prescribed for Miss Salvatori for
   a.____muscular contracture.
   b.____✓stimulation of the circulation.
   c.____✓muscular atrophy.
   d.____debilitation.
   e.____removal of exudates.

7. Flexion contractures of the left arm may be prevented by
   a.____✓supporting the arm on a pillow in the position of abduction.
   b.____supporting the arm on a pillow high in the axilla.
   c.____using rolls of gauze to keep the fingers extended.
   d.____using traction to keep the fingers extended.
   e.____using a splint to keep the fingers extended.
   f.____✓using passive exercises.

8. Outward rotation of the leg is prevented by

    a. ✓ using a sand bag to the outer aspect of the leg, from above the hip to well below the knee.

    b.____using a sand bag to the outer aspect of the leg, from the mid-thigh to the ankle.

    c.____using a smaller sand bag along the inner aspect of the thigh to the ankle.

    d.____using a smaller sand bag along the inner aspect of the thigh to below the knee.

    e.____using traction.

Questions for Discussion and Student Projects

1. What precautions should be initiated to prevent contractures, foot- and wristdrop and rotation of the legs, in the event Miss Salvatori developed spastic paralysis of an extremity? Outline the specific instructions you would give the family in regard to proper body alignment, placement of hands and fingers, etc., to prevent unnecessary deformities.

2. Outline a plan for the family which will suggest practical measures to assist Miss Salvatori when she returns home. Include a plan for a day's activities, prevention of accidents, requirements for diet and physical and occupational therapy. How would you advise the family to cope with (a) uncontrolled emotionalism and (b) the need for diversion and social contacts?

3. How could the problem of incontinence of urine and stools be handled if Miss Salvatori developed loss of sphincter control? What suggestions might be made to her family? How may she be spared embarrassment from this condition and still associate with others and be a member of her family group? How may she assist herself in overcoming this difficulty?

4. Compare the neurologic findings for Miss Salvatori with the typical findings for patients with multiple sclerosis.

5. Investigate current research findings on the use of drugs to overcome muscle spasm.

6. How would you answer Miss Salvatori if she asks you if there are any "cures" for her disease? How would the family be informed of the prognosis? By whom?

7. Discuss the purpose, activities and financial support of the National Mutiple Sclerosis Society. What value would this organization have for Miss Salvatori?

8. Discuss the difference between the customs of an Italian-born family and those of a family who has been in this country for a generation. What adjustment problems do you think a second-generation Italian young person might have in her contacts with the family and the outside world?

9. Do you think Miss Salvatori should marry? What should her fiancé be told about her illness?

Section 10. Nursing Care of Patients with Disorders of the Eye and the Ear[*]

STUDY SUGGESTIONS: Before beginning the study of this Section, the student will find it helpful to

A. Review
1. Anatomy and physiology: eye and ear.
2. Physics: sight and hearing.

B. Study
1. In pharmacology texts: drugs affecting the eye.
2. In surgical nursing texts: disorders of the eye and ear.

C. Read the additional References listed before attempting to answer the questions relating to each patient study.

THE OLD LADY WITH FAILING EYESIGHT
Background Review Questions

1. The uveal tract is made up of the
   a._____anterior and posterior chambers.
   b._____choroid, cornea and sclera.
   c._____rods and cones.
   d._____lens, cornea and iris.
   e._____choroid, iris and ciliary body.

2. The lens is a
   a._____transparent body with concave surfaces and lies between the pupil and the vitreous body.
   b._____colorless, opaque body with convex surfaces and lies posterior to the pupil.
   c._____transparent body with convex surfaces and lies anterior to the vitreous body.
   d._____colorless, translucent body with concave surfaces and is sandwiched between the iris and the vitreous body.

3. The function of the lens is to
   a._____refract rays of light so that they will be focused on the retina.
   b._____filter out those rays of light which distort optimum vision.
   c._____become thick or thin (with the aid of the ciliary muscle) so that dark- or light-colored objects may be seen clearly.
   d._____provide substance in the anterior chamber which prevents a prolapse of the iris.

4. The white portion of the eye as viewed anteriorly is the
   a._____sclera.   c._____cornea.
   b._____iris.   d._____lens.

[*] Disturbances of sight and hearing related to injury to the brain are treated in Section 9, Neurologic Disorders.

5. Which one of the following possesses no direct blood supply?

   a._____sclera.   c._____cornea.
   b._____iris.   d._____choroid.

6. Cones are found only in the

   a._____optic disc.   c._____fovea centralis.
   b._____orra serrata.   d._____cornea.

7. The area of the retina where the optic nerve leaves the eyeball is called the

   a._____orra serrata.   c._____fovea centralis.
   b._____optic disc.   d._____macula lutea.

8. When an image cannot be focused clearly on the retina, the condition is described as

   a._____myopia.   d._____ametropia.
   b._____emmetropia.   e._____presbyopia.
   c._____hyperopia.

9. When the rays of light are focused in front of the retina because the eyeball is too long in its anteroposterior diameter, the condition is referred to as

   a._____miosis.   d._____hyperopia.
   b._____mydriasis.   e._____presbyopia.
   c._____myopia.

10. Argyrol is the same as

   a._____silver nitrate.   d._____atropine sulfate.
   b._____silver proteinate.   e._____Mercurophen.
   c._____Protargol.

11. As one grows older, he may become farsighted due to the lens' losing its elasticity. This condition is called

   a._____presbyopia.   d._____anopia.
   b._____hyperopia.   e._____diplopia.
   c._____myopia.

12. Atropine sulfate 1 per cent as eyedrops produces

   a._____dilatation of the pupil.
   b._____contraction of the pupil.
   c._____increased power of accommodation.
   d._____paralysis of the power of accommodation.
   e._____increased intra-ocular pressure in the normal eye.
   f._____increased intra-ocular pressure when there is a tendency to increase, e.g. glaucoma.
   g._____decreased intra-ocular pressure in the normal eye.
   h._____decreased intra-ocular pressure when there is a tendency to increase, e.g. glaucoma.

13. The anesthetic of choice in most eye surgery is

    a._____cocaine.   d._____ether.
    b._____Avertin.   e._____Pentothal Sodium.
    c._____cyclopropane.

14. The reason for the choice of the anesthetic in question 13 is that this drug

    a._____allows the patient to fall into an apparently natural sleep and can be administered easily per rectum.
    b._____is rapid-acting, pleasant to take and particularly non-irritating for patients who have respiratory complications.
    c._____produces anesthesia within 30 seconds; the onset of anesthesia is extremely pleasant and postoperative nausea and vomiting are almost negligible.
    d._____produces complete relaxation, has a wide margin of safety and constricts the pupils.
    e._____produces a loss of sensation, causes a contraction of the capillaries and dilates the pupils.

15. Fluorescein solution is a common eye medication used to

    a._____inhibit the growth of staphylococci and streptococci.
    b._____reduce the power of accommodation by paralyzing the circular muscle of the iris.
    c._____limit the flow of tears when the lacrimal duct is infected.
    d._____detect corneal abrasions because it produces a bright green stain.

16. Eserine sulfate is an eye medication which

    a._____is a myotic.
    b._____is a mydriatic.
    c._____can be kept in a colorless transparent bottle because it does not deteriorate readily.
    d._____must be kept in a dark bottle because it darkens and becomes more irritating.
    e._____allows the aqueous humor to escape more easily into the lymph channels.
    f._____prevents the aqueous humor from escaping into the lymph channels.

17. Match the following (there may be more than one correct answer):

    a._____miotic.   (1) homatropine.
    b._____mydriatic.   (2) eserine sulfate.
                            (3) pilocarpine.
                            (4) atropine sulfate.
                            (5) Euphthalmine.
                            (6) physostigmine.
                            (7) Paredrine.
                            (8) Neo-synephrine.

18. Match the following:

    a._____chalazion.
    b._____hordeolum.
    c._____presbyopia.
    d._____keratitis.
    e._____strabismus.
    f._____pterygium.
    g._____ptosis.
    h._____esotropia.
    i._____entropion.
    j._____exotropia.

    (1) "cross eyes."
    (2) turning out of one or both eyes.
    (3) drooping of the lid.
    (4) meibomian cyst.
    (5) "stye."
    (6) accommodation loss in old age.
    (7) corneal inflammation.
    (8) inversion of the eyelid.
    (9) squint.
    (10) triangular thickening of the conjunctiva on the cornea.

19. Match the following:

    a._____left eye.
    b._____both eyes.
    c._____right eye.
    d._____either eye.

    (1) O.D.
    (2) O.S.
    (3) O.U.

20. Match the following:

    a._____hyperopia.
    b._____myopia.
    c._____cannot use powers of accommodation.
    d._____must use powers of accommodation.
    e._____corrected with a concave lens.
    f._____corrected with a convex lens.
    g._____converging, positive lens.
    h._____diverging, negative lens.

    (1) nearsightedness.
    (2) farsightedness.

21. Match the following:

    a._____one skilled in optics, the nature and properties of light. (Not a doctor of medicine.)
    b._____one who grinds, fits and supplies glasses and instruments.
    c._____one who specializes in the diagnosis and alleviation of eye diseases by the aid of medicine, surgery and optics. (A doctor of medicine.)

    (1) optician.
    (2) optometrist.
    (3) oculist.
    (4) ophthalmologist.
    (5) ophthalmic physician.

      d._____one who prescribes and
dispenses glasses but is not
trained to recognize and
treat ailments of the eye.
(Not a doctor of medi-
cine.)

THE OLD LADY WITH FAILING EYESIGHT—PATIENT STUDY

Since Agatha Bronson was now 80 years old, she considered herself too old to have to go through a surgical operation. Her periodic visits to the Eye Clinic during the past 4 years revealed a progressively lessening of vision in the right eye and a definite senile cataract in the other.

When she met the nurse upon arrival on the Eye Ward, she said, "Why can't they give me medicine for my eyes instead of wanting to operate on me? They used to give me eye drops that helped." True, Miss Bronson had been receiving Dionyn eye drops at bedtime because it was hoped that the irritation produced in the eye would bring about an improvement in nutrition and circulation and perhaps slow up the process of opacification. However, the only help available now was to do an intracapsular extraction of the cataract in the left eye.

Miss Bronson lives with her only close relative, another spinster, and they make their home in the family homestead. During the past several years, they have taken in boarders for financial assistance since neither of the old ladies is employed. This source of income, plus interest from some family investments, have allowed them to live modestly and independently. Miss Agatha is, however, not prepared financially to meet a serious or long illness, but at present her chief concern is a real fear of blindness and possibly a fear of death.

The Bronsons have a small circle of acquaintances but no close friends. They enjoy their radio and would have considered getting a television set, had Miss Agatha's eyesight been better. Miss Agatha likes to knit squares for afghans because it keeps her busy and she can do it without straining her eyes.

On the evening of her first day in the hospital, she was convinced by the physician that the only possible help for her sight was to have surgery. When she realized that she did not have to take ether, she seemed greatly relieved. She was told by the nurse some of the things to be expected on her return from the operating room, such as lying in one position, having both eyes bandaged, etc. However, the nurse made a notation in her notes that she doubted whether this information had really been assimilated by Miss Agatha.

Medical orders can be summarized as follows: The night before surgery, she received chloral hydrate 0.6 Gm. The next morning the nurse administered penicillin solution eye drops gtts. iv in each eye; later Miss Agatha had a cleansing enema. On call to the operating room she received Neo-synephrine 10 per cent gtts. ii. O.S. since this was the eye to have surgery.

Immediately postoperatively, and for 24 hours, Miss Bronson was kept flat in bed with instructions not to turn, cough or strain. She was allowed a soft diet the next two days and the head of her bed was elevated 25°. On the third p.o. day, a peep-hole window was made in the mask, allowing her unoperated eye to see. By the fifth day she was allowed out of bed and had just a patch over the operated eye. A week after her admission she was ready for discharge with careful instructions for her follow-up care. In a month both she and the surgeon were pleased to note that sight was gradually improving in the eye that had been operated on.

References

Chace and Shaw: Treatment and nursing care of patients with cataract, Am. J. Nursing **48**:150, 1948.
Preu, P. W., and Guida, F. P.: Psychoses complicating recovery from extraction of cataract, Arch. Neurol. and Psychiat. **38**:818, 1937.
Smith, E. K.: When shadows fall, Sight-Saving Rev., **8**: No. 4, December 1938.
Weiss, M. O.: Psychological aspects of nursing care for eye patients, Am. J. Nursing **50**:218, 1950.

Questions Relating to the Patient Study

1. If Miss Bronson had had a senile cataract in one eye and normal vision in the other, would the cataract have been removed? Why?
   a.____Yes, for otherwise there is a possibility that vision in the remaining good eye might become impaired.
   b.____No, because binocular single vision will not be allowed and diplopia will result.
   c.____Yes, because cataracts have a tendency to grow progressively worse.
   d.____No, because any surgical intervention tends to weaken total visual acuity.

2. Intracapsular extraction of a cataract is the removal of the
   a.____lens plus the anterior capsule.
   b.____lens but not the capsule enveloping it.
   c.____cataract from the lens.
   d.____mature or ripe cataract with the lens to which it is attached.
   e.____immature cataract with the lens but not the capsule.

3. The best reply to Miss Bronson's query, "Why do I have to have an enema this morning?", is
   a.____"Because you may have a general anesthetic and it is routine for those patients."
   b.____"So that you will not have to 'go to the bathroom' during your operation. That would be embarrassing."
   c.____"This will eliminate the possibility of your straining yourself for a couple of days after surgery. Any strain can produce serious complications in your eye."
   d.____"In order that you will not have to use the bedpan so frequently after your operation. We want you to conserve your strength."

4. During the first 24 hours postoperatively, every effort should be made by the nurse to
   a._____keep the patient comfortable by allowing her to turn on her side for a few minutes every 6 hours.
   b._____make her independent by letting her feed herself.
   c._____explain why a flat position must be maintained without exception.
   d._____provide a paper and pencil for Miss Bronson to write any messages since she should not talk.
   e._____encourage deep breaths for proper lung expansion following her anesthetic.

5. Immediate postoperative care is directed primarily toward preventing
   a._____prolapse of the iris.   d._____hemorrhage.
   b._____decubitus ulcer.   e._____retinal detachment.
   c._____infection of the cornea.   f._____migraine headache.

6. The best method of treatment for a senile cataract is
   a._____to use drugs to dissolve the cloudy film.
   b._____to use dark glasses for a prescribed period of time.
   c._____an iridectomy which should be followed by the wearing of proper glasses.
   d._____surgical removal of the cloudy film leaving the lens intact.
   e._____surgical removal of the lens.

7. "Needling" or discission is a surgical method for treating congenital or traumatic cataract. In this technic
   a._____a needle is inserted into the lens capsule and the cataract is aspirated.
   b._____the lens is pierced several times by a needle and the broken fragments of lens eventually are absorbed by the aqueous humor.
   c._____a piece of cataract tissue is aspirated for biopsy purposes; the results of this test will determine the course of treatment.

Questions for Discussion and Student Projects

1. How can you help Miss Bronson overcome her fear of blindness and fear of death? Be more specific than simply using the term "reassure."
2. Postoperative complications are prevented by keeping the patient's head immobile with the eyes facing the ceiling. Any activity which may cause increased pressure within the eye must be avoided. How can you, as a nurse, handle the following problems most effectively?
   a. Miss Bronson tells you she is about to sneeze.
   b. On the first postoperative night, Miss Bronson awakens and is about to raise herself to the sitting position. When she is reminded that she must lie quietly, she insists that she must get out of bed to go to the bathroom.
   c. Miss Bronson refuses mouth care because the last time she used the curved basin, some fluid escaped and got the back of her neck and hair wet.

3. Imagine that you are blindfolded, lying flat in bed, and that you are about to be served a semi-soft lunch. List the things you would want to be told by the nurse as she feeds you. What information could you as a patient give to the nurse which would help her in allowing you to enjoy your meal to the fullest?

4. While Miss Bronson had both eyes bandaged, the nurse tried to encourage her to chat with other patients. However, when a patient was introduced, Miss Bronson discouraged conversation by not speaking except in direct reply to a question. Later, when asked why, Miss Bronson replied, "But I don't know how he looks." How can you develop such a means of diversional therapy?

   a. Preliminary preparation of Miss Bronson.
   b. Preliminary preparation of the visitor.
   c. What topics of conversation might be introduced?

5. List other forms of recreational or diversional therapy which might appeal to Miss Bronson. How and when would you introduce them?

6. One way of making Miss Bronson conscious of avoiding those activities which produce strain is to play a "Quiz" game with her. Have her enumerate all the physical activities she can recall which made her strain. List the answers that you would expect.

7. Prepare a list of all the environmental factors which are important to consider in promoting a quiet atmosphere for a postoperative eye patient who has both eyes bandaged and must lie perfectly quiet for several days.

8. What is the incidence of postoperative psychoses in patients who have had surgery for senile cataracts? What safeguards can be employed to lessen this problem?

9. How successful are operations for cataracts with reference to future vision for the individual patient?

10. Miss Bronson will have to learn how to use glasses as her sight improves in her left eye. How can she be helped to overcome the following difficulties:

    a. objects will seem to be displaced; hence the hazard of going up and down stairs or crossing the street.
    b. when shifting her gaze from one plane to another, a feeling of dizziness may prevail and she may think that she is falling.
    c. a tendency to hold her head in a stiff and angular position.

LIVING IN THE DARK—PATIENT STUDY

Mr. Bonoma, who is 64 years old, arrived on the eye ward in a wheelchair. It was immediately obvious that he could not see and that he was under great emotional tension.

Fortunately, Mr. Bonoma was well known to the hospital personnel. His distress was so great that a coherent history was impossible. All one could gather was that he had buried his wife 2 days ago, and on the day following her funeral had awakened completely sightless and with pain and swelling in his right eye. His distress over his wife's death was aggravated by the fact that he felt that, had she better understood her condition (diabetes), she might have cared for herself more adequately.

Mr. Bonoma's hospital history was voluminous. For 25 years he had been a patient in the out-patient department and had had 4 previous admissions.

At the time of his first admission he came to the hospital stating that "I suddenly realized that I could see nothing with my left eye." The diagnosis at that time was chronic glaucoma and the treatment was iridectomy. However, no sight returned to this eye. At the same time, the vision in the right eye was much reduced. The use of pilocarpine 1 per cent eye drops and glasses brought the vision almost to normal.

One day 10 years ago Mr. Bonoma left his glasses off while he was chopping wood. A chip flew up and hit him in the right eye, and the sight in this remaining "good" eye was much impaired.

Mr. Bonoma was forced to give up his work as a bricklayer. His married son and family live with him in a small house in the country where they have a large vegetable garden and a few chickens. In this way, and with financial help from the Society for Aid to the Blind, the Bonomas have been able to live comfortably.

Although Mr. Bonoma's vision has been hazy, he was, until today, able to see doorways, furniture, etc., and since he has lived in the same house for years, has been able to get around very well.

Mr. Bonoma was put on bed rest for 5 days, with the following orders:

> Procaine penicillin 300,000 U q.d. (I.M.).
> Nupercaine solution 1:5,000 gtts. ii O.D. t.i.d.
>   Follow in 5 minutes with an irrigation of 3–5 cc. of penicillin eye
>   drops (1 cc.–2,000 U).
> Atropine sulfate 1 per cent gtts. ii O.D. b.i.d. for pain and tension.
> Aspirin gr. x. p.r.n., or
> Demerol 50 mg. q. 3 h. p.r.n. for pain.
> Chloral hydrate 4 cc. h.s. p.r.n. for insomnia.

After 3 days up and about, Mr. Bonoma was discharged with the following prescription for home use:

> Sodium sulfacetimide 30 per cent gtts. ii. O.D. q. 3 h.
> Sodium sulfacetimide 10 per cent ointment to be used O.D. h.s.
> Atropine sulfate 1 per cent gtts. ii. O.D. b.i.d.

It was felt that pilocarpine would no longer be of any help since Mr. Bonoma's sight is now permanently gone. He was discharged with the understanding that he would continue to be seen in the Eye Clinic. Plans were made for him to adjust to the fact that he would be blind permanently.

References

Blake, Eugene M.: Glaucoma, Am. J. Nursing 52:451, 1952.
Weiss, M. O.: Psychological aspects of nursing care for eye patients, Am. J. Nursing 50:218, 1950.

Eye Health, The National Society for the Prevention of Blindness, Pub. 447, 1947.

The Newly Blinded, pamphlet published by the Seeing Eye, Inc., Morristown, N.J.

Questions Relating to the Patient Study

1. Panophthalmitis is considered to be a very serious condition because
   a._____the outcome usually is phthisis bulbi (shrunken eyeball) with entire loss of vision.
   b._____there is intense suppuration and the process goes on to complete destruction of the eye.
   c._____it is an inflammatory condition affecting the entire eye; however, with proper chemotherapy, the prognosis is excellent.
   d._____it affects the bony eye socket but not the eyeball; it has a tendency to destroy bone as does osteomyelitis.

2. Glaucoma is more common among
   a._____men.
   b._____women.
   c._____those who use their eyes to do close work.
   d._____those who do little reading or sewing.
   e._____darker races.
   f._____Jewish and other white races.
   g._____those who worry, over-eat, etc.
   h._____those who are more placid.
   i._____those whose parents, grandparents or relatives have had it.
   j._____those with no familial tendency toward it.

3. Symptoms of acute glaucoma are
   a._____frequent headaches, pain, dilated pupil, diminished peripheral vision.
   b._____no headaches, cloudiness of vision, hardening of the eyeball, diminished central vision.
   c._____frequent headaches, contracted pupil, "steaming," greenish-looking cornea, diminished central vision.
   d._____no headaches, no pain, contracted pupil, diminished peripheral vision.

4. A drug which contracts the pupil is recommended in the symptomatic relief of acute glaucoma because it
   a._____does not affect the aqueous humor; relaxes smooth muscle.
   b._____prevents aqueous humor from draining into the canal of Schlemm.
   c._____allows aqueous humor to drain into the canal of Schlemm.

5. An instrument used in measuring intra-ocular pressure is a (an)
   a._____tentatome.
   b._____tenotomy knife.
   c._____tonometer.
   d._____oculometer.
   e._____ophthalmeter.
   f._____ophthalmoscope.

6. An increased pressure within the eyeball is a significant diagnostic aid. Match the following:

Pressure Readings	*Probable Condition*
a. 0–15 mm.	(1)_____normal eye.
b. 17–28 mm.	(2)_____chronic glaucoma.
c. 25–35 mm.	(3)_____acute primary glaucoma.
d. 35–40 mm.	
e. 45–100 mm.	

7. The most frequent operative procedure for glaucoma is

a._____enucleation.   c._____iridectomy.
b._____extraction of the lens.   d._____trephining.

8. The following practices are recommended for helping a blind person:

a. When walking with a blind person,

(1)_____allow him to walk ahead of you as you hold his elbow.
(2)_____let him follow you by lightly touching your elbow.

b. Let him use a light-weight walking stick

(1)_____for tapping on the sidewalk so that people will clear his path.
(2)_____to act as an extended hand to give warning of things unseen.

Questions for Discussion and Student Projects

1. Discuss glaucoma, using the following headings:

a. The nature of the symptoms. Do they encourage the patient to seek early medical advice?
b. The incidence of blindness caused by glaucoma.
c. The various medical and surgical treatments; the anticipated results of each of these.
d. The relationship of this disease to other systemic difficulties, such as

(1) allergy.   (2) hypertension.   (3) emotional disturbances.

2. Since a patient with glaucoma must learn to live with what is definitely a chronic disease, what should he know about the disease? What health measures does he need to follow?

3. Mr. Bonoma was a modest man who found it difficult to be on an open ward and to be taken care of by women. Because he was blind, he was never sure that his bed curtains shielded him from the rest of the ward or that the nurse would not come in without his realizing it. What suggestions can you make to develop the ease of mind which Mr. Bonoma needs? How would you handle visits from other personnel, such as laboratory technicians, kitchen maids, etc.?

4. On two occasions, Mr. Bonoma was found rubbing his eyes with a

rough washcloth. What dangers are involved in this act? How would you teach him to care for itchiness, burning or pain in his eyes?

5. Is there any relationship between the emotional impact of his wife's death and Mr. Bonoma's subsequent complete loss of sight? Substantiate your position.

6. The hardest nursing task of all was that of preparing Mr. Bonoma for the fact that he was now totally and permanently blind. He had had much the same experience years ago, and, after 6 months had passed, he had recovered as much sight as he had had before. He expected this to occur again. He had been placed next to another eye patient who was also "whistling in the dark" to keep up his courage. The two kept telling each other that what the doctor had said was not true, and it was difficult to try to tell Mr. Bonoma the truth without stepping on the hopes of the other patient who had a good chance of recovering some of his sight. How can this situation be handled most effectively to the benefit of these two individuals?

7. Would you let Mr. Bonoma do the following activities? If so, list the steps you would follow in teaching him each function.

   a. Use a fork and knife.   c. Eat a piece of pie.
   b. Light his own cigarette.   d. Shave.

8. Outline specifically what Mr. Bonoma should be told upon discharge with respect to physical and emotional activity. What reasons would you give for each recommendation? What instructions should be given to Mr. Bonoma's daughter-in-law, who will be caring for him?

9. How prevalent is blindness in this country? What are the chief causes? What is the relation of venereal diseases to the incidence of blindness?

10. What facilities are there in your community for teaching the blind? What is the function of the Society for Aid to the Blind?

11. What are the functions of the National Society for the Prevention of Blindness? How do they receive funds? Of what help can this organization be to Mr. Bonoma?

12. Describe the program at Morristown, N.J., where they train seeing-eye dogs. How could arrangements be made for Mr. Bonoma to benefit by this program? What is the cost and how is it borne?

Nursing Care of Patients with Other Eye Disorders

References

Flitter, H.: An Introduction to Physics in Nursing, pp. 127–132, "The Physics of Vision," St. Louis, Mosby, 1948.

Kuhn, H. S.: Emergency nursing care of the eyes in industry, Am. J. Nursing 47:24, 1947.

Lancaster, W. B.: Crossed eyes in children, Am. J. Nursing 50:535, 1950.

Power, Adolph: Why dark glasses?, Sight-Saving Rev. 14: No. 3, Winter, 1944.

Shields, M.: Contact lenses, Hygeia 25:674, 1949.
First Aid Textbook, American Red Cross, Washington, D.C., 1945.
Eye Health, The National Society for the Prevention of Blindness, Pub. 447, 1947.

1. Acceptable first-aid treatment for a foreign body in the eye is as follows:

   a._____when the object can be seen on or near the pupil, to carefully use the clean corner of a handkerchief and wipe it out.
   b._____to instruct the patient to rub the affected eye gently so that the lacrimal duct is stimulated to secrete fluid. This will produce the desired flushing of the eye.
   c._____to remove any visible object on the lower lid with a pair of fine-tooth forceps (tweezers).
   d._____for objects on the lining of the eyelid, to grasp the upper lashes gently, having the victim look upward as you pull the eyelid forward and downward over the lower lid.

2. An acid burn of the eye can be treated best by

   a._____flushing well with large quantities of clean water.
   b._____flushing well with large quantities of an equally strong base.
   c._____leaving it alone and calling the doctor immediately.

3. A retinal detachment can often be remedied by

   a._____having the patient lie flat on his back for several days with his eyes bandaged.
   b._____irrigating the affected eye with penicillin solution every 4 hours.
   c._____removing a wedge from the iris (iridectomy).
   d._____drainage of the solution caught behind the retina and cauterization.

4. One of the few pathologic eye conditions in which the use of contact lenses is justified is

   a._____cataract.
   b._____keratoconus.
   c._____interstitial keratitis.
   d._____keratocele.
   e._____keratoma.

5. To safely introduce eye drops the nurse should hold the lower lid down with the left index finger and with the right hand hold the dropper

   a._____at right angles to the eye; direct the patient to look down; express the drop of drug on the cornea.
   b._____parallel to the eye; direct the patient to look up; express the drop of drug into the cup made by the everted lower lid.
   c._____at right angles to the eye; direct the patient to look up; express the drop of drug into the cup made by the everted lower lid.
   d._____parallel to the eye; direct the patient to look down; express the drop of drug on the cornea.

6. The use of the Snellen chart is a standard test of central visual acuity for distance. When the resultant reading is 20/40, it means that

a._____at 40 feet, one can read the 20-foot size letter.
b._____at 20 feet, one can read the 40-foot size letter.
c._____the individual has very poor reading vision.
d._____the individual has better than average vision.

7. Desirable characteristics of reading materials to promote good eye hygiene are:

a._____Glossy paper and ink are to be avoided because of reflected glare.
b._____Green paper is "easier on the eyes" than dull-finished white or cream-tinted paper.
c._____Wide margins are not desirable.
d._____Lines of print are read more easily if not over 4½ inches in length.
e._____Typed lines should not exceed 6 inches.
f._____Plain type with sharp edges is the most distinct.

Questions for Discussion and Student Projects

1. What aspects of the anatomy of the eye are to be taken into consideration in order to do eye procedures with the greatest safety?
2. Demonstrate the method of introducing an ointment into the conjunctival sac from an ophthalmic tube which has a small lip and opening. What precautions must be observed, and why?
3. How important a problem are errors of refraction? What types of eye defects cause eyestrain? Why?
4. List the precautions which are being taken in the industrial plants of your community to safeguard against eyestrain and injury. Are they adequate? How frequently are the plants inspected? By whom? What teaching is being done? How effective is it? What more can be done?
5. Crossed eyes is a condition which is not only a cosmetic problem but also a problem of abnormal binocular vision. How soon in infancy can it be detected? When is the best time to initiate treatment? Is surgery necessary? What is orthoptics and what place does it have in treating crossed eyes?
6. Corneal transplantation (keratoplasty) can now be done with a measure of success for certain conditions. The transplant may be obtained from the same individual or from another individual. If the transplant from a patient in your hospital is to be used in another hospital, how would such an enucleated eye be packaged for delivery? Is there any factor involved in getting the eye to its destination? Suppose a patient you were caring for knew he was going to die and made a request to you to have his eye (or eyes) preserved for corneal transplantation. What would you do about it?
7. What types of prosthetics are available for patients following enucleation? How can they be cared for? What are the psychologic problems involved and how can you help in their solution?

8. What problems does a patient encounter in adjusting to bifocal glasses? What assistance can you give to such a person?
9. A former high-school classmate is interested in getting contact lenses. Because you are a nurse, she asks for your frank opinion. These are her questions:

How expensive are they?
Are they easy to insert?
How often must they be changed and cleaned?
Are they painful to wear?
Can they break?
Are there any hazards involved?
Am I justified in getting them? Why?

10. The use of sunglasses has become very popular in the past few years. Is one justified in wearing his favorite color in sunglasses? Is there any difference in brownish gray green, or blue glasses from the point of view of safe vision? Of what value are lenses with polarizing properties? Is it possible to burn a hole in one's retina with very dark glasses? Why? What is "snow blindness" and can it be controlled?

Nursing Care of Patients with Disorders of the Ear

References

Flitter, H.: An Introduction to Physics in Nursing, pp. 133–137, "The Physics of Sound and Hearing," St. Louis, Mosby, 1948.
Lewis, D. K.: Deafness, Am. J. Nursing 52:575, 1952.
Rosenberger, H. C., and Bukovina, E.: Fenestration, Am. J. Nursing 47:730, 1947.

Review Questions

1. The eustachian tube connects the pharynx with the

    a.____external ear.   b.____middle ear.   c.____inner ear.

2. The perception of pitch is dependent upon the structure and vibration of

    a.____Reissner's membrane.   c.____the basilar membrane.
    b.____the oval window.   d.____the round window.

3. Permanent deafness which cannot be relieved by any type of hearing aid would result from

    a.____fusing together of the ossicles.
    b.____immobility of the stapes.
    c.____destruction of the vestibular branch of the auditory canal nerve.
    d.____destruction of the organ of Corti.

4. The tympanic membrane forms a partition between the

   a._____external and middle ears. c._____middle and inner ears.
   b._____external and inner ears. d._____middle and oral pharynx.

5. The perception of intensity (or loudness) of a sound is dependent upon the

   a._____vibrations of the basilar membrane.
   b._____location of the hair cells that are stimulated.
   c._____depth of the excursion of the round window.
   d._____depth of the excursion of the stapes into the oval window.

6. The unit for expressing the energy of a sound wave is the decibel.

   a. The sound for average speech is

      (1)_____0–10 decibels.
      (2)_____10–20 decibels.
      (3)_____20–40 decibels.
      (4)_____40–60 decibels.
      (5)_____70–100 decibels.

   b. The sound of riveting is about

      (1)_____0–10 decibels.
      (2)_____10–20 decibels.
      (3)_____20–40 decibels.
      (4)_____40–60 decibels.
      (5)_____70–100 decibels.

7. The average range of human audibility is

   a._____0 to 100 vibrations.
   b._____10 to 10,000 vibrations.
   c._____0 to 50,000 vibrations.
   d._____20 to 20,000 vibrations.
   e._____100 to 1,000 vibrations.

8. Medically, the middle ear is a very significant part of the anatomy of the head because

   a._____it is the area where sound waves are transmitted from the external to the internal ear.
   b._____one cannot hear if the incus, malleus and stapes are not in proper working order.
   c._____it is a connecting pathway from the nasopharynx and eustachian tube to the mastoid area and the thin bone plate separating it from the meninges.
   d._____the paranasal sinuses are connected one to another and to the middle ear, which makes it a vulnerable spot for infection.

9. A. Indicate safe methods of removing the following substances from the external auditory canal by placing the number of the method(s) in the space preceding the name of the object or substance.

Substance	Method
a.＿＿seeds (beans, peas).	(1) irrigate with warm sterile saline solution.
b.＿＿insects (fleas, ants).	
c.＿＿beads or buttons.	(2) removal (by physician) with hook or forceps.
d.＿＿cerumen (wax).	(3) instillation of 1 or 2 drops of warm oil.

B. Give the reason for your selection of each method.

a.＿＿＿＿＿＿＿＿＿＿＿＿＿＿＿＿

b.＿＿＿＿＿＿＿＿＿＿＿＿＿＿＿＿

c.＿＿＿＿＿＿＿＿＿＿＿＿＿＿＿＿

d.＿＿＿＿＿＿＿＿＿＿＿＿＿＿＿＿

10. In irrigating the ear, the following points should be observed:

a. The temperature of the solution should be

(1)＿＿105°–110°F.
(2)＿＿115°–130°F.

b. The height of the irrigation can should be from

(1)＿＿1 to 2 feet.
(2)＿＿4 to 6 feet.

c. In an adult, the pinna is

(1)＿＿lifted upward and forward.
(2)＿＿lifted upward and backward.
(3)＿＿pulled gently downward and forward.
(4)＿＿pulled gently downward and backward.

d. In a child, the pinna is

(1)＿＿lifted upward and forward.
(2)＿＿lifted upward and backward.
(3)＿＿pulled gently downward and forward.
(4)＿＿pulled gently downward and backward.

11. Because air in the middle ear is affected by changes in atmospheric pressure during ascent and descent, the individual must keep equalizing the pressure in his middle ear to avoid aero-otitis media. Some ways of doing this are by

a.＿＿chewing gum.
b.＿＿placing the head between one's knees.
c.＿＿yawning.
d.＿＿blowing one's nose.
e.＿＿breathing through one's mouth.

12. Dramamine is used to

a.＿＿inhibit a feeling of faintness.
b.＿＿treat Ménière's disease.

    c._____prevent aero-otitis media.
    d._____combat motion sickness.
    e._____induce hypnosis.

13. The most common side reaction from Dramamine is

    a._____earache.   d._____nausea.
    b._____dizziness.   e._____nystagmus.
    c._____drowsiness.

14. A myringotomy is a surgical procedure in which an incision is made into the

    a._____ear lobe to drain a subcutaneous abscess.
    b._____eardrum to drain pus from a middle-ear infection.
    c._____partition between the middle and the inner ear to facilitate hearing in otosclerosis.
    d._____petrous portion of the temporal bone to allow for drainage in mastoiditis.

15. In preparing the patient for a mastoidectomy, the following method should be used in each case:

    a. simple postaural mastoidectomy.   (1)_____shave the head for a distance of about 2 inches around the auricle.
    b. radical postaural mastoidectomy.
    c. simple endaural mastoidectomy.
    d. radical endaural mastoidectomy.
    (2)_____clean the auricle thoroughly but no shaving of hair is necessary.

16. About which of the following functions will a surgeon be most concerned in a patient who has just had a radical mastoidectomy?

    a._____speaking.   d._____seeing.
    b._____hearing.   e._____smelling.
    c._____smiling.

17. The reason for the surgeon's concern in question 16 is that a nerve may be accidentally injured or severed. This nerve is the

    a._____glossopharyngeal.   d._____optic.
    b._____auditory.   e._____olfactory.
    c._____facial.

18. Characterize each of the following descriptions by indicating the type of deafness it describes:

    a. conduction deafness.   (1)_____"bone" deafness.
                          (2)_____"nerve" deafness.
                          (3)_____the patient hears his own voice rather loudly and consequently tends to speak quietly.
    b. perception deafness.   (4)_____the patient's voice is apt to be

quite loud since he tries to raise it to the intensity at which he can hear.

(5)_____the patient hears better in a noisy environment.

(6)_____the patient tolerates excessive loudness poorly—he does not like to be shouted at.

(7)_____the patient hears poorly over the telephone.

(8)_____the patient hears well over the telephone.

(9)_____the patient benefits only moderately from a hearing aid.

(10)_____the patient wears a mechanical hearing aid with ease and comfort.

19. Immediate postoperative nursing care of a patient who has had a fenestration operation for otosclerosis would include the following:

a._____Watch the breathing rate carefully, because with heavy postoperative medication it may be low.

b._____Expect nausea, vomiting and vertigo; give any medications which are ordered to alleviate these symptoms.

c._____Allow the patient to turn on his unoperated side so that pressure will be released on the operated side.

d._____Encourage the patient to get out of bed as soon as he recovers from the general anesthetic so that dizziness will be averted.

Questions for Discussion and Student Projects

1. How would you instruct a parent in applying moist heat or dry heat to the ear? List the principles of chemistry and physics involved.

2. Are there any schools for the "deaf and speechless" in your community? Where is the nearest school? How extensive is its program? How is it financed? If you had such a patient in your hospital, what part could you play in getting her enrolled in such a school?

3. Assume that you are a school teacher or school nurse of pre-school and primary-age children. Several children have hearing and speech defects. How would you handle the following problems?

a. The defects are ignored by the parents.
b. Personality, behavior and delinquency problems have resulted.
c. Isolation and withdrawal of some children has been noted.
d. There is evidence of retardation in school work.

4. Investigate 3 or 4 companies who supply hearing aids.

a. For what type of patient do they advocate their product?
b. How does the hearing aid operate?
c. Is it equipment which would be unduly conspicuous when worn?

    d. How expensive is it?

    e. On the average, what are the upkeep costs?

5. Imagine that an aunt, now living with your family, is becoming progressively deaf. As the nurse member of the family, how can you help her, and your family, with the following problems?

    a. Your aunt refuses to accept the handicap.

    b. She seems to be excessively worried.

    c. She has become irritable, unpleasant and sometimes unfair to her friends and relatives.

6. What is the function of the American Society for the Hard of Hearing? (1537 35th St., N.W., Washington, D.C.)

Section 11. Nursing Care of Patients with Disorders of the Female Reproductive System[*]

STUDY SUGGESTIONS: Before beginning the study of this Section, the student will find it helpful to

A. Review
  1. Anatomy and physiology: female reproductive tract.
B. Study
  1. In medical nursing or gynecologic texts: the endocrines (gonad), the menopause.
  2. In pharmacology texts: drugs affecting the reproductive tract, hormones (sex glands).
  3. In surgical or gynecologic nursing texts: surgery of the female reproductive system.
C. Read the additional References listed before attempting to answer questions relating to each patient study.

THE CHILDLESS SCOTSWOMAN

Background Review Questions

1. The female sex gland is the

   a._____uterus.
   b._____ovary.
   c._____ovum.

   d._____corpus luteum.
   e._____graafian follicle.

2. The usual number of sex cells which a female secretes each month is

   a._____not known.
   b._____millions.
   c._____hundreds.

   d._____two.
   e._____one.

3. Ovulation occurs when

   a._____there is a flow of blood from the uterine cavity.
   b._____the ova begins to ripen or mature, enlarging as a sort of cyst.
   c._____the graafian follicle enlarges, ruptures and discharges an ovum into the peritoneal cavity.
   d._____an ovum meets a spermatozoon and union takes place.

4. When a spermatozoon and ovum unite, they form a one-celled individual called a (an)

   a._____embryo.
   b._____zygote.
   c._____fetus.

   d._____morula.
   e._____chromosome.

[*] Additional gynecologic problems are treated in the obstetric nursing section.

5. Match the following:

   a. dysmenorrhea. (1)____appearance of blood between periods or
   b. amenorrhea.   after the menopause.
   c. menorrhagia.   (2)____painful menstruation.
   d. metrorrhagia.   (3)____whitish or yellowish vaginal discharge.
   e. leukorrhea.   (4)____absence of menstrual flow.
                        (5)____excessive bleeding at the time of regular
                              menstrual flow.

6. The purpose of a cytologic test is to detect early

   a.____pregnancy.   d.____involution.
   b.____benign tumor.   e.____carcinoma.
   c.____venereal disease.

7. The advantages of the Papanicolaou test over a biopsy to detect cancer are as follows:

   a.____The type and origin of the cell usually is clear.
   b.____It takes less time to do a microscopic examination than that for biopsy.
   c.____It may show cancer cells in the incipient stage even before a lesion is clinically evident.
   d.____It is less expensive, simple and more convenient to do.
   e.____The grade of malignancy usually is detectable.

8. The most effective area from which to aspirate vaginal secretions is the

   a.____external cervical os.   c.____anterior fornix.
   b.____endocervical canal.   d.____posterior fornix.

9. A method(s) for determining ovulation is (are)

   a.____the vaginal-smear test.   d.____the frog test.
   b.____the Rubin test.   e.____endometrial biopsy.
   c.____charting the daily basal temperature.

10. A Rubin test is a method of

    a.____determining the time of ovulation.
    b.____determining tubal patency.
    c.____detecting early carcinoma.
    d.____detecting fetal heart sounds.
    e.____determining the position of the uterus.

11. The purpose of menstruation is to

    a.____throw off waste products from the uterus; this provides space for a potentially fertilized ovum.
    b.____discharge excess or impure blood which accumulates in the female body monthly.

    c._____rid the uterus of its lining; it was prepared for a fertilized ovum which did not develop.

    d._____expel the unfertilized ovum; if this were not done, the lining of the uterus would become irritated.

12. The gynecologist who is about to do a pelvic examination will need gloves, lubricant and

    a._____double tenaculum forceps, speculum forceps, uterine sound and probe, tampons.

    b._____long dressing forceps, tampons, assorted specula, tenaculum forceps, uterine probe and sound.

    c._____speculum forceps, tenaculum forceps, assorted uterine curets, uterine sound, tampons.

    d._____tenaculum forceps, Hegar dilators, assorted uterine curets, sound probe, tampons.

13. The purpose of glycogen which is present in the vaginal epithelium is to

    a._____lubricate the walls.

    b._____protect from infection.

    c._____decrease the possibility of pregnancy.

    d._____increase the possibility of pregnancy.

14. The amount of glycogen is apt to be low or lacking

    a._____before puberty.

    b._____immediately before menstruation.

    c._____immediately after menstruation.

    d._____during pregnancy.

    e._____after the menopause.

15. Therapeutic purposes of a dilatation and curettage include removal of

    a._____diseased endometrium, to reduce bleeding.

    b._____myomata uteri without abdominal incision.

    c._____postpartum residual placenta.

16. The diagnostic purpose of a dilatation and curettage is to

    a._____obtain endometrial tissue for examination.

    b._____determine the patency of the fallopian tubes.

    c._____determine pregnancy.

17. A dilatation and curettage should be performed in the

    a._____patient's room, no special precautions necessary.

    b._____physician's office or gynecologic clinic.

    c._____operating room, under aseptic conditions.

18. When a patient is placed in lithotomy position on the operating table and given general anesthesia, it is essential that

    a._____shoulder braces be used.

    b._____the patient's arms be restrained.

c.____soft pads such as foam rubber be placed under the flexed knees (which are resting on the angulated table attachment).

d.____the table be tilted to the Trendelenburg position.

e.____the feet be placed in stirrups in such a way that footdrop is prevented.

19. If a single fibroid is enucleated from the uterus, this is called a

a.____myomectomy.
b.____myotomy.
c.____hysterectomy.
d.____myoplasty.
e.____myorrhaphy.

20. Match the following:

Surgical Removal of the

a. subtotal hysterectomy.
b. total hysterectomy.
c. panhysterectomy.
d. vaginal hysterectomy.

(1)____uterus including the cervix.
(2)____uterus including the cervix and the vagina.
(3)____uterus excluding the cervix.
(4)____uterus including the tubes and the ovaries.
(5)____uterus via the cervical canal.
(6)____uterus via the vaginal canal.

21. The possibility of benign myomata of the uterus developing into a sarcoma is

a.____1 per cent. b.____5 per cent. c.____10 per cent. d.____25 per cent. e.____50 per cent.

22. The incidence of myomata uteri is greater in

a.____the white race.
b.____the Negro race.
c.____the 30–40 age group.
d.____the 40–60 age group.
e.____women who have borne children.
f.____women who have never borne children.

THE CHILDLESS SCOTSWOMAN—PATIENT STUDY

The nurses enjoyed Emily MacDundee from the moment she entered the hospital. The petite, 48-year-old wife of a machinist had lived in Scotland for the first 20 years of her life. She still had a delightful Scotch accent, possessed a warm sense of humor and both before and after surgery, while up and about, took care of her own and other patients' flowers, passed out evening nourishment and kept up the morale of the ward with her commonsense and wit.

Mrs. MacDundee's recovery from a subtotal hysterectomy was relatively uneventful. There was a momentary concern when, returning from the operating room, she had symptoms of acute respiratory distress. Her nurse knew how to handle this problem and in a short while Mrs. Mac-Dundee resumed peaceful breathing. During the first few postoperative hours the nurse was concerned about Mrs. MacDundee's inquiries about her children (the couple were childless) and whether they had found cancer.

The patient had some postoperative discomfort from abdominal distention, relieved by Prostigmin, and some difficulty in voiding, necessitating catheterization. Other postoperative orders included Demerol for pain, an oil-retention enema on the second day and a daily douche after the second day.

In spite of the outward show of well-being, the observant nurse recognized that Mrs. MacDundee was cloaking some worry with an air of over-optimism. She recalled the patient's mumblings about "children" and "cancer" while she was coming out of ether.

The nurse checked with the surgeon regarding the microscopic study of the fibroids removed to learn that they were benign. The surgeon said that he did not believe Mrs. MacDundee was really worried about cancer because she had never asked him about it (nor had he specifically told her that the tumor mass was not malignant).

The patient's chart revealed that 3 years ago she had come to the psychiatric clinic because of episodes of depression. There was a record of only two interviews and the comment "good response."

Mrs. MacDundee left the hospital on the ninth day. But her nurse continues to wonder if her helpful patient is having mental problems.

References

Baer, J., Barnett, M., and Myers, N.: Carcinoma of the reproductive organs in women, Am. J. Nursing 49:78, 1949.
McClain, M. E.: Scientific Principles in Nursing, "Treatments of Vaginal Canal," pp. 244–250, Mosby, St. Louis, 1950.
McLaughlin, E.: Nursing care in hysterectomy, Am. J. Nursing 50:295, 1950.
TeLinde, R. W.: Hysterectomy, Am. J. Nursing 50:293, 1950.
Walker, E.: Cytologic test for cancer, Am. J. Nursing 49:43, 1949.

Questions Relating to the Patient Study

1. The respiratory obstruction which Mrs. MacDundee experienced immediately postoperatively was due to the blocking of her airway. This may be caused primarily by

   a._____a relaxation of the muscles of the larynx.
   b.___/__the tongue falling backward.
   c.___✓__a falling back of the lower jaw.
   d._____a high concentration of ether in the respiratory tract.
   e._____a lack of oxygen in the proper concentration.

2. Obvious symptoms of such a respiratory problem are

   a._____extreme flushing of the face.
   b.__✓__choking and irregular respirations.
   c.___/__a drop in blood pressure.
   d.__✓__cyanosis of the skin.
   e._____a marked drop in the pulse rate.

3. Immediate treatment for respiratory obstruction which the nurse can do for patient en route from the operating room is to

    a.✓ push forward on the angle of the lower jaw.
    b.✓ grasp the tongue and pull it forward.
    c.____aspirate secretions with a catheter and suction set-up.
    d.____place an emergency call for the anesthetist (state that a tracheotomy set is necessary).
    e.____administer oxygen therapy.
    f.____administer carbon-dioxide inhalations.

4. The nurse may be successful in getting Mrs. MacDundee to void postoperatively if she

    a.____places a chilled bedpan under the patient.
    b.____lets water fall from a faucet, drop by drop.
    c.____shows her the types of catheters which can be used.
    d.✓ allows warm water to flow over the vulva.
    e.____presses on the lower abdomen of the patient.
    f.✓ lets her run her fingers through water in a basin.

5. The first day postoperatively, Mrs. MacDundee asked for the bedpan frequently and voided a few cubic centimeters each time. The nurse should know that this is indicative of a

    a.____craving for attention and should be disregarded.
    b.____craving for attention and the patient should be pacified.
    c.✓ symptom of bladder distention and the patient should be catheterized.
    d.____symptom of bladder distention but the patient should be encouraged to wait until pain is severe.
    e.____normal result of having been catheterized on the previous day.

6. A serious postoperative complication of hysterectomy, the incidence of which has been reduced by early ambulation, is

    a.____wound evisceration.   c.✓ pulmonary embolus.
    b.____postoperative hernia.   d.____prolapsed uterus.

7. Postoperative pulmonary complications may be prevented by the following technics:

    a.____Report to the surgeon only the most obvious signs of U.R.I. in preoperative patients.
    b.____Place postoperative patients who have had abdominal surgery in an oxygen tent for the first 6 hours.
    c.____Give all surgical postoperative patients CO_2 inhalations for 10 minutes of each hour during the first 12 hours.
    d.✓ Insist that a fresh postoperative patient take 10 deep breaths every hour for the first day, even if he complains of pain.

8. Carbon-dioxide inhalations are given for the purpose of

    a.____depressing rapid respirations.
    b.✓ stimulating respirations during depression.

c.___✓___inhibiting singultus.

d._____preventing pulmonary emboli.

9. The best method when administering CO_2 inhalations is to

a._____place a mask over the nose and mouth of the patient; administer 100 per cent CO_2 for 3 minutes; repeat every 20 minutes if necessary.

b._____insert a nasal oxygen catheter while the CO_2 is flowing freely; leave it in place for 10–15 minutes.

c.___✓___flow carbon dioxide over the face of the patient, holding the delivery tube at least 4 inches above the nose; discontinue if not effective in 3 minutes.

10. Indicate the methods recommended for each type of abdominal distention:

a. gastric dilatation.　　(1)___c___rectal tube.

b. small intestinal　　　(2)_b c_Prostigmine.
   dilatation.　　　　　(3)_a c_turpentine stupes.

c. large intestinal　　　(4)___c___colonic irrigation.
   dilatation.　　　　　(5)___a___Wangensteen suction with Levin tube.

　　　　　　　　　　　(6)_b_Pitressin.

　　　　　　　　　　　(7)___c___small cleansing enema.

　　　　　　　　　　　(8)_b, c_glycerin or oil-retention enema.

11. The following characteristics differentiate the retention enema from the cleansing enema:

a._____The amount of solution used is greater.

b.___✓___The catheter is left in place after the solution is given and clamped.

c._____The fluid is not retained as long.

d.___✓___The size of the catheter is smaller.

e._____The patient may lie on his right side during the inflow of fluid.

12. The vagina is the normal habitat for

a.___✓___rod-shaped gram-positive Döderlein bacilli.

b._____*Staphylococcus albus* and *aureus*.

c._____colon bacillus.

d._____*Streptococcus pyogenes*.

13. Infection in the vagina can be introduced by

a.___✓___drawing toilet tissue toward the front after defecation.

b._____failing to sterilize (by steam under pressure) personal douche equipment before each use.

c._____using a catheter rather than a douche nozzle when taking a douche.

d._____not changing a perineal pad frequently enough during menstruation.

14. When a patient is lying flat in bed with the knees flexed, the proper way of inserting a douche nozzle is to direct it
    a._____into the vagina in a straight path parallel to the bed for a distance of 5 cm.
    b._____upward toward the abdomen for about 3 cm. and then backward.
    c._____downward for about 3 cm. and then backward.

15. The height of the irrigating can or bag determines the amount of pressure of the liquid. Ordinarily, the pressure should not be more than
    a._____½ pound.
    b._____1 pound.
    c._____5 pounds.
    d._____10 pounds.
    e._____14½ pounds.

16. Elevation of an irrigating can to 1 foot creates a pressure of
    a._____¼ pound.
    b._____½ pound.
    c._____2½ pounds.
    d._____5 pounds.

17. Unless otherwise ordered, a hot douche should not exceed a temperature of
    a._____105°. b._____110°. c._____115°. d._____120°. e._____130°.

18. When a vinegar douche is ordered, the following amount of vinegar is added to 2 liters of water:
    a._____1–2 teaspoons.
    b._____30 cc.
    c._____4–6 teaspoons.
    d._____1 cup.
    e._____1 pint.

19. When the surgeon arrives to remove the steel alloy stitches from Mrs. MacDundee's abdominal wound, the nurse will have the following equipment sterile: Sterile gloves and a sterile tray containing alcohol sponges, dressings, and
    a._____plain forceps, scissors, grooved director, hemostat.
    b._____tooth forceps, plain forceps, wire cutters.
    c._____plain forceps, clip remover.
    d._____scalpel, 6 hemostats, scissors, plain forceps, silk sutures, suture needles.

20. Three days postoperatively, Mrs. MacDundee complained of frequent and painful voiding. The nurse noticed that the urine was cloudy. Following urinalysis, a diagnosis of cystitis was made. This infection could have been caused by
    a._____poor surgical technic.
    b._____over-distention of the bladder → injury to the mucous membrane.
    c._____contamination from catheterization.
    d._____either (a) or (b).
    e._____either (b) or (c).

21. The intern ordered soda bicarbonate gr. x t.i.d. The purpose of this was to

    a._____increase thirst, resulting in greater fluid intake.
    b._____alkalize the urine, to decrease irritation.
    c._____act as a mild urinary disinfectant.
    d._____act as a placebo, to satisfy the patient.

22. The attending physician ordered sulfathiazole 1 Gm. q. 4 hours. The sulfonamides are effective in treating infections of the urinary tract because they are

    a._____specific for all organisms.
    b._____excreted in urine and therefore act locally.
    c._____less toxic than the antibiotics.

23. When the sulfathiazole is ordered the nurse should know that the soda bicarbonate should be

    a._____discontinued.
    b._____continued.
    c._____continued only if specifically re-ordered.

24. During the administration of the sulfathiazole, the fluid intake should be

    a._____increased to the patient's tolerance.
    b._____decreased to as little as possible.
    c._____maintained at a specific prescribed level.

25. Toxic symptoms of sulfathiazole related to the urinary tract include

    a._____hematuria.   c._____polyuria.
    b._____oliguria.   d._____tenesmus.

26. A toxic reaction to sulfathiazole which is not common to the sulfonamides is

    a._____a condition resembling "pink eye."
    b._____an urticaria resembling erythema.
    c._____crystals in the urine.
    d._____cyanosis.

Questions for Discussion and Student Projects

1. Mrs. MacDundee had one tube and ovary removed. Will she be able to menstruate? Will she need supplementary hormones? Why?
2. "As soon as fibroids of the uterus are diagnosed, the patient should plan to have a hysterectomy." Discuss the pros and cons of this statement.
3. Although a certain nurse recognized that sometimes warmth is needed to reduce tension which keeps a patient from urinating, she admitted that the application of heat did not always work. She suddenly re-

membered from her course in physics that cold contracts tissue. Thereafter, she always made a practice of chilling her hands with ice and
then placing them directly on the abdomen of a patient who could not
void postoperatively. She rationalized that cold would contract the
bladder muscle and produce urination. Discuss the effectiveness of her
technic.

4. Is the following practice in giving a douche acceptable? Give reasons
for your opinion: After the douche nozzle is inserted, tighten the labial
folds around it as the solution is running into the vagina. This will
enhance the effect of the douche.

5. Why would the nurse anticipate that Mrs. MacDundee will be depressed after her operation? How might the anticipated depression have
been alleviated?

6. How might the nurse get Mrs. MacDundee to express her feelings in
regard to the operation?

7. What are some of the fears that Mrs. MacDundee may have in regard
to the loss of the reproductive organs?

THE BRIDE WHO LONGED FOR BABIES—PATIENT STUDY

Mrs. Martin is 18 years old and a bride of a year. When I first peeked
into the cubicle to which she was assigned in the Admitting Room, I could
see that she was very upset, and was dabbing her eyes furiously in an
attempt to stem the tide of tears that just had to come.

"This has been an upsetting experience for you, hasn't it?" I said. She
bit her lower lip and nodded.

This would be the second abortion for this girl, if it became inevitable.
Just six months before she had lost her first pregnancy. Now with a
"threatened abortion" at 2 months she was doubly upset because she
began to doubt her ability to carry a baby to term.

This pregnancy had been uneventful until this present illness except
for such minor complaints as slight nausea, occasional urinary frequency,
and a white-yellow leukorrhea. Two days ago the patient noted the onset
of a slight amount of red-brown vaginal discharge and mild low backache;
no cramps. When she reported to the out-patient department, she was
advised to go to bed and to take stilbestrol 5 mg. b.i.d., and thyroid gr. i
daily. The bleeding had increased slightly this morning with the passage
of small clots, but no tissue. She had a severe headache and dizziness on
rising, but no fever. A sterile pelvic examination revealed a small amount
of old blood in the vagina. The cervical os was slightly open and oozing
dark bloody mucus. In an attempt to save her pregnancy, the physician
advised hospital admission, bed rest, phenobarbital, stilbestrol, thyroid,
Nembutal and a clear liquid diet.

The physician was not overly optimistic but assured her that losing this
second pregnancy would not mean she could not carry a third to term. At
this juncture, she broke down and cried again and explained that her husband was in the state penitentiary for a term of 2 to 4 years for stealing
and she wanted this baby desperately for it would give her something of
his until he got back.

Questions Relating to the Patient Study

1. The most dangerous time of pregnancy in which spontaneous abortion occurs as incomplete abortion is the

   a.✓___second half of the first trimester.

   b.___first half of the second trimester.

   c.___second half of the second trimester.

   d.___first half of the third trimester.

2. Abortion occurring after the following period of time usually terminates completely:

   a.___first month.

   b.___second month.

   c.✓___first trimester.

   d.___second trimester.

3. Match the following:

   a. threatened
   b. inevitable
   c. complete
   d. incomplete
   e. missed.

   (1)_d__the fetus has died and some of the products of conception have been expelled.

   (2)_b__there are more severe cramps and increased bleeding, associated with passing of chorionic tissue.

   (3)_e__no products of conception have been passed; the uterus still contains the dead fetus.

   (4)_a__a woman who is pregnant complains of slight cramps and scanty bleeding.

   (5)_c__the fetus and chorionic tissue are expelled.

4. After admission to the ward, one of the first procedures which the nurse should do for Mrs. Martin is to

   a.___give her a hot bath for relaxation.

   b.___give her an enema.

   c.___give her a saline douche.

   d.✓___get her into bed and keep her quiet.

Questions for Discussion and Student Projects

1. What are the possible causes of Mrs. Martin's threatened abortion?
2. What can the nurse do to "reassure" such a patient? Be specific.
3. When the nurse was bathing Mrs. Martin the first day, she shied away from soaking her feet in the tub because "it will make my baby come." Was her remark justified? Substantiate your answer.
4. What are some of the reasons why Mrs. Martin may want her baby? Are there any reasons to indicate that she may be ambivalent about wanting her baby?
5. If Mrs. Martin does not abort, what social agencies may be able to help her care for her child while her husband is in prison?
6. Investigate the recent findings on the relationship of hormones to the maintenance of pregnancy. What is stilbestrol? What is the desired reaction of this drug?

Nursing Care of Patients with Other Gynecologic Disorders

References

Ernst, E. C.: Probable trends in the irradiation of carcinoma of the cervix uteri with the improved expanding type of radium applicator, Radiology 52:46, 1949.
Peck, E.: Perineal care, Am. J. Nursing 47:170, 1947.
Pratt, J.: Care of patients with vesicovaginal fistulas, Am. J. Nursing 48:239, 1948.
Williams, M.: Precautions in working with radium, Am. J. Nursing 47:226, 1947.

THE WOMAN WITH CERVICAL CARCINOMA—PATIENT STUDY

Mrs. McNair had radium implanted in her cervix for the treatment of carcinoma. This was done in the operating room. Three capsules containing radium were encased in rubber tubing and inserted in the cervix. An indwelling catheter was inserted and the vagina was packed with gauze. A red card was attached to the patient's chart indicating the time of insertion, the amount of radium used and the time for withdrawal.

Questions Relating to the Patient Study

1. The chief reason for using an indwelling catheter is to

   a._____prevent the patient from contaminating the packing in her vagina.
   b._____prevent the bladder from becoming distended; this may shift the position of the bladder into the path of radium rays.
   c._____keep the bladder collapsed for the comfort of the patient; the presence of radium and packing are uncomfortable enough.
   d._____prevent cystitis from frequent catheterizations which would inevitably be necessary in a patient receiving radiation.

2. Early symptoms of radium sickness are

   a._____temperature elevation, nausea and vomiting, anorexia.
   b._____pallor, a general state of apathy, a drop in temperature.
   c._____itchiness of the vulva, generalized urticaria, headache.
   d._____a burning sensation in the perineal area, pain in the lower abdomen, apprehension.

3. Nursing activities to safeguard the radium are

   a._____to keep all soiled linen in a special hamper in the patient's unit until carefully checked.
   b._____to allow the patient to get out of bed once a day only, to prevent circulatory complications.

    c._____not to allow the patient to move or turn for fear of dislodging the radium.

    d._____to serve a low-residue diet and to encourage the patient to take fluids.

4. Equipment which should be available for the removal of radium includes sterile gloves and long

    a._____scissors, long forceps, speculum, waste basin.

    b._____forceps, packing, waste basin.

    c._____forceps, cervical dilator, long applicator sticks, probe, waste basin.

5. After removal, radium should be

    a._____returned to the Radiology Department uncleaned; they usually have better cleaning facilities there.

    b._____washed in soapy water using long forceps and handling the element behind a lead shield.

    c._____measured and checked by the Radiology Department before the nurse leaves.

    d._____not necessarily checked by the Radiology Department since the doctor checked it at the time he removed it from the patient.

Questions Relating to the Section in General

1. Gonorrhea of the female genital tract can be acquired easily by

    a._____taking a bath after the tub has been used by an infected person.

    b._____sexual contact with an infected person.

    c._____sitting on a contaminated toilet seat or bedpan.

    d._____receiving a douche in a hospital from equipment which was used by an infected person the previous day.

2. A nurse may acquire a venereal disease from a patient by

    a._____handling bedpans without wearing rubber gloves.

    b._____pricking herself with a safety pin which was used to hold a sanitary pad on an infected person.

    c._____handling contaminated dressings with an unprotected tiny cut on her finger.

    d._____taking care of infected patients when she was "run down" and feeling unusually tired.

    e._____splashing a drop of irrigating fluid from the vaginal area into her eye when giving a douche to a patient with gonorrhea.

3. A gynecologic problem is often presented when an infection of Bartholin's gland occurs. These glands are located

    a._____on each side of the vaginal orifice.

    b._____below the bladder encircling the urethra.

    c._____lateral to the ovary on either side.

    d._____below the base of the uterus encircling the cervix.

4. Match the following:

a. *Trichomonas vaginalis.*
(1)_____caused by a yeast infection.
(2)_____caused by a protozoan flagellate.
(3)_____produces small, patchy white membranous areas in the vagina.

b. *Monilia albicans.*
(4)_____produces a white, yellowish or greenish frothy discharge.
(5)_____an organism inhibited in an acid medium provided by such medications as Floraquin
(6)_____treated successfully with applications of 1 per cent aqueous solution of gentian violet

5. Kraurosis vulvae is a disease characterized by marked atrophy of the skin of the vulva.

a. The chief symptom is

(1)_____a burning sensation.
(2)_____a foul-smelling discharge.
(3)_____frequency of urination.
(4)_____pain on defecation or urination.
(5)_____marked itching.

b. The chief danger is that it

(1)_____is often precancerous.
(2)_____is highly infectious.
(3)_____is a social problem because of the foul odor.
(4)_____may cause sterility.
(5)_____produces ulcers.

c. Therapy includes

(1)_____vitamin A.
(2)_____vitamin-B complex.
(3)_____radium.
(4)_____antihistaminics and estrogens.
(5)_____eventually surgery.

6. A downward displacement of the anterior wall toward the vaginal orifice is called

a._____cystocele.
b._____rectocele.
c._____condylomata.
d._____kraurosis.
e._____cystadenoma.

7. A pessary is

a._____a contraceptive device worn in the vaginal canal.
b._____a type of instrument used to dilate the vagina during a D.&C.
c._____a hard rubber instrument worn in the vaginal canal to treat retroversion of the uterus.

8. A repair of a laceration of the cervix is called

a._____colpotomy.
b._____colporrhaphy.
c._____episiotomy.
d._____trachelorrhaphy.
e._____Manchester operation.

Questions for Discussion and Student Projects

1. Miss White, aged 23, was menstruating, and while we were discussing the respective values of pads *vs.* tampons, she shyly asked me "If it were an old wives' tale that there was a membrane across the vagina, and that if a husband found it ruptured in his wife, then he knew that she wasn't a virgin, and that is why tampons ought not to be used until after marriage." How would you answer this girl?
2. "Most patients having symptoms of dysmenorrhea can be cured by taking prescribed perineal exercises." Comment on this statement after discussing the following aspects of dysmenorrhea:

   a. clinical characteristics.
   b. causes.
   c. present accepted methods of treatment.

3. Perineal exercises are often prescribed for postoperative patients to help strengthen muscles. Describe how you would teach a patient to take these exercises effectively.
4. It has been said that applicator swabs of antibiotic and chemotherapeutic jellies eventually will replace all need for vaginal douching. What is the latest information on this in current literature?
5. Is there any way of adjusting "gracefully" to the menopause? Why does one have "hot flashes"?
6. How would you meet the following problems in caring for gynecologic patients?

   a. A patient finds a pelvic examination repulsive and refuses to consent to it.
   b. A tendency on the part of a patient to talk constantly about her marital problems.
   c. A mood swing in a patient from sensitivity and embarrassment regarding any gynecologic treatment or examination to the opposite extreme of complete lack of modesty.
   d. A patient who has a dread of sterilization.
   e. A patient who threatens to leave the hospital because the gynecologist implied that her illness is not so grave as she herself feels it is.

Section 12. Nursing Care in Emergency Situations*

STUDY SUGGESTIONS: Before beginning the study of this Section, the student will find it helpful to

A. Review

1. Emergency situations in each Section of the Guide.
2. In pharmacology texts: The treatment of poisoning.
3. The American Red Cross First Aid Handbook.

B. Read the additional References listed before attempting to answer questions relating to each patient study.

THE DESPONDENT COLLEGE BOY—PATIENT STUDY

Paul Prentice is an attractive 20-year-old college senior. He was brought to the university hospital on Sunday afternoon in a deep coma. The police also brought an empty bottle labeled "phenobarbital gr. 1½" which had been found by his bedside.

Because of his comatose state and the evidence of the empty bottle, the admitting room physician instigated prompt emergency treatment for phenobarbital poisoning.

As soon as Paul's respirations had improved and he had begun to show slight signs of response, he was transferred to the medical ward.

By the second day, Paul had responded enough to tell his story. He seemed eager to talk to the doctors and nurses. Although a good student until this year, Paul had failed several examinations this term. He had planned to become a chemist, but found some of the advanced courses difficult. The failure on examinations at this stage of his education seemed to him to be an unfaceable disgrace. After brooding for several days, he broke into the college office and changed the records. This act, of course, was discovered, and Paul was asked to resign from the university.

For several days Paul brooded, considering suicide as "the only way out." He felt that he had no one to turn to. Although a Roman Catholic, he had not established close contact with a local priest and hesitated to go to the parish for help. The teachings of his religion did make him hesitate, for a while, from taking his own life.

Paul had no close family ties. His mother had died at his birth and Paul had been raised by an aunt. His father, a post-office clerk, had assumed little responsibility, other than financial, for the boy.

On Saturday night Paul attempted to forget his problems by attending

* For other emergency treatment, see eye and ear nursing, musculoskeletal section (fractures), neurologic section (head and spine injuries, convulsions), pediatric section (burns).

an undergraduate party with a casual date. He was unable to shake off his depression, although he drank more than usual in an attempt to cheer up. At 2 A.M. he took his date to her home and returned to the fraternity house greatly depressed. He remembered a bottle of phenobarbital on the bathroom shelf, and suddenly this was the answer. He swallowed as many pills as he could—"probably about 20"—and remembered nothing else until he awakened in the hospital.

Paul's recovery was complicated by the development of bronchopneumonia which responded well to penicillin therapy.

Mr. Prentice was contacted. He visited the boy and spent long hours with the psychiatrist. Paul expressed the feeling that "Dad and I are closer than ever since this episode."

The Catholic priest who visited Paul regularly was able to establish a firm feeling of confidence in the lad. The psychiatrist had the impression that Paul's act was an impulsive attempt brought on by feelings of discouragement and guilt and aggravated by alcohol. He believed that there were no personality disturbances evident at the present time.

In 13 days Paul seemed to be completely recovered and anxious to be discharged. His only difficulty is insomnia, for he has "a lot on his mind." He seems eager to continue to work with his psychiatrist in an attempt to make good. He hopes to return to college next year and is already planning to change to a less-demanding major field of study.

Questions Relating to the Patient Study

1. When the nurse on the medical ward was notified of Paul's admission, she should prepare to have at his bedside
   a._____an airway.   d._____oxygen.
   b._____a tracheotomy set.   e._____oxygen and helium.
   c._____amyl nitrate.

2. The physician would have been able to initiate many life-saving measures even without the evidence of the empty phenobarbital bottle. The outstanding symptom which Paul presented, which would facilitate the choice of an emergency drug, was
   a._____shallow respirations.
   b._____weak, rapid pulse.
   c._____persistent vomiting.
   d._____hectic flush.

3. The drugs which probably would be ordered for immediate emergency treatment for Paul would be
   a._____atropine sulfate.   d._____picrotoxin.
   b._____strychnine.   e._____whisky.
   c._____caffeine sodium benzoate.

4. The most immediate danger to Paul's life that must be averted is
   a._____cerebral edema.   d._____coronary occlusion.
   b._____respiratory failure.   e._____bronchopneumonia.
   c._____convulsions.

5. The drug action desired, to prevent death, is

    a.___✓___stimulation of the respiratory center.
    b._____stimulation of the vagus.
    c._____stimulation of the autonomic nervous system.
    d._____an emetic, to produce vomiting.

6. The characteristic reaction which can be used to distinguish morphine poisoning from phenobarbital poisoning is

    a._____shallow respirations.   c._____coma.
    b.__✓__pin-point pupils.   d._____delirium.

7. The sale of barbiturates is restricted by

    a._____the Harrison Drug Act.
    b.__/__the Federal Food, Drug and Cosmetic Act.
    c.__✓__state or local regulations.
    d._____uniform regulations throughout the state.
    e._____the pharmacists' and druggists' ethical code.

8. Compare the common poisons by completing the following table:

Drug	Symptoms of Over-dosage	Antidote	Emergency Treatment
Atropine sulfate.......			
Barbiturates..........			
Mercuric chloride.....			
Opium...............			
Phenol..............			

Questions for Discussion and Student Projects

1. Suppose that you had found Paul Prentice unconscious in his room. What measures would you have instigated while waiting for the physician or ambulance?
2. Assume that Paul was given all the nursing care recommended for the prevention of bronchopneumonia. Why did this condition develop? Do you believe it could have been prevented?
3. Outline a nursing-care plan for Paul's first evening and second day in the hospital, including

    a. observation for "danger" signals.
    b. suicide precautions.
    c. prevention of complications.
    d. methods of supplying fluids and nourishment.
    e. nursing responsibility for probable medical treatment.
    f. possible emergency procedures.

4. Attempt to visualize Paul's problems as he returns to normal life. How do you think his friends will accept him? If you were one of his college friends, how could your attitude help him?

5. What factors may have been responsible for Paul's college failure? Discuss the desirability of change of one's vocational goals when one discovers that the first choice is not always the suitable one.
6. Discuss the nurse's responsibility in the administration of sedative drugs. What dangers are inherent in the practice of leaving an "h.s. medication" at the bedside for the patient to take if necessary?
7. What precautions are taken with sedative (non-narcotic) drugs in your institution to prevent accessibility of them to personnel? What do you think of the practice of night workers taking sedatives?
8. How is the sale of sedative drugs controlled in your state? How widespread is the use of these drugs without medical supervision? What proportion of suicides and attempted suicides are with the use of sedatives?

SITUATION STUDY I

On an unusually hot summer day, two patients were brought to the emergency room in a state of collapse.

Mr. O'Reilly, the policeman who patrols the area near the hospital, collapsed as he entered the door. His skin was pale and cold and clammy, and his pulse was weak.

Mr. Karsky was brought to the hospital by car from the nearby steel factory. The patient was comatose, the skin hot and dry. His rectal temperature was 105.8°F.

Questions for Discussion and Student Projects

1. Mr. O'Reilly probably is suffering from
   a._____heat exhaustion.
   b._____heat stroke.
   c._____either of the above.

2. Mr. Karsky probably is suffering from
   a._____heat exhaustion.
   b._____heat stroke.
   c._____either of the above.

3. If a choice is necessary, emergency measures will be initiated first for the patient whose condition is most critical. The patient to be treated first is
   a._____Mr. O'Reilly.   b._____Mr. Karsky.

4. Treatment of Mr. Karsky is directed primarily toward
   a._____reduction of body temperature.
   b._____reduction of shock.
   c._____stimulation of the central nervous system.
   d._____replacement of body fluids.

5. Treatment of Mr. O'Reilly is directed primarily toward
   a._____reduction of body temperature.
   b._____reduction of shock.

c.＿＿＿stimulation of the central nervous system.

d.＿＿＿replacement of body fluids.

SITUATION STUDY II

A young motorcyclist while speeding failed to make a curve and collided with the stone wall of a bridge. You have arrived on the scene to find that he is unconscious, lying face down; blood is spurting from a laceration of his occipital scalp. His right leg is deformed with a wide gash visible. Upon further examination, you find that he has a hissing puncture wound of his chest and multiple scattered first- and second-degree burns from the ignited gasoline.

Questions for Discussion and Student Projects

1. After making a rapid general inspection of the victim, in what order would you care for each of the following injuries:

    a.＿＿＿unconsciousness.

    b.＿＿＿bleeding from a lacerated scalp.

    c.＿＿＿a deformed right leg.

    d.＿＿＿a wide gash in the leg.

    e.＿＿＿a hissing wound of the chest.

    f.＿＿＿multiple first- and second-degree burns.

2. A hissing wound of the chest usually means that

    a.＿＿＿the patient is still alive.

    b.＿＿＿the patient is dying.

    c.＿＿＿air is entering the arterioles.

    d.＿＿＿air is escaping from the lung.

    e.＿＿＿air is entering the pleura.

3. The chief danger of any puncture wound is

    a.＿＿＿that the wound will heal from the surface first.

    b.＿＿＿the possibility of developing tetanus.

    c.＿＿＿the danger of concealed hemorrhage.

    d.＿＿＿the likelihood of aerobic growth.

4. If the following articles were available, which should be selected as a tourniquet?

    a.＿＿＿a rope.   d.＿＿＿a man's leather belt (1 inch in width).

    b.＿＿＿a stocking. e.＿＿＿a woman's cotton dress belt (2 inches in

    c.＿＿＿wire.   width).

5. Any tourniquet should be left in place

    a.＿＿＿continuously, until the bleeding can be stopped by some other means.

    b.＿＿＿for 15 to 20 minutes, then loosened and reapplied.

    c.＿＿＿for 2 hours, then loosened.

6. Digital pressure to arteries leading to the head and neck should be applied.

   a._____just in front of the ear, against the skull.
   b._____just in back of the ear, against the skull.
   c._____on both sides of the windpipe, against the backbone.
   d._____about an inch forward from the angle of the jaw.

7. For a gash in the lower leg, a tourniquet should be applied

   a._____at the knee.
   b._____below the knee.
   c._____about a hand's breadth from the groin.

8. In dressing a wound or burn, absorbent cotton

   a._____should never be used because it sticks and is hard to remove.
   b._____is better than a gauze dressing because it is soft and less traumatizing.
   c._____is undesirable because it prevents air exchange.
   d._____is ideal because its thickness can be adjusted easily to meet any need.

9. In the Emergency Ward, the patient will receive tetanus antitoxin. This is used to prevent

   a._____lockjaw.   d._____anaerobic infection.
   b._____gas gangrene.   e._____aerobic infection.
   c._____tetany.

10. Tetanus antitoxin is administered

    a._____subcutaneously. b._____intramuscularly. c._____intravenously.

11. If a victim has had tetanus antitoxin injections and later sustains a "dirty" wound, he should

    a._____receive an additional dose of tetanus antitoxin.
    b._____receive a small booster dose of tetanus toxoid.
    c._____not receive any additional injections since he now has an immunity.

Questions for Discussion and Student Projects—(*Continued*)

1. Should you remove his burned clothing? Why? If yes, how?
2. In the crowd which gathered, someone offered a bottle of whisky to help revive the injured one. Would you administer it to the patient? Why?
3. In what position should he be placed? Why?
4. What initial observations which you might make on approaching the injured motorcyclist would be significant to the physician later? Why?
5. There may be an interval of time before an ambulance arrives. If a basin of warm water, soap and towels are available from a roadside house, would you attempt to clean the wounds of the victim to minimize infection? Why? If yes, how?

Nursing Care in Other Emergency Situations

1. The following materials can create static electricity, therefore, they should not be worn near combustible anesthetic gases:

   a._____sharkskin. d._____nylon.
   b._____cotton. e._____cotton and wool.
   c._____silk.

2. If a thumb is amputated, the tourniquet should be applied

   a._____at the wrist.
   b._____near the elbow.
   c._____about a hand's breadth from the shoulder.

3. In emergency care of a wound with intestine protruding

   a._____do nothing but rush the patient to a physician.
   b._____cover the intestine with a dry clean cloth such as a man's handkerchief.
   c._____cover the intestine with a warm, moist cloth, moistened preferably with a solution of 1 tablespoon of salt to a pint of water.
   d._____push back the intestine with a dry cloth, bandage tightly and call for a physician.

4. A special danger from animal bites is the possibility of

   a._____claustrophobia. b._____hydrophobia. c._____hypochondria.

5. When a dog bites a human, the dog should be

   a._____killed immediately so that others will not be harmed.
   b._____tied to a secure pole so that he has an amount of freedom.
   c._____confined to escape-proof quarters and observed.

6. First-aid for a snake bite consists of

   a._____suction, bandage, immobilization.
   b._____disinfections, dressing, elevation.
   c._____constriction, incision, suction.
   d._____bleeding, irrigation, dressing.

7. Sally Galt swallowed some drain-pipe cleaner. This mixture contains lye. Emergency treatment would be

   a._____gastric lavage.
   b._____any emetic which might be available.
   c._____a drink of diluted lemon or orange juice.
   d._____a drink of soda bicarbonate.

8. Don Roberts, a 4-year-old, was playing in the garden when his father was spraying DDT as an insecticide on his plants. Don had inhaled the spray for a few minutes before his father noticed him. Emergency treatment would include

a._____a tablespoonful of castor oil.
b._____a sedative to control tremors or convulsion.
c._____the ingestion of protein material, such as milk and eggs.
d._____gastric lavage.

Questions for Discussion and Student Projects

1. A young housewife received second-degree burns of her face, arms and chest when the lid of her pressure cooker blew off, causing her to be spattered with hot stew. What first aid would you give to this woman who is about to faint from the intense pain?

2. Tommy Rathbun, a daring 8-year-old, decided to ride his new bicycle down hill with his hands off the handle bars. He was progressing proudly when suddenly his front wheel was jarred by a stone. Tommy was hurled over his bicycle. You rush to help him and find that he is unconscious. Blood is oozing from his left ear; his face is cut and his right arm and leg appear deformed. What first aid will you administer to Tommy?

3. A high wind and rainstorm knocked down a high-tension wire. In an attempt to clear the sidewalk, a highway department man accidentally touched the electric wire and received severe burns of his body when his clothes ignited. The man was not breathing when you arrived. What would you do?

4. Mr. Jackson was sitting in the grandstand watching the Giant-Dodger baseball game when he let out a hoarse cry, had convulsive movements, drooled bloody saliva, and lapsed into unconsciousness. What emergency care should be given to this man? Qualify your suggestions.

5. Imagine you are walking down the street in a residential area when cries of anguish force you to investigate. You discover a housewife who obviously has been washing clothes and is now in agony because her hair has been caught in the wringer of the electric washing machine. You note scalp bleeding and the woman on the verge of unconsciousness. Describe your method of handling the situation.

6. Four-year-old Billy, a newcomer to the housing project by the dock, was fascinated by all the birds. In attempting to capture a sea gull which was sitting on the dock's edge, Billy fell into 3 feet of water. You happened to be near by. After rescuing the youngster, what would you do if he were apneic and unconscious?

7. Prepare a list of safety rules for the following departments in your hospital:

   a. operating rooms.   d. x-ray and laboratories.
   b. dietary.   e. maintenance.
   c. housekeeping.

8. What is meant by red, white, and blue unconsciousness? Give an example of each as well as its emergency treatment.

9. Make a list showing how you would improvise splints and bandages from articles ordinarily found on a man or woman, for the following possible injuries:

a. finger.
b. wrist.
c. head.

d. hip.
e. ankle.

10. Demonstrate the application of the following bandages:

a. a four-tail bandage for the nose.
b. a spiral bandage to cover the end of the finger.
c. a pressure bandage for the palm.
d. a sprained ankle bandage.
e. a shoulder bandage using muslin triangles.

11. Demonstrate the application of a half-ring traction splint using cravat bandages. Assume the victim has a broken hip.
12. Demonstrate two methods of administering artificial respiration. Discuss the advantages of each.

Nursing Care in Mass Disaster

References

Freeman, Ruth: Nursing care following exposure to ionizing radiation, Am. J. Nursing 51:86, 1951.
First Aid Handbook, American Red Cross. 1945.
Medical aspects of atomic weapons, prepared for N.S.R.B. by Dept. of Defense and the U.S. Atomic Energy Commission.
The nurse in civil defense, TM-11-17, published by the Federal Civil Defense Administration.

Background Review Questions

1. The greatest damage from an atomic explosion occurs when the bomb is detonated

a._____in the air.   b._____on the ground.   c._____under water.

2. In an atomic explosion which has occurred on the ground, the greatest damage occurs from

a._____heat.   b._____blast.   c._____radiation.

3. In an atomic explosion occurring under water, the greatest damage occurs from

a._____heat.   b._____blast.   c._____radiation.

4. At the periphery of an area where there has been an atomic blast, there are many injured persons. The rôle of the litter bearer would include the following essential functions:

a._____stop bleeding.
b._____wash and clean wounds.
c._____cover wounds.

f._____tag individuals for location and urgency.
g._____immobilize fractures.

d._____administer fluids by vein.
e._____give sedatives or nar-
    cotics.

h._____remove dirty clothing.
i._____apply petrolatum to burned
    areas.
j._____transport victims.

5. The highest incidence of wounds following an atomic explosion occurs as

   a._____fractures.
   b._____lacerations.
   c._____contusions.

6. Tissue damage resulting from atomic flash burns can be lessened by wearing

   a._____thin, black garments.
   b._____heavy, black garments.
   c._____thin light-colored garments.
   d._____heavy light-colored garments.

7. Factors which can modify the effect of flash burns are

   a._____atmospheric conditions, e.g. humidity.
   b._____thick application of cold cream.
   c._____dark pigment in the skin.
   d._____the angle of incidence of radiant energy.

8. A lethal dose of radiation for the human body is

   a._____60 r (roentgen).
   b._____100 r.
   c._____300 r.
   d._____600 r.
   e._____1,000 r.

9. The typical radiation syndrome experienced by an individual is

   a._____shock reaction → latent period → infection and toxicity → hemorrhage → anemia and malnutrition.
   b._____nausea and vomiting → hemorrhage → toxicity latent period → anemia and malnutrition.
   c._____general malaise → bloody diarrhea → nausea and vomiting → latent period → rapid emaciation.

10. Penetrating ionizing radiation means that every cell in the body receives an equal amount of radiation providing there is no shielding wall. Number the following structures in the order of their sensitivity to radiation (greater to lesser).

   a._____skin.
   b._____intestinal epithelium and germ cells.
   c._____lymphatic system.
   d._____epiphyseal (growing) bone.
   e._____bone marrow.

11. "Nerve gas" which was developed in Germany in World War II is considered one of the major threats in chemical warfare. The symptoms of nerve-gas poisoning are

    a._____pupillary dilatation, occipital headache, malaise, anorexia, excessive thirst, localized convulsions.

    b._____pupillary constriction, dimming of vision, pain in back of the eyeball, intermittent bronchoconstriction with dyspnea, coughing, watery discharge from the nose, circulatory disturbances.

    c._____ipsilateral dilatation of the pupils, reddening and watering of the eyes, pain in the chest, excessive salivation, Cheyne-Stokes respirations.

12. First-aid treatment for a victim of nerve-gas poisoning is the administration of

    a._____morphine sulfate.
    b._____atropine sulfate.
    c._____phenobarbital.
    d._____caffeine sodium benzoate.

Questions for Discussion and Student Projects

1. How should casualties be labeled? Why?
2. What is recommended by the Medical Division of the Federal Civilian Defense Administration as emergency treatment of burns?
3. What is the difference between flash and flame burns? Is there any difference in the treatment of each? If so, what?
4. Discuss the effects of ionizing radiation under the following headings:

    a. as a cause of cancer.
    b. producing baldness in men.
    c. rendering individuals sterile.
    d. producing mentally deficient children in succeeding generations.
    e. changing the color and nature of hair.

5. Following the atomic attack on Hiroshima, statistics point out that a considerable number of patients have developed keloid formation and that many have developed cataracts. Can these developments be avoided? How?
6. Why is meticulous care of wounds of special significance when a victim has also been exposed to radiation?
7. What type of indicator do individuals in your x-ray department wear to show the amount of roentgen exposure? What amount is considered unsafe? What inexpensive indicators are available for common use in the event of a threatened atomic attack?

LET'S BE READY—SITUATION STUDY

The hospital in which you are employed is in a suburban community several miles from a large industrial center. The city has been notified that possible enemy planes have been detected and alerted for possible bombing. Your hospital is alerted to receive casualties.

The following questions relate to the situation study:

1. What facilities are available for the care of the dead, seriously injured and those sustaining minor injuries? Estimate the number of patients who can be evacuated to make room for the disaster victims.
2. What kind of casualties would you expect to receive? What proportion of the total casualties would be expected of each type?
3. Outline the first-aid treatment for each type of casualty which is to be done in the admitting room.
4. Indicate the type of equipment and supplies, including emergency drugs, etc., you will try to have available in large quantities.
5. What responsibilities, other than medical and nursing treatment of injured patients, will need to be delegated to admitting-room personnel?
6. What are the symptoms of radiation sickness? How soon may they be expected to appear? What diagnostic technic may be employed to distinguish radiation sickness from similar symptoms caused by hysteria? Discuss the medical and nursing care of patients with radiation sickness, including the prevention of complications.
7. How long will your hospital personnel need to be "mobilized" for the emergency? For how long a period may you expect to have a large patient census as a result of the disaster?

References

Beyond the Line of Duty, the Nursing Services. (Portfolio), American Red Cross, June 1952.
First Aid Handbook, American Red Cross, 1945.
Handbook for Physicians and Nurses, American Red Cross 1640E, Feb. 1952.
In the Wake of Disaster, American Red Cross 969.
Mass Care in Disaster, American Red Cross 1540.
When Disaster Strikes, American Red Cross 209.

Community Planning for Mass Disaster

1. One of your friends is an active member of a parent-teachers association. The group has been planning a program on civilian defense. How would you answer the following questions?

   a. What training should the housewife and mother plan to take so that she may be most helpful? Where may she receive this training?
   b. What will persons trained in first aid be asked to do in the event of enemy attack?
   c. How can a household plan be designed to be self-sufficient and reasonably safe in the event of an attack?
   d. What information should be included in a program of civilian defense in the schools?

2. Discuss the factors to be taken into consideration in handling the following community problems in the event of an atomic attack:

    a. supervision of first-aid activities.

    b. management of panic-stricken survivors.

    c. radiologic safety including decontamination of persons and clothing.

    d. collection and distribution of blood for transfusion.

    e. treatment of casualties including perhaps 20,000–30,000 burns, a similar number of traumatic injuries, and 5,000–15,000 radiation injuries.

    f. supervision of public health activities including water and food supplies, burial of dead, control of waste.

3. Analyze the statement "the better prepared the citizen is, the less apt he is to 'panic' in the event of enemy attack." What psychologic factors are involved? What would you do with a mildly hysterical uninjured person who appears in the admitting room after a disaster? With a severely hysterical uninjured person?

4. Emotional response in a group of people can be markedly affected by an atomic explosion. Describe mass hysteria and what responses can be expected. How can these reactions be averted or modified?

5. When a large disaster occurs, emergency lodgings must be set up to provide for displaced persons. Outline a program for the nurse assigned to supervise the housing of a group of displaced families assigned to a school building, considering the following problems:

    a. prevention of the spread of disease.

    b. care of ambulatory individuals with chronic diseases such as cardiac, diabetes, etc.

    c. care of gastric upsets, diarrhea, upper respiratory infections, etc.

    d. sanitation problems, because of inadequate or clogged plumbing, insufficient or contaminated water.

    e. care of infants, bathing, provision of formula, diaper laundering, etc.

6. Investigate the program of the nearest chapter of the American Red Cross.

    a. What is the rôle of the A.R.C. in civilian defense? Differentiate this rôle from the one the A.R.C. plays in disaster from natural sources.

    b. What training programs are offered by the local chapter of the A.R.C.? Which of these are being emphasized to meet civilian defense needs?

    c. In what types of disaster does the A.R.C. assume responsibility? What functions does it perform in these disasters? What types of assistance are available to a hospital when a large number of patients are admitted because of a local major disaster?

    d. How does a nurse become enrolled in the Red Cross? In what types of activities may she engage?

Section 13. Nursing Service Problems

STUDY SUGGESTIONS: In the previous Sections you have been concerned with learning to meet the needs of individual patients. This Section is concerned with planning to meet these same needs when you have the responsibility of caring for groups of patients. Before attempting to answer the questions raised in each student project it will be necessary to

A. Review

1. The patient study of each patient in the "assignment."
2. In medical and surgical nursing texts: the nursing care of each patient assigned.

B. Read the additional References listed before attempting to answer the questions relating to the assignment of functions to non-professional workers and the nursing service team.

References

Berger, N., and Johnson, M.: Developing the nursing team at St. Luke's, Chicago, Am. J. Nursing 49: 442, 1949.
Bradenberg, V. C.: Nursing Service Research, Experimental Studies with the Nursing Service Team.
Kuntz, M., and Rogers, M.: Planning assignments for nursing teams, Am. J. Nursing 50:526, 1950.
Strure, M., and Lindblad, A.: Nursing teams in the hospital, Am. J. Nursing 49:5, 1949.
Criteria for the assignment of the nursing aide, (N.L.N.E.), Am. J. Nursing 49:331, 1949.
Practical Nurses and Auxiliary Workers for the Care of the Sick, American Nurses' Association, New York City, 1947.

STUDENT PROJECT I

A. Assume that the beds in the 17-bed men's surgical unit pictured in Figure 1, p. 304 are occupied as follows:

Ward B: occupied by convalescent industrial compensation cases.
Ward A: Bed #1, John Black, 1 week following toe amputation.
Bed #2, unoccupied.
Bed #3, unoccupied.
Bed #4, Mr. Bonoma, glaucoma, third day of hospitalization.
Bed #5, Mr. Smedley, scheduled for tracheotomy this morning.
Bed #6, unoccupied.
Room #1 (single), Patient convalescing from thoracoplasty; to return to the sanatorium this afternoon.

300

Room #2: Bed #1, Mr. Boling, fractured skull, seventh day of hospitalization.

Bed #2, Jim Dougherty, laminectomy, 2 weeks postoperative.

Room #3, Mr. Epstein, fifth day of hospitalization.

Room #4, Jack Donay, admitted from O.R. two nights previously, appendectomy.

You are notified that Jasper Jones is to be transferred from the medical unit following an ileostomy this morning.

Make the best possible placement of the patients, using the following criteria

a. prevention of cross-infection.
b. observation of the patients.
c. economy of nursing care.
d. needs of the patients for socialization or absolute rest.

B. 1. Assume that you are assigned the care of the following patients. You have a nurse's aide to assist you. You are on duty from 8–11 A.M., have classes from 1–3 P.M. and return to the ward from 5–7 P.M. The nurse's aide is on duty from 8–4:30. Make out a detailed plan in sequence indicating how you will allocate the available time to the care of these patients including physical care, treatments and medication, provision for planned teaching, diversional therapy and observation.

2. What duties would you assign to the nurse's aide? What criteria, other than the patient's physical condition and orders, would use in assigning these duties?

3. What responsibility do you have to see that these patients are cared for during your periods at class and off duty?

Patient Assignment:

Mr. Boling, fractured skull, fifth day of hospitalization.
Jim Dougherty, laminectomy, 1 week postoperative.
Jack Donay, appendectomy, third day postoperative.
Mr. Bonoma, glaucoma, third day of hospitalization.
John Black, Buerger's disease, 1 week following toe amputation.

C. 1. You are assigned to evening duty on the male surgical unit. The patients are placed as you planned in A. A graduate staff nurse is in charge of the ward. You are assigned the patients in Ward A and Rooms 3 and 4. Make out a nursing care plan for this evening period, making provision for the nursing aspects listed in B.

2. The graduate staff nurse suggests that you would "save time" by passing all p.r.n. sedatives at one time, leaving the medication on the bedside of those patients who felt they "might not need a sleeping pill." How would you react to this suggestion?

3. The evening supervisor made the following statements: "I have noticed that the nurses who spend the most time in the evening making their patients comfortable finish their work earlier" and

"The best way to judge the work of the evening nurse is to make rounds at 2 A.M." Comment on these statements. Do you agree or disagree?

STUDENT PROJECT II

A. Assume that the beds in the 17-bed men's medical unit pictured in Figure 1, p. 304 are occupied as follows:

Ward A: Bed #1, Mr. Pasha, peptic ulcer, eighth day of hospitalization.

Bed #2, unoccupied.

Bed #3, Mr. John Black, Buerger's disease.

Bed #4, unoccupied.

Bed #5, Mr. Bonoma, glaucoma.

Ward B: Bed #1, convalescent diabetic patient (to be discharged in 3 days).

Bed #2, unoccupied.

Bed #3, unoccupied.

Bed #4, unoccupied.

Bed #5, Mr. Muller, diabetes, third day of hospitalization.

Room #1, Mr. Keith, cardiac failure, third day of hospitalization.

Room #2: Bed #1, Mr. Adams, pneumonia, third day of hospitalization.

Bed #2 unoccupied.

Room #3, Mr. Harris, cerebrovascular accident, fifth day of hospitalization.

Room #4, Jasper Jones, ulcerative colitis, fourth day of hospitalization.

You are notified by the admitting room that Mr. Clark, coronary occlusion, and Mr. Keller, glomerular nephritis, are to be admitted. Make the best possible placement of these patients, using the following criteria:

a. prevention of cross-infection.

b. observation of the patients.

c. economy of nursing care

d. needs of the patients for absolute quiet or social contact.

B. 1. You are a senior student, team leader of a group consisting of yourself, a graduate practical nurse, and a nurse's aide. The patients assigned to your team are:

Mr. Adams, pneumonia, seventh day of hospitalization.

Mr. Muller, diabetic, seventh day of hospitalization.

Mr. Pasha, peptic ulcer, to be discharged in 2 days.

Mr. Keith, cardiac failure, seventh day of hospitalization.

Mr. Jasper Jones ulcerative colitis, eighth day of hospitalization.

Mr. Black, Buerger's disease.

Mr. Clark, coronary occlusion, fourth day of hospitalization.

Mr. Keller, glomerular nephritis, fourth day of hospitalization.

Mr. Gaines (case not described in this guide), uncomplicated diabetes, admitted for control, to be discharged in 3 days.

Make a day's assignment of duties for your team. What is your responsibility for the patients whose care you assign to the non-professional workers? Who should check your plan?

2. If there is a school of practical nurses in your community, investigate their program. What duties assigned to them have not been taught? What nursing functions, which they have been taught, are they not permitted to do in your hospital?

3. How can you, as team leader, plan so that the non-professional worker will be interested? So that her job will be challenging and not routine? What is her attitude toward graduate nurses? Students? Why?

4. How are nurse's aide in your institution prepared for their duties? What duties may be assigned to them?

C. Assume that you are assigned to this medical ward (with the patient census described in A) for the period 11 P.M. to 7 A.M. You have a nurse's aide to assist you. Make out a nursing care plan for your duties and the duties of the nurse's aide, including provision for scheduling (a) observation of patients, (b) treatments and medications, (c) charting and reporting, (d) assigned "housekeeping" functions.

Assume that an emergency occurred which took approximately 2 hours' nursing time. Readjust your original plan to allow for this interruption.

STUDENT PROJECT III

A. The 12-bed unit pictured in Figure 2, p. 304 has 5 double rooms and 2 single rooms. The single rooms have private baths. Medical and surgical women patients are admitted to this unit. Assume that the beds are occupied as follows:

Room #1: Bed A, Janet Tabor, to have surgery for hallux valgus.
           Bed B, unoccupied.
Room #2: Bed A, unoccupied.
           Bed B, Mrs. Allen, tuberculosis, transferred from sanatorium for thoracoplasty.
Room #3: Bed A, Mrs. Archer, pernicious anemia, third day of hospitalization.
           Bed B, Mrs. Miller, to have thyroidectomy in a few days.
Room #4: Bed A, Mary Salvatori, multiple sclerosis, third day of hospitalization.
           Bed B, unoccupied.
Room #5: Patsy Hall, student nurse, hepatitis, admitted 1 week ago.
Room #6: unoccupied.
Room #7: Bed A, unoccupied.
           Bed B, Miss Evans, epilepsy, third day of hospitalization.

The room clerk calls you in the evening and tells you that the following patients are to be admitted:

Miss Andrews, amebic dysentery
Mrs. MacDundee, for hysterectomy.

Miss Flossner, for mouth surgery.
Mrs. Anderson, asthma.

All of the patients have requested private rooms, but have been told that such accommodations may not be available. Which patient(s) would you assign to a private room? In which rooms would you place the others? Would it be necessary to move any of the patients previously admitted to make the best placement? Which ones?

B. Investigate the benefits of the Blue Cross plan. To what extent does it meet the costs of private and semi-private rooms in your hospital? What are the other costs of illness, not met by Blue Cross, for the patients in this unit?

C. How are the costs of a student's hospitalization met in your school? Estimate the approximate cost of Patsy Hall's hospitalization (for this illness).

D. How are private-duty nurses employed? How is their practice controlled? To whom are they responsible? Who would be legally liable if the private-duty nurse made an error?

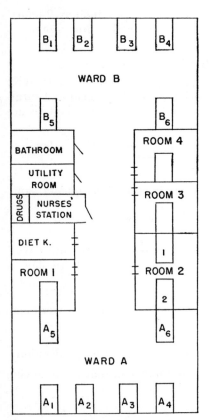

FIG. 1   FIG. 2

Part Two

Nursing Care of Children

Section 1. Nursing Care During Infancy

STUDY SUGGESTIONS: Before beginning the study of this Section, the student
will find it helpful to

A. Review

1. In nutrition texts: nutritional needs of infants (from birth to 18
   months).
2. In orthopedics texts: congenital deformities, the care of casts.
3. In pediatrics texts: (a) child development (from birth to 18 months),
   and (b) nursing procedures for infants: the cleansing enema, the collection of specimens, the administration of fluids, gastric suction, restraints.
4. In pharmacology texts: atropine, aureomycin, codeine sulfate, computing
   dosages.

B. Study

1. In pediatrics texts: the units relating to the nursing care of infants with
   the specific disease condition under consideration.

C. Read the additional References listed before attempting to answer the questions relating to each patient study.

THE TINY BABY WITH PYLORIC STENOSIS—PATIENT STUDY

Dickie Harrison was 3½ weeks old when he was admitted to the pediatric unit. The chief complaint was vomiting and the tentative diagnosis
was pyloric stenosis. Medical history showed that his birth weight was 7
pounds and his present weight was 8 pounds. He had been receiving a
formula of evaporated milk, water and Karo syrup, 2 tablespoonfuls of
orange juice and 5 drops of Oleum Percomorphum daily. The vomiting
had started 5 days previous to admission.

Dickie was given an intravenous infusion of 300 cc. of normal saline
solution through a scalp vein. He was taken in his crib to the x-ray department where a flat plate of his abdomen was made. A small amount of
barium was introduced by gavage into the stomach and a fluoroscopic examination showed definite evidence of pyloric stenosis. The next morning,
Dickie was taken to the operating room for surgical correction of the
defect. He remained in the hospital for a total of 8 days. Mrs. Harrison
was given instruction for his care at home and an appointment to return
with him to the physician's office in 1 week.

Questions Relating to the Patient Study

1. From your knowledge of pyloric stenosis you would expect that Dickie
   developed symptoms of this condition

   a.____gradually over a period of 2 or 3 days.
   b.__✓__gradually with regurgitation of occasional feedings.

c.____abruptly with projectile vomiting as the first symptom.

d.____abruptly at the time orange juice was started.

2. In observing Dickie's behavior before surgery, you would expect him to be

a.___✓__fretful, hungry, easily startled.

b.____drowsy, irritable, thirsty.

c.____comatose, irritable, convulsive.

d.____contented, happy, active.

3. In the early postoperative period as feedings are started, vomiting may be prevented by

a.___✓__holding the baby for feedings, giving feedings by bottle, giving small amounts.

b.____leaving the baby in bed, feeding with a medicine dropper, giving small amounts.

c.____restraining the baby in a blanket, giving feedings by spoon, giving small amounts.

d.____moving baby as little as possible, feeding with a spoon, giving small amounts.

4. In the report from the x-ray department following a flat plate of Dickie's abdomen, you would expect

a.___✓__thickening of the pyloric musculature.

b.____gaseous distention of the lower bowel.

c.____that the position of the stomach appears more nearly horizontal than vertical.

d.____widening of the pyloric lumen.

5. You would expect the report of the fluoroscopic examination with the introduction of barium into the stomach to show

a.____rapid emptying of the stomach.

b.___✓__active, vigorous, peristaltic waves.

c.____relaxed cardiac sphincter.

d.____hypertrophy of the cardiac sphincter.

e.____constriction of the entire stomach.

6. Orange juice was given to Dickie to prevent

a.____rickets.

b.____beriberi.

c.____otitis media.

d.___✓__scurvy.

e.____pellagra.

7. Oleum Percomorphum (a vitamin-D preparation) was given to Dickie to prevent

a.___✓__rickets.

b.____beriberi.

c.____otitis media.

d.____scurvy.

e.____pellagra.

8. Dickie weighed 7 pounds at birth and only 8 pounds at 5 weeks of age when he was released from the hospital. Assuming that he might be expected to weigh around 10 pounds, which one of the formulae shown below comes nearest to filling his caloric requirements?

   a._____evaporated milk   12 ounces
          water   18 ounces
          Karo syrup   1 tablespoonful
   b._____whole milk   21 ounces
          water   7 ounces
          Karo syrup   2 tablespoonfuls
   c._____evaporated milk   18 ounces
          water   12 ounces
          Dextri-Maltose   2 tablespoonfuls

9. When the surgeon talked with Mr. and Mrs. Harrison he told them that

   a._____Dickie could be expected to show gastrointestinal symptoms for the next 2 or 3 years.
   b._____Dickie probably would return to health in another 2 or 3 weeks with no undesirable after effects from the present illness.
   c._____if untreated, Dickie might have lived only a few days.
   d._____other children born to this family will be prone to develop pyloric stenosis.

Questions for Discussion and Student Projects

1. When admitting Dickie to the hospital, what should the nurse do to help the mother feel comfortable about leaving the baby?
2. Prepare a list of the questions you should ask Mrs. Harrison to get the kind of information you would need to give good nursing care to Dickie. How do you think the mother feels when you ask such questions?
3. Describe methods effective in teaching Mrs. Harrison the preparation of artificial feedings. Plan a classroom demonstration on formula making, using home equipment.
4. Assume you are the nurse responsible for Dickie during his hospitalization. Under the general headings "preoperative" and "postoperative" periods show what you think should be included in the nurse's notes. Be prepared to explain your reasons for including each item.
5. List the important points to include when teaching Mrs. Harrison to care for Dickie at home. Include emotional as well as physical care.

Questions Relating to the Section in General

1. Symptoms observed in infants with pyloric stenosis include

   a._____projectile vomiting, diarrhea, visible peristaltic waves.
   b._____bile-stained vomitus, constipation, projectile vomiting.
   c._____dehydration, visible peristaltic waves, diarrhea.
   d._____irritability, hunger, bile-stained vomitus.
   e._____projectile vomiting, visible peristaltic waves, constipation.

2. Pyloric stenosis occurs more frequently in

   a.___males, during the first 4 to 6 months of life, in the white race.
   b.___first born, males, during the first 6 weeks of life.
   c.___females, under the first 2 weeks of life, in the white race.
   d.___all races alike, males, over 6 months of age.
   e.___premature infants, males, in the white race.

3. Symptoms of dehydration in infancy are

   a.___diarrhea, irritability, depressed anterior fontanel.
   b.___constipation, irritability, bulging anterior fontanel.
   c.___loss of weight, depressed anterior fontanel, dry skin.
   d.___dry skin, irritability, diarrhea.

4. The operation for pyloric stenosis is known as the

   a.___Ramstedt-Hollet.
   b.___Fredet-Ramstedt.
   c.___Hand-Schüller.
   d.___Olivier-Fredet.

5. Instructions to mothers are most effective when teaching is

   a.___done by only one person.
   b.___carried on out of the baby's presence.
   c.___spaced over as much time as possible.
   d.___done only under a doctor's order.
   e.___given only as the mother asks questions.

6. In the treatment of pylorospasm, thickened feedings are ordered because

   a.___extra calories are needed in the diet.
   b.___thickened feedings are vomited less readily.
   c.___vitamin B is provided in its natural state.
   d.___the infant's appetite is improved.

7. The purpose of administering atropine solution to an infant with pylorospasm is to

   a.___produce general relaxation.
   b.___reduce the amount of fluid lost by perspiration.
   c.___relax the pyloric sphincter.
   d.___increase the baby's appetite.

8. Atropine is given to the baby

   a.___with his feeding.
   b.___15 or 20 minutes before feeding.
   c.___15 or 20 minutes after feeding.
   d.___1 hour before feeding.
   e.___1 hour after feeding.

9. The dosage of atropine solution is determined by the infant's response. Usually the medication is started by giving 1 drop of 1:1,000 solution or 10 drops of 1:10,000 solution, increasing by 1 drop at each dose until one of the following reactions is observed in the baby:

   a._____pupils are dilated, vomiting is lessened, face is flushed.
   b._____fever is present, pupils are dilated, face is flushed.
   c._____diarrhea is present, pupils are dilated, fever is present.
   d._____face is flushed, fever is present, diarrhea is present.
   e._____vomiting is controlled, baby is constipated, pupils are dilated.

10. Following the above reaction one of the plans listed below is carried out:

    a._____atropine is discontinued.
    b._____the dose is decreased gradually until it is eliminated entirely.
    c._____the dose is decreased gradually and maintained at the dose which controls vomiting but which does not produce flushed face or fever.
    d._____the dose is maintained at the level reached when the reaction was first observed.

11. Atropine solution to be given a small infant should be mixed with

    a._____the formula.
    b._____1 ounce of water.
    c._____1 teaspoonful of orange juice.
    d._____a few drops of water.
    e._____1 teaspoonful of thickened cereal feeding.

12. The most effective method of giving atropine solution to the infant is by

    a._____gavage.
    b._____medicine dropper.
    c._____teaspoon.
    d._____medicine glass.
    e._____nursing bottle.

13. Following surgery for pyloric stenosis, the feedings usually are started about

    a._____12 hours postoperatively, offered at 4-hour intervals.
    b._____12 hours postoperatively, offered at 2-hour intervals.
    c._____24 hours postoperatively, offered at 4-hour intervals.
    d._____24 hours postoperatively, offered at 2-hour intervals.

14. The feeding usually offered in the postoperative period is

    a._____an evaporated milk, water and Karo syrup formula in amounts determined by the infant's caloric needs.
    b._____an evaporated milk, water and Karo syrup formula in amounts determined by the infant's tolerance.
    c._____skim milk in amounts determined by the infant's caloric needs.
    d._____skim milk in amounts determined by the infant's tolerance.

15. The best size of the hole in the nipple is
    a.____large. b.____small. c.____determined by the infant's eagerness.

16. The best feeding "plan" is to
    a.____hold the baby in your arms, stop feeding between each ½ ounce.
    b.____hold the baby in your arms, "bubble" only after the entire feeding.
    c.____leave the baby in the crib, "bubble" only after the entire feeding.
    d.____leave the baby in the crib, stop feeding between each ½ ounce.

17. After the feeding the baby should be placed on his
    a.____right side; defer changing the diaper until his stomach is more nearly empty.
    b.____right side; change the soiled diaper before leaving the baby.
    c.____left side; change the soiled diaper before leaving the baby.
    d.____left side; defer changing the soiled diaper until his stomach is more nearly empty.

Questions for Discussion and Student Projects—(*Continued*)

1. Describe the type of restraint used for a 3-week-old baby receiving fluids by scalp vein. Plan a classroom demonstration using a practice doll to show this method of restraint.
2. In your pediatric unit are mothers permitted to take infants out of cribs? What are the advantages and disadvantages of this activity from the standpoint of the child, the mother and the nurse?
3. In your pediatric unit are parents permitted to make telephone calls directly to the wards? What are the advantages and disadvantages to the parents and to the nurses of such telephone calls?
4. How are parents notified that a surgical procedure is to be carried out? Describe specific ways of giving this type of information and try to anticipate the kind of questions parents might ask. Do you think they should be notified the night before or on the morning of the operation?
5. In your hospital do the parents sign an operative permit? What are the nurse's legal responsibilities in regard to operative permits?
6. Describe the nursing care for an infant with a diagnosis of pylorospasm.

THE 3-MONTH-OLD BABY WITH CLEFT LIP—PATIENT STUDY

You are assigned to a 4-bed unit to which Susie, aged 3 months, has been admitted for repair of a congenital cleft lip, left side. Susie also has a cleft palate. The head nurse has explained to you that surgery is planned for the following day and that you will care for Susie during the postoperative period. From the chart you learn that the parents are from a very low economic level and that Susie is the tenth child in the family. Later, during the afternoon visiting hours, you notice that the mother is thin and pale. She tells you she is too tired to come to see Susie at every visiting hour, but has brought a plastic rattle from the 10-cent store.

Reference

Mitchell-Nelson: Textbook of Pediatrics, ed. 4, p. 570, 1945; ed. 5, p. 765. Philadelphia, Saunders, 1950.

Questions Relating to the Patient Study

1. The incidence of cleft lip and cleft palate is approximately 1 per
    a._____1,000 population.
    b._____100 population.
    c._____5,000 population.
    d._____10,000 population.

2. The age of the infant at the time of surgical repair varies by weeks or months. Some of the factors which determine the proper time for treatment are the
    a._____weight of the infant, the availability of a plastic surgeon, the type of feedings the infant can take.
    b._____presence of other congenital defects, the general condition of the infant, the attitude of the parents.
    c._____age of the infant, past development history, the absence of infection.
    d._____general condition of the infant, the absence of infection, the availability of a plastic surgeon.

3. When feeding Susie during the preoperative period, the most successful methods to follow would be to use
    a._____a medicine dropper, a nipple with a small hole, a small glass.
    b._____a teaspoon, gavage, a bulb syringe.
    c._____a medicine dropper, a nipple with a large hole, a small spoon.
    d._____gavage, a small cup, a medicine dropper.

4. While feeding Susie, the nurse should
    a._____hold the baby on her lap, bubble frequently, take plenty of time.
    b._____leave the baby on the bed, pick her up at the end of the feeding, restrain her arms at the side.
    c._____hold the baby on her lap, restrain her arms, feed her rapidly.
    d._____feed the baby slowly, leave her in bed, leave her arms free.

5. When Susie's mother gives you the plastic rattle you should
    a._____tell her such a toy is not suitable for the baby.
    b._____wash the rattle in soap and water and give it to Susie to hold.
    c._____show her that toys are provided by the hospital.
    d._____wash the rattle in soap and water and tie it to the crib side.
    e._____discard the rattle after the visiting hour.

6. While talking with the mother, she told you that she believed that it was her fault that Susie had this condition. The mother described to

you how she was startled by a rabbit during the sixth month of pregnancy and said she guessed she had "marked" her baby. You should reassure the mother by telling her that

a._____it is old-fashioned to believe babies are "marked" prenatally.
b._____no one understands the cause of cleft lip and palate.
c._____she shouldn't feel guilty about the baby's defect.
d._____the condition was present before the sixth month of pregnancy.

7. Nursing care for Susie in the preoperative period should be directed toward

a._____maintenance of adequate nutrition, a description of the stools, the prevention of infection.
b._____prevention of infection, maintenance of adequate nutrition, picking baby up when she cries.
c._____recording intake and output, maintenance of adequate nutrition, the prevention of infection.
d._____a description of the stools, recording weight, adjustment to feeding technics to be used after surgery.

8. On the day of operation, specific preparation includes

a._____Omit feedings for about 4 hours before surgery, cleanse the nostrils by using cotton swabs moistened with water, cleanse the mouth by giving sterile water after the last feeding.
b._____Omit feedings for about 8 hours before surgery, cleanse the mouth with cotton applicators moistened with boric acid solution, cleanse the nostrils with moistened cotton swabs.
c._____Omit feedings for about 2 hours before surgery, cleanse the nostrils with a cotton applicator moistened with boric acid solution, cleanse the lip and the mouth with a cotton sponge moistened with Zephiran Chloride solution 1:10,000.

9. Upon return from surgery, Susie should be placed in a warm crib in the following position:

a._____arm restraints tied to the bar of the crib side, prone position, foot of the bed elevated.
b._____arm restraints pinned at the sides of the diaper, Fowler's position, no pillow under her head.
c._____arm restraints pinned at the sides of the diaper, baby on her side with a rolled pad at the back, mattress flat.
d._____arm restraints tied to the bar of the crib side, dorsal recumbent position, one pillow under her head.

10. Check those observations of Susie's in the immediate postoperative period which should be reported at once:

a._____pulse rate of 120 beats per minute, dilated pupils, flushed face.
b._____difficulty in breathing, bleeding around the suture line, violent crying.

c.____respiratory rate of 36, pulse rate of 120 beats per minute, failure to urinate.

d.____flushed face, dilated pupils, failure to urinate.

11. Susie's adjustment to hospitalization would be made easier by

   a.____gentle handling, feeding when hungry, providing for soft music in the room.
   b.____removing restraints frequently, leaving in crib at all times, feeding on schedule.
   c.____gentle handling, feeding when hungry, removing restraints frequently.
   d.____feeding on schedule, leaving in crib at all times, placing a small toy in each hand.

Questions for Discussion and Student Projects

A. Related to Patient Study

1. Plan a classroom demonstration using a practice doll to show the care of the suture line as it is carried out in your hospital. Include arm and body restraints as used on a young infant, a Logan Bow or other lip guard if used, and a tray containing the articles necessary to care for the lip while sutures are present.
2. In caring for Susie after operation, how often and under what conditions should you remove the arm restraints? Describe measures to be provided while restraints are off to add to the baby's comforts.
3. What is the responsibility of hospital personnel toward a mother who is pale, thin and too tired to visit her baby? How do you think Susie's care after discharge would be affected by the mother's health? What information would you want about the father and other 9 children when planning for Susie's care at home? What facilities exist in your hospital and community for helping families with health problems?
4. Prepare a plan for teaching Susie's mother to care for her at home following the cleft lip repair, including

   a. feedings at the time of discharge and foods to be added later.
   b. physical care, such as bathing, dressing, care of the hair, sleeping, exercise and play.
   c. personality development, such as avoidance of overprotection while preventing possible exposure to upper respiratory infections, attitudes of the entire family toward cleft palate, the value of handling Susie as near normally as possible.
   d. prevention of disease, such as immunization facilities in the community, vitamins needed daily, avoidance of all communicable diseases.
   e. plan for future health supervision, such as preparation of Susie and entire family for later hospitalization for repair of cleft palate, referral to speech therapist by surgeon, nurse or social worker before Susie begins to talk and use of social agencies for financial help if necessary.

B. Related to Cleft Palate in General

   1. The chief objective of nursing care in the postoperative period in
      cleft lip repair is to assure optimum healing of the suture line. List
      about 6 ways in which this objective is realized, and be prepared to
      explain in detail how your proposed methods should be carried out.
   2. What would be the precautions to protect a child's mouth, while
      removing restraints, for a 6-months-old child, a year-old child, a
      2-year-old child? Suggest appropriate play or toys for each of these
      3 age groups while the arms are restrained, and during free periods.
   3. Assume you are caring for a 4-year-old child in your hospital who
      has had a cleft palate repair. The parents ask you how they can find
      a speech therapist who will work with the child over a long period
      of time. They also need to know the approximate cost of such a
      service. State how you would obtain this information for them.

THE ACUTELY ILL 4-MONTH-OLD INFANT—PATIENT STUDY

Johnnie Keller, a 4-month-old infant, was admitted to the pediatric unit
at midnight. His mother stated that he fell asleep after his 10 P.M. feeding but awakened screaming and vomiting an hour later. The family
physician was called; he advised hospitalization immediately.

A blood count was ordered stat and reported as follows:

Hemoglobin	13.2 Gm. per 100 cc. of blood
Erythrocytes	4,820,000
Leukocytes	17,250
Polys	53
Lymphs	45
Monocytes	22

A urine specimen was obtained for laboratory examination and showed
the following results:

Color	Light yellow
Appearance	Flocculent
Reaction	5.5
Albumen	Trace
Sugar	Negative
Acetone	Negative
Specific gravity	1.020
Casts	Few

A cleansing enema of soap solution was ordered and given by the nurse
on duty. Physical examination by the doctor, observations by the nurse,
and results of laboratory tests established the diagnosis of intussusception
and Johnnie was prepared for surgery.

A preoperative medication of codeine sulfate gr. $\frac{1}{24}$ and atropine sulfate gr. $\frac{1}{600}$ was given. Under ether anesthesia it was found that an upper
segment of the bowel had invaginated into the part distal to it, resulting
in about 1 inch of gangrenous bowel. This was resected and the abdomen
closed.

Postoperative orders were as follows:

Continuous gastric suction
5 per cent glucose in physiological saline solution parenterally—100 cc. q. 4 h. for 5 hours. (Repeat for next 2 days.)
S. R. Penicillin U. 200,000 b.i.d.
Nothing by mouth

On the second postoperative day gastric suction was discontinued; the parenteral fluids were discontinued on the third day. Johnnie was given 5 per cent glucose water 3 ounces every 3 hours by mouth for 12 hours, then offered an evaporated milk formula.

Reference

Gesell, Arnold, and Ilg, Frances: The Infant and Child in the Culture of To-day, pp. 100–107, New York, Harpers, 1943.

Questions Relating to the Patient Study

1. Nurse's notes most helpful to Johnnie's physician in making a diagnosis of intussusception include the

   a.———position the child assumes in bed, the past feeding history, the description of stools.
   b.———response to being picked up, the description of stools, the description of vomiting.
   c.———record of fluid intake and output, the record of hourly temperature, pulse and respiration, the position the child assumes in bed.
   d.———description of stools, the position the child assumes in bed, the frequency and amount of vomiting.

2. Abdominal pain was suspected in this baby because he

   a.———drew his knees up toward his abdomen.
   b.———cried violently when handled.
   c.———rolled his body from side to side.
   d.———refused all attempts at feeding.

3. In giving an enema to Johnnie the following points of procedure should be observed:

   a.———child resting on back, use size 10 French catheter, give about 500 cc. of solution.
   b.———child resting on left side, use size 10 French catheter, give about 200 cc. of solution.
   c.———child resting on right side, use size 14 French catheter, give about 300 cc. of solution.
   d.———child resting on back, use size 10 French catheter, give about 300 cc. of solution.

4. You would expect results from the cleansing enema given Johnnie to show

    a._____a large amount of soft formed stool.
    b._____no fecal material.
    c._____a small amount of fecal material with blood-tinged mucus.
    d._____a small amount of green watery stool.

5. In case the mother asks you to tell her what caused Johnnie's sudden illness, you would tell her that

    a._____she may have fed him too much or too rapidly.
    b._____she should ask her physician to answer this question.
    c._____the cause of this condition is not clearly understood.
    d._____you will give her some literature to read on the subject.

Questions for Discussion and Student Projects

1. Describe ways in which you would give kind, sympathetic nursing care to Johnnie while he is restrained for parenteral fluids and gastric suction.
2. Suppose Mrs. Keller is permitted to remain with Johnnie most of the time. Would you ask her to leave the room when intramuscular injections are given? How would you answer her questions concerning the purpose of gastric suction?
3. Prepare a written nursing care plan for Johnnie during the postoperative period. Include information you would wish to give to the nurse caring for Johnnie while you are off duty.
4. Do you think that Johnnie should be referred to the Visiting Nurse Association when he is ready to go home? If so, what information should you include on the referral form?

Questions Relating to the Section in General

1. Intussusception occurs most frequently in

    a._____males, between 2 and 6 months of age, healthy babies.
    b._____males, over 1 year of age, undernourished babies.
    c._____males, under 1 year of age, healthy babies.
    d._____females, under 1 year of age, healthy babies.
    e._____females, over 1 year of age, undernourished babies.

2. Outstanding symptoms of intussusception are

    a._____abdominal pain, vomiting, blood in stools.
    b._____vomiting, elevation of temperature, abdominal pain.
    c._____blood in stools, diarrhea, elevation of temperature.
    d._____abdominal pain, constipation, vomiting.
    e._____elevation of temperature, restlessness, prostration.

3. From the laboratory values given below underline those you consider to be nearest normal for small children:

a. Blood:

   (1)____erythrocytes per cubic millimeter:____4,100,000;____
      4,440,000;____4,680,000.

   (2)____leukocytes per cubic millimeter:____18,000;____9,000;
      ____14,000.

   (3)____Hemoglobin expressed in grams per 100 cc. of blood:____
      12.8;____16.1;____14.5.

b. Urine:

   (1)____Reaction   ____6.0   ____4.0   ____8.5
   (2)____Specific gravity   ____1.010   ____1.001   ____1.035
   (3)____Casts   ____many   ____few   ____none

4. The prognosis in intussusception may be described as

  a.____generally poor.
  b.____excellent if reduction is accomplished during the first 12 hours.
  c.____always fatal.
  d.____generally favorable if surgery is performed on the second day following the onset of symptoms.

5. Intussusception occurs more frequently in infants than in adults because of

  a.____lack of roughage in the diet.
  b.____swallowing of air during feedings.
  c.____hypermobility of the lower intestinal tract.
  d.____frequent feedings.

6. Areas in the intestinal tract most commonly affected are

  a.____the small intestine.
  b.____the ileocecal junction.
  c.____the colon.
  d.____all part of the intestinal tract equally affected.

7. The average dose of codeine for a 4-month-old infant is

  a.____$\frac{1}{2}$ grain.
  b.____$\frac{1}{24}$ grain.
  c.____$\frac{1}{4}$ grain.
  d.____$\frac{1}{8}$ grain.

8. The average dose of atropine for a 4-month-old infant is

  a.____$\frac{1}{600}$ grain.
  b.____$\frac{1}{300}$ grain.
  c.____$\frac{1}{150}$ grain.
  d.____$\frac{1}{250}$ grain.

9. Match the following table of apothecary measures to their metric equivalents:

   (1)____1 grain.   a. 0.6 mg.
   (2)____5 grains.   b. 30 mg.

(3)_____15 grains.   c. 0.06 Gm.
(4)_____¾ grain.   d. 0.2 mg.
(5)_____½ grain.   e. 0.3 Gm.
(6)_____¼ grain.   f. 1 Gm.
(7)_____⅛ grain.   g. 15 mg.
(8)_____1/100 grain.   h. 0.06 mg.
(9)_____1/300 grain.   i. 45 mg.
(10)_____1/600 grain.   j. 8 mg.
(11)_____1/1000 grain.   k. 12 mg.
                                    l. 0.25 mg.
                                    m. 0.1 mg.

[Questions 10, 11, 12 and 13 have more than one correct response.]

10. At 4 months the average baby

  a._____recognizes his mother by sight.
  b._____shifts a toy from one hand to the other.
  c._____coos, babbles, laughs aloud.
  d._____shows fear of strangers.
  e._____picks up small objects with his fingers.

11. Sleep habits of the 4-month-old infant are described as:

  a._____sleeps approximately 12 hours at night (6 P.M. to 6 A.M.).
  b._____remains awake all morning.
  c._____takes a short morning nap and a longer afternoon nap.
  d._____cries loudly for a feeding upon awakening.
  e._____plays alone for 10 or 15 minutes upon awakening before he
         fusses to eat.

12. Feeding characteristics at 4 months are as follows:

  a._____there are usually from 3 to 5 feedings per day.
  b._____solid foods are rejected unless placed on the back of the tongue.
  c._____there is no discrimination of foods by taste.
  d._____sucking demand is very strong.
  e._____the average fluid intake per day is about 50 ounces.

13. Socially the 4-month-old infant

  a._____shows an awareness of other children.
  b._____prefers solitary play.
  c._____tends to demand social stimulation at the end of the day.
  d._____prefers his own crib to his carriage.
  e._____cries when people leave him.

Questions for Discussion and Student Projects—*(Continued)*

1. Consider how you should advise parents in the home who resist early
   medical care when the diagnosis is possible intussusception.
2. Suppose you are ordered to administer codeine sulfate gr. 1/24 and you
   have on hand codeine sulfate tablets gr. ⅛. How is the dose calculated

and prepared? Solve the same problem for atropine sulfate using a tablet of gr. $\frac{1}{100}$ to obtain the desired dose of gr. $\frac{1}{600}$. What is the total amount of solution you should give hypodermically to a 4-month-old infant?

3. Prepare a list of foods suitable for a healthy 4-month-old baby and plan a menu showing the time of day certain foods should be offered.

THE 5-MONTH-OLD BABY WITH ECZEMA—PATIENT STUDY

Margaret Green was taken to the family physician at 5 months of age for a routine check-up. She was found to be in good health and her first injection of Tri-Immunol was given. Three weeks later Mrs. Green returned with Margaret to the doctor stating that during the past week the baby had developed a rash over her face, arms and legs and for the past 3 days had had a fever of 102 degrees F. Since Mrs. Green was very distressed about the condition, the doctor advised hospitalization and Margaret was admitted to a Children's Hospital the next day. Admission orders were as follows:

1. C.B.C. and differential.
2. Nasal smear for eosinophils.
3. Elixir Luminal gtt. xv q. 4 h. p.r.n.
4. Nothing by mouth for 12 hours, then glucose water 2½ per cent, offer 1 ounce q. 2 h.
5. Omit soap and water, cleanse daily and as necessary with mineral oil.
6. Restrain arms if child is scratching.

In obtaining the history, the resident found that Margaret's father had been given a medical discharge from the Army because he was allergic to wool, breaking out in blisters every place it touched his skin.

The following day the baby's skin lesions had become more moist and had extended to the chest and back. Continuous wet dressings of normal saline solution were used for the next 3 days. Crystalline vitamins in aqueous solution were started and a Mulsoy formula 6 ounces was offered every 3 hours. When the wet dressings were discontinued, coal tar ointment was applied daily to the lesions. Rapid progress was made and at the end of Margaret's tenth hospital day restraints were removed and she was playing happily.

Six weeks had passed since the first injection of Tri-Immunol and the doctor gave her a second dose of 0.5 cc. During the next 24 hours the skin lesions reappeared and it was necessary to repeat the procedures as for the first 10 days.

Total hospitalization continued over a period of 21 days. Margaret was discharged with the following orders:

1. Use mineral oil for cleansing, no soap or water.
2. Multi-vitamin preparation in aqueous solution.
3. Infant soft diet, omitting wheat, eggs, orange, and substituting Mulsoy for milk.

The head nurse instructed Mrs. Green in the care of Margaret at home and sent a referral to the Visiting Nurse Association.

References

Cooke, Robert A.: Allergy in Theory and Practice, Philadelphia, Saunders, 1947.

Gesell, Arnold, and Ilg, Frances: The Infant and Child in the Culture of Today, pp. 108–115, New York, Harpers, 1943.

Lofthouse, Eleanor M.: Infantile eczema, Am. J. Nursing 49:500, 1949.

Questions Relating to the Patient Study

1. Tri-Immunol was given to Margaret to prevent

   a._____diphtheria, tetanus, pertussis
   b._____tetanus, smallpox, pertussis.
   c._____pertussis, typhoid, diphtheria.
   d._____diphtheria, typhoid, tetanus.
   e._____pertussis, diphtheria, scarlet fever.

2. The nursing care for Margaret was directed primarily toward

   a._____maintaining adequate nutrition.
   b._____keeping the baby contented.
   c._____preventing upper respiratory infections.
   d._____applying ointments to lesions.
   e._____preventing skin infections.

3. The nurse responsible for feeding Margaret during the acute phase should

   a._____leave her in bed, remove both arm splints, feed quickly.
   b._____remove both arm splints, hold the baby on her lap, feed slowly.
   c._____remove one arm splint, hold the baby on her lap, feed slowly.
   d._____hold the baby on her lap, feed quickly, leave both arm splints on the baby's arms.

4. Crystalline vitamins in aqueous solution rather than in the usual oily base were ordered for Margaret because there

   a._____is a tendency for oils to produce diarrhea.
   b._____is more rapid assimilation of the aqueous solution.
   c._____is less danger of aspiration of oil into the lungs while the infant is restrained.
   d._____are fewer ingredients to which the baby might be sensitive.

5. Daily vitamin requirements for Margaret at the age of 6 months are

   a._____vitamin C 100 mg., vitamin D 500 I.U., vitamin A 1,000 I.U.
   b._____vitamin C 50 mg., vitamin D 800 I.U., vitamin A 5,000 I.U.
   c._____vitamin C 150 mg., vitamin D 1,500 I.U., vitamin A 2,000 I.U.
   d._____vitamin C 15 mg., vitamin D 100 I.U., vitamin A 5,000 I.U.
   e._____vitamin C 50 mg., vitamin D 500 I.U., vitamin A 3,000 I.U.

6. Margaret probably will

   a._____have chronic eczema but no other allergic conditions.
   b._____have chronic eczema and other allergic conditions.

c._____recover completely from eczema but have other allergic conditions later.

d._____recover from eczema and have no later allergic conditions.

Questions for Discussion and Student Projects

1. What should you do about physician's orders which seem contradictory, as those for Margaret: nothing by mouth and elixir Luminal gtt. xv p.r.n.?

2. Describe ways in which you should plan for Margaret's physical comfort while wet dressings are used. How will she be kept warm? How often is the normal saline solution reapplied? How often are the dressings changed completely? What method is used to maintain dressings in place if ordered for cheeks and/or scalp? What protection is used over the mattress?

3. Describe Margaret's emotional needs while restrained. How often and at what times may restraints be removed? Do you think that the mother should be encouraged to pick Margaret up and hold her during visiting hours? What toys are appropriate for Margaret to look at and to hold? Do you believe that the nurse caring for Margaret is justified in using additional time talking and singing to her?

4. In using coal tar ointment, what measures should you take to conserve hospital linens? Do you feel less inclined to pick up babies and hold them for feedings when coal tar ointment is used?

5. In view of the father's allergy to wool, would you expect Margaret to show a similar sensitivity? If so, what adjustments should you make in her nursing care?

6. Discuss the importance of continuing the immunization program for Margaret. Would the third dose of Tri-Immunol be essential for her protection?

7. Prepare a daily diet for Margaret at home based on the discharge instructions. Estimate the cost per day, including a multi-vitamin preparation in aqueous solution and the Mulsoy formula (or similar milk substitute used in your community).

8. Prepare a summary of instructions you think should be given to Mrs. Green for Margaret's care at home. When should such teaching be started during the hospitalization period?

9. In order to secure completely satisfactory care of this baby in the home, what information about her and the family should you include when making referral to the Visiting Nurse Association?

Questions Relating to the Section in General

1. The type of skin lesion which produces the moist or weeping phase of eczema is the

a._____macule.

b._____papule.

c._____vesicle.

d._____pustule.

2. While infants may be allergic to a variety of substances, the most common offenders in infantile eczema are

  a._____eggs, milk, wheat cereals.
  b._____fruits, eggs, chocolate.
  c._____woolens, house dust, dander.
  d._____cottons, soaps, powders.

3. Eczematous lesions most commonly occur on the infant's

  a._____abdomen, cheeks, scalp.
  b._____cheeks, forehead, flexor surfaces of the arms and the legs.
  c._____buttocks, abdomen, scalp.
  d._____elbows, knees, back.

4. Skin testing is rarely done in infantile eczema because infants

  a._____are usually sensitive to foods only.
  b._____tend to show positive reactions to all skin testing.
  c._____tend to show negative reactions to all skin testing.
  d._____with a history of allergy in the family may show positive reactions to allergens though they never show clinical manifestations.

5. In a family in which both parents have some form of allergy, of 4 children you would expect allergic manifestation in

  a._____2 of the children.
  b._____all of the children.
  c._____3 of the children.
  d._____none of the children.

6. Eosinophils are blood cells of the leukocyte series. Underline the correct response.

  a._____the normal range is 2–5, 6–9, 15–20 per cent.
  b._____the number of eosinophils is increased in allergic states, in pneumonia, in peritonitis.

7. From the following list, check the methods effective in preventing or delaying symptoms of allergy in infants having a family history of allergy:

  a._____introducing new foods gradually.
  b._____giving very small amounts of new foods.
  c._____leaving the infant alone as much as possible.
  d._____removing substances known to produce allergic manifestations in the parents.
  e._____providing sincere love for and acceptance of the child.
  f._____withholding all vitamin preparations.
  g._____delaying immunization procedures.

8. Infantile eczema is more common in

  a._____breast-fed, overweight babies.
  b._____bottle-fed, overweight babies.

c.____bottle-fed, underweight babies.
d.____breast-fed, underweight babies.

9. Exposure to strong sunlight tends to

    a.____produce resistance to eczema.
    b.____improve the lesions of eczema.
    c.____produce eczema in infants disposed to the condition.
    d.____have no effect on eczema.

10. In the treatment of eczema, the antihistamine drugs have been shown to be

    a.____useful.   b.____of little value.   c.____detrimental.

[Questions 11, 12, 13 and 14 have more than one correct response.]

11. At 6 months the average baby

    a.____holds his head erect.
    b.____shifts a toy from one hand to the other.
    c.____picks up small objects with his fingers.
    d.____prefers toys which do not make noise.
    e.____pushes with his feet when held in a standing position.

12. Sleep habits of the 6-month-old infant are as follows:

    a.____sleeps approximately 12 hours at night (6 P.M. to 6 A.M.).
    b.____cries when put to bed for the afternoon nap.
    c.____shows a desire to be rocked to sleep at night.
    d.____awakens in a happy frame of mind from his naps.
    e.____needs a cuddly toy in his crib while sleeping.

13. Feeding characteristics at 6 months are as follows:

    a.____prefers solid foods to milk preparations.
    b.____expresses impatience to be fed.
    c.____takes liquids from a cup or glass.
    d.____develops dislikes for many foods.
    e.____eats better alone than at the family table.

14. Socially the 6-month-old infant

    a.____plays happily alone for 20 to 30 minutes at a time.
    b.____shows no awareness of strangers.
    c.____enjoys splashing in tub while being bathed.
    d.____cries easily when taken for a stroll in his carriage.
    e.____responds to more than one person at a time.

Questions for Discussion and Student Projects—(*Continued*)

1. What is the nurse's responsibility in relation to an order for a nasal smear? What report would you expect from the laboratory?
2. How do you think a mother feels toward her baby who has weeping, itching skin lesions and who is fretful much of the time?

3. Prepare a report for class (suggested assignment for one student) giving the names and ingredients of various commercially prepared foods used for infants with allergic conditions.

THE 9-MONTH-OLD BABY WITH DIARRHEA—PATIENT STUDY

One hot summer day a public health nurse was called to the home to see Shirley Mae, a 9-month-old infant. The mother told the nurse that the baby had been vomiting and having large watery stools for the past 24 hours. The nurse conferred with the mother, then reported her observations to the family physician, who advised hospitalization.

Shirley Mae was admitted to the pediatric ward of a general hospital on the same day. Her admission orders were:

1. Nothing by mouth.
2. 500 cc. of 2½ per cent glucose solution subcutaneously.
3. C. B. C. and differential.
4. CO_2 combining power.
5. Agglutinations for typhoid and paratyphoid.
6. Stool specimen to laboratory for culture.
7. Urinalysis.
8. Vollmer patch test.
9. Penicillin 400,000 units daily.
10. Record intake and output.
11. Bedside isolation.

Liquid stools continued over a period of 5 days. Vomiting decreased markedly on the second day and Shirley Mae was permitted 1 ounce of 5 per cent dextrose solution by mouth every hour when awake. Intravenous fluids were given each day until the stools became more nearly normal. A total of 1,000 cc. of either 5 per cent glucose and water or 5 per cent glucose in normal saline was given daily through an open vein in the ankle. The stool culture was reported to be negative for infectious organisms and agglutinations were negative for typhoid and paratyphoid.

At the end of 5 days, Shirley Mae's orders were changed as follows:

1. Discontinue I.V. fluids.
2. Discontinue penicillin units 400,000 daily.
3. Offer boiled skimmed milk ounces 6 q.4 h.
4. Multi-vitamins in aqueous solution.
5. Aureomycin 50 mg. q.4 h.
6. Sterile water as tolerated in addition to 5 per cent dextrose solution.
7. C. B. C. and Hgm.
8. If red count below 4,000,000, type for blood transfusion.

Shirley Mae retained fluids and medications by mouth and on the following day whole milk and gelatin were added to her diet. The laboratory examination showed a red blood count of 3,900,000 and hemoglobin of 51 per cent. A transfusion of 500 cc. of whole blood was given and Shirley Mae was discharged on the tenth day.

Discharge orders were:

1. Return gradually to infant diet.
2. Provide for daily afternoon nap and at least 10 hours' sleep at night.
3. A.B.D.E.C. drops 10 daily.
4. Return to family physician in 1 week.

The head nurse sent a referral form to the Visiting Nurse Association and called the agency by telephone to tell them the day that Shirley Mae would be home.

References

Clifford, Martha L.: Well babies and hot weather, Am. J. Nursing 50:459, 1950.

Gesell, Arnold, and Ilg, Frances: The Infant and Child in the Culture of Today, pp. 116–140, New York, Harpers, 1943.

Jeans, Phillip, Rand, Winifred, and Blake, Florence: Essentials of Pediatrics, ed. 4, pp. 540–46, Philadelphia, Lippincott, 1946.

Mitchell-Nelson: Textbook of Pediatrics, ed. 4, pp. 611–616, 1945; ed. 5, pp. 808–814, 1950; Philadelphia, Saunders.

Background Review Questions

1. Match the descriptive phrase from the column on the right with its corresponding term in the column on the left:

    a._____hemoconcentration.
    b._____cations.
    c._____anions.
    d._____parenteral.
    e._____enteral.
    f._____anhydremia.
    g._____salmonella.

    (1) elements which maintain alkaline stability.
    (2) elements which maintain acidity.
    (3) decrease in water content of the blood.
    (4) decrease of red blood cells in the total blood volume.
    (5) outside the gastrointestinal tract.
    (6) pertaining to the intestinal tract.
    (7) a species of organisms causing gastrointestinal infections.
    (8) increase in red blood cells in the total blood volume.

2. The column on the left shows the names of veins through which fluids may be administered to infants. Match the location of these veins from the column on the right with the corresponding name in the column on the left:

    a._____popliteal.
    b._____internal saphenous.
    c._____median cephalic.
    d._____longitudinal sinus.
    e._____femoral.
    f._____external jugular.

    (1) inner aspect of the ankle.
    (2) inner aspect of the elbow.
    (3) in the area of the anterior fontanel.
    (4) in the anterior surface of the groin.
    (5) lateral surface of the neck.
    (6) posterior aspect of the knee.
    (7) outer aspect of the ankle.

Questions Relating to the Patient Study

1. Shirley Mae's mother asked the public health nurse how diarrhea might be prevented. The nurse should have told her to

   a._____keep the baby out of circulating air.
   b._____give 2 or 3 times the usual amount of water.
   c._____add salt to the formula.
   d._____add carbohydrates to the diet.

2. The nurse gave the following advice regarding the clothing Shirley Mae should wear on very warm days:

   a._____a diaper is sufficient.
   b._____a flannelette gown should be used in addition to the diaper.
   c._____cotton stockings, gown and diaper are necessary.
   d._____light-weight wool and cotton shirt and diaper are necessary.

3. The purpose of the bedside isolation order was to

   a._____protect Shirley Mae from other infections.
   b._____prevent illness among hospital personnel.
   c._____prevent the spread of diarrhea to other patients.
   d._____prevent contamination of hospital linens used in the pediatric unit.

4. Isolation technics indicated by the nature of Shirley Mae's illness include

   a._____use of isolation gown while giving care, handwashing.
   b._____boiling all articles used in the room, soaking diapers in 5 per cent Lysol solution.
   c._____handwashing, wearing of face mask.
   d._____wearing of rubber gloves while giving care, restriction of all visitors.

5. Penicillin was given to Shirley Mae

   a._____to treat the diarrhea.
   b._____to prevent infection from hospital sources.
   c._____to combat infection already present.
   d._____since oral antibiotics were contraindicated because of vomiting.

6. Aureomycin was ordered later because

   a._____it is beneficial in the treatment of viral infections.
   b._____intramuscular injections are disturbing to an infant.
   c._____infants do not become allergic to aureomycin.
   d._____it combats infection in the intestinal tract.

7. Skimmed milk was ordered for Shirley Mae because

   a._____vomiting may be caused by whole milk.
   b._____fats are not well tolerated in diarrhea.
   c._____skimmed milk has a higher protein content than whole milk.
   d._____skimmed milk has a low sugar content.

8. You would expect Shirley Mae to show signs of discomfort during the acute phase due to increased peristalsis. Such signs include

   a._____fretfulness, sleep disturbances, irritability.
   b._____violent crying, holding the hands over the abdomen, irritability.
   c._____finger sucking, a weak fretful cry, sleep disturbances.
   d._____violent crying, sleep disturbances, thumb sucking.

9. Shirley Mae's abdominal discomfort may be relieved by placing her on her abdomen over a hot-water bottle at a temperature of

   a._____115°.
   b._____95°.
   c._____120°.
   d._____105°.

10. Measures recommended to prevent excoriated buttocks while Shirley Mae was in the hospital are to

    a._____change the diaper frequently, cleanse the buttocks with oil.
    b._____bathe the buttocks frequently with soap and water, apply dusting powder after each stool.
    c._____change the diaper frequently, cleanse the buttocks with 70 per cent alcohol.
    d._____use cotton padding inside the diaper, cleanse the buttocks with oil.

Questions for Discussion and Student Projects

1. Suppose you are the public health nurse who is called to visit Shirley Mae in the home before hospitalization. Describe how you would answer the mother when she asks you these questions:

   a. What should I give the baby to eat or to drink?
   b. Should I give her orange juice and cod-liver oil today?
   c. How about giving her a dose of paregoric?
   d. A neighbor told me to give the baby a dose of milk of magnesia to get rid of whatever is causing this trouble. Do you think I should give it?
   e. Is there any danger of the other children catching this from Shirley Mae?

   In reporting your observations to the physician, what specifically would you include as to Shirley Mae's symptoms? Describe how you would explain to the mother the value of hospitalization. What information would you include when preparing a referral form for hospital personnel?

2. Describe your plan of nursing care for Shirley Mae in the hospital including

   a. Special nursing measures:
      (1) care of the skin, especially excoriated buttocks.
      (2) types of restraints used during administration of fluids parenterally.

   (3) method of maintaining a record of intake and output.
   (4) position of the infant in bed for maximum comfort and prevention of orthopedic deformities.
   (5) technics indicated by order for bedside isolation.

b. Nursing observations, especially in relation to:

   (1) stools.
   (2) behavior, such as irritability, stupor and response to adults.
   (3) type of pulse and respirations.
   (4) color of skin.
   (5) signs of dehydration.

c. Relationships with her mother:

   (1) explanation of Shirley Mae's daily progress.
   (2) explanation of visiting regulations.
   (3) information as to suitable items her mother may bring to the hospital.
   (4) plan for the mother to confer with the doctor as she expressed need.
   (5) plan for continued care following dismissal.

d. Nursing associated with medical treatment:

   (1) preparation for and responsibility in assisting with the administration of fluids.
   (2) method of controlling the rate of flow of fluids.
   (3) reason for giving penicillin and aureomycin.
   (4) size of the needle used in giving I.M. injections to a 9-month-old infant.
   (5) body area most suitable for I.M. injections.

e. Nursing care associated with feeding:

   (1) technics of feeding a baby while restrained.
   (2) desirable amount of feeding and time spent taking each ounce.
   (3) size of the hole in the nipple.
   (4) methods useful to relieve abdominal distress if present.
   (5) stage of illness at which baby may be picked up for feedings.

f. Emotional needs:

   (1) response of a 9-month-old infant to separation from her mother.
   (2) frustrations resulting from restraints.
   (3) anxiety shown at not being fed when hungry.
   (4) provision for diversional activities.
   (5) interpretation of signs as head rolling, finger sucking and severe apathy after a few days' hospitalization.

3. Describe a plan of care for Shirley Mae at home, including

a. Activities of the public health nurse who is able to make 3 home visits per week during the first 2 weeks:

(1) teaching indicated for the physical comfort of the infant.
(2) teaching around the nutritional needs of the entire family, with emphasis on Shirley Mae.
(3) measures taken to prevent a recurrence of the diarrhea.
(4) assurance needed by the entire family that Shirley Mae gradually will regain her weight loss.

b. Type of foods you would provide for this baby:

(1) total nutritional needs, including vitamins and minerals.
(2) number of feedings per day.
(3) amounts of food given at any one time.

c. Future plan for health supervision, as

(1) child health conference.
(2) family physician.
(3) hospital clinics.

Questions Relating to the Section in General

1. Diarrhea tends to occur more frequently in infants who are

a.____breast fed, poorly nourished, underfed in calories.
b.____artificially fed, poorly nourished, overfed in amount.
c.____well nourished, breast fed, given insufficient water.
d.____fed at the family table, given too much water, poorly nourished.

2. Diarrhea tends to occur more frequently in

a.____hot weather, in high humidity, in the presence of a parenteral infection.
b.____cool weather, in high humidity, in infants dressed too warmly.
c.____hot weather, in low humidity, in infants otherwise healthy.
d.____cool weather, in low humidity, in the presence of parenteral infection.

3. The leading causes of diarrhea in infancy are

a.____overfeeding in hot weather, the use of unripe fruits in the diet, an excess of protein in the diet.
b.____underfeeding in hot weather, bacterial contamination, an excess of carbohydrate in the diet.
c.____upper respiratory infection, contaminated drinking water, underfeeding in hot weather.
d.____overfeeding in hot weather, bacterial contamination of the formula, an excess of fat in the diet.

4. The outstanding symptoms in infantile diarrhea are

a.____frequent watery stools, a fever of 105°F., projectile vomiting.
b.____blood and mucus in the stools, abdominal pain, flushed face.

    c.____frequent watery stools with mucus, dehydration, irritability.
    d.____projectile vomiting, a fever of 101°F., dehydration.

5. In severe diarrhea you would expect laboratory reports to show the following changes:

    a.____Hemoconcentration, low specific gravity of urine, CO_2 combining power 30 volumes per cent.
    b.____High specific gravity of urine, stool culture negative for bacterial growth, low hemoglobin level.
    c.____CO_2 combining power 50 volumes per cent, high leukocyte count, agglutination positive for typhoid O.
    d.____High specific gravity of urine, hemoconcentration, CO_2 combining power 30 volumes per cent.

6. The Vollmer patch test is used to determine

    a.____an individual's susceptibility to tuberculosis.
    b.____whether or not an individual has active pulmonary tuberculosis.
    c.____whether or not an individual has or has had any type of tuberculosis.

7. Diarrhea in infants may be prevented by

    a.____breast feeding when possible, maintaining adequate nutrition, keeping the baby dressed warmly at all times.
    b.____breast feeding when possible, keeping the baby dressed lightly in hot humid weather, avoiding infections of all types.
    c.____sterilization of all ingredients used in artificial feeding, allowing infants plenty of water in hot humid weather, early immunizations.
    d.____storing formulae in refrigerators, restricting fluid intake during hot weather, maintaining adequate nutrition.

8. An agglutin is a substance which causes bacteria to

    a.____decrease in number.
    b.____increase in number.
    c.____scatter throughout the body.
    d.____stick together in clumps.

9. During an infection in the body, agglutins are

    a.____decreased in number.
    b.____increased in number.
    c.____unchanged in number.

10. The purpose of the laboratory examination called CO_2 combining power is to

    a.____determine the carbon dioxide content of the blood plasma.
    b.____determine the hemoglobin content of the blood.

c._____measure the oxygen content of the blood.

d._____measure the sugar content of the blood.

11. The normal range for the carbon dioxide content of blood plasma is

    a._____30–50 vols. per cent.

    b._____45–70 vols. per cent.

    c._____50–80 vols. per cent.

    d._____40–55 vols. per cent.

12. Paregoric may be ordered for the relief of colic in the acute phase of infantile diarrhea. Paregoric is a derivative of

    a._____belladonna.

    b._____coal tar.

    c._____opium.

13. Paregoric is administered

    a._____intramuscularly.

    b._____rectally.

    c._____hypodermically.

    d._____orally.

14. The dose of paregoric for a 9-month-old baby is

    a._____20 minims.

    b._____2 cc.

    c._____10 cc.

    d._____10 minims.

[The following multiple-response items in questions 15, 16 and 17 refer to the development of the average baby at 9 months.]

15. Physically the baby is able to

    a._____sit alone unsupported.

    b._____stand alone.

    c._____feed himself using a spoon.

    d._____grasp a rattle by its handle.

    e._____pull himself up to a standing position.

16. Sleep habits may be described as

    a._____shows the need for sleep by fussing and wiggling.

    b._____resists being put down to sleep.

    c._____prefers sleeping outdoors to indoors.

    d._____needs only one nap during the day.

    e._____cries violently if disturbed during the night.

17. Socially the baby

    a._____plays alone for 30 to 40 minutes.

    b._____shows no fear of strangers.

    c._____responds to his own name.

    d._____demands a frequent shift of toys.

    e._____adjusts equally well to care given by the father or by the
           mother.

[The following multiple-response items in questions 18, 19, 20 and 21
refer to the development of the average baby at 15 months.]

18. Physically the child is able to
    a._____walk alone.
    b._____climb down a flight of stairs.
    c._____put his shoes on.
    d._____place a small pellet in a bottle.
    e._____build a tower of 3 blocks.

19. Feeding characteristics may be described as

    a._____demands to feed himself.
    b._____shows definite food preferences.
    c._____gives up bottle of own accord.
    d._____adjusts well when fed at the family table.
    e._____shows impatience if not fed immediately when hungry.

20. Socially the infant

    a._____shows evidence of affection toward members of family.
    b._____plays happily with another baby of the same age.
    c._____displays an interest in animals, especially dogs.
    d._____relaxes in the carriage when taken for a stroll.
    e._____responds to rhythmic music.

21. Mental development is shown by the ability to

    a._____comprehend the time of day.
    b._____point to his nose, ears, hair or mouth.
    c._____fit a round block into a round hole.
    d._____use sentences of 3 or more words.
    e._____memorize short nursery rhymes.

THE 18-MONTH-OLD CHILD WHO HAS NOT WALKED—PATIENT STUDY

Jane Kay was brought to the orthopedic clinic when she was 18 months
old. Her parents had noticed that she did not kick with her left leg and
stated that it seemed shorter than the right one. Following is a brief
summary of the history and physical examination.

History of Pregnancy. Full term; delivery unattended because the
mother did not tell anyone she was in labor and the doctor was called after
Jane was born. Estimated birth weight, 8 pounds.

Developmental History. Baby held up her head at 3 months, has not
tried to sit alone, to stand or to pull herself up, and has made no attempt
to talk—makes unintelligible vocal sounds.

Feeding History. Formula of evaporated milk, water and Karo syrup
since birth. Solid foods started at 7 months—all refused by baby. Also
refused orange juice and refused cup. Concentrated cod-liver oil was given

irregularly about once or twice weekly until the baby was 17 months old, when it was started daily.

Medical History. Frequent colds and tonsillitis, no immunizations.
Physical Examination:

Heart and lungs normal.
Abdomen distended.
Anterior and posterior fontanels closed.
Red moist skin eruption present over the lower abdomen and genito-anal region.
Weight on admission 16 pounds, 10 ounces.
Height on admission 29 inches.
Head circumference 17 inches.
Chest circumference 16¾ inches.
Length of left leg 11¼ inches from anterior superior spine to medial malleolus.
Length of right leg 11¾ inches from anterior superior spine to medial malleolus.

Diagnosis: Congenital dislocation, left hip.

Upon completing the examination, the orthopedic resident told Jane's mother that he would like to admit her to the hospital. Mrs. Kay replied, "Go ahead and keep her as long as you want to—my husband's company insurance will pay for it."

Nurses' notes described Jane on admission as having a weak, fretful cry and a most disagreeable odor. One nurse stated that the child seemed to shrink from contact with the nurses and doctors. Buck's extension was used on Jane's left leg for 3½ weeks. A hip spica was then applied and she was returned to her home with instructions to return to clinic in 6 weeks.

Six months later Mrs. Kay returned with Jane. The cast was wet and soft, and the baby weighed 13 pounds. Her abdomen was distended and she was having large, frothy, foul-smelling stools. Mrs. Kay reported that Jane had been taking only milk and that she refused all other foods. Again she was admitted to the hospital where she remained 2 months.

Because of the type of stools, a duodenal drainage was done which proved to be negative for cystic fibrosis of the pancreas. A blood count showed 3,500,000 erythrocytes, 15,200 leukocytes and a hemoglobin of 7 Gm. per 100 cc. of blood. Three transfusions of 250 cc. of whole blood were given.

During the second hospitalization, nurses' notes included a description of fearful behavior the first few days. Later she smiled, then came to demand almost constant attention from the nurses.

As Jane gained weight and her skin became healthier, another hip spica was applied. After 6 weeks, x-ray films showed the head of the left femur to be in a satisfactory position in the acetabular cavity. The cast was removed and Jane was dismissed with instructions to return to physiotherapy once weekly and to the orthopedic clinic in 1 month. Her age at this time was 27 months.

References

Gibbs, Gordon E., and Smith, Kathryn: Cystic fibrosis of the pancreas, Am. J. Nursing **50**:783, 1950.

Ribble, Margaret A.: The Rights of Infants, pp. 35–42, 60–71, 81–91, New York, Columbia, 1943.

Background Review Questions

1. The anterior fontanel is expected to close at the age of 18mo and the posterior fontanel at the age of 2mo.

2. The average circumference of the baby's head is
   a. at birth 13½ inches; 35 cm.
   b. at 4 months ____ inches; ____ cm.
   c. at 1 year ____ inches; ____ cm.
   d. at 2 years ____ inches; ____ cm.

3. The average circumference of the baby's chest is
   a. at birth 13½ inches; 35 cm.
   b. at 4 months ____ inches; ____ cm.
   c. at 1 year ____ inches; ____ cm.
   d. at 2 years ____ inches; ____ cm.

4. The average length of the baby is
   a. at birth 20 inches.
   b. at 4 months ____ inches.
   c. at 1 year ____ inches.
   d. at 2 years ____ inches.

5. The number of teeth expected in the average baby is
   a. at 8 months 2.
   b. at 1 year 6.
   c. at 2 years 18.
   d. at 2½ years 20.

6. Match the following orthopedic terms and definitions:
   a. _5_ abduction.
   b. _1_ adduction.
   c. _8_ perineum.
   d. _3_ hyperextension.
   e. _9_ extension.
   f. _7_ flexion.
   g. _2_ lordosis.
   h. _10_ scoliosis.
   i. _6_ gluteal fold.
   j. _4_ gluteal muscles.
   k. _14_ acetabulum.
   l. _13_ anterior superior spine.
   m. _12_ medial malleolus.

   (1) the drawing of a part toward the median line of the body.
   (2) curvature of the spine with a forward convexity.
   (3) extreme or excessive extension.
   (4) the muscles of the buttocks.
   (5) the withdrawing of a part away from the median line of the body.
   (6) the fold of skin between the thigh and the buttocks.
   (7) the movement which bends a part of the body.
   (8) an area of the body between the thighs, buttocks and genitalia.
   (9) the movement which brings a part of the body into a straight line.
   (10) lateral curvature of the spine.
   (11) the head of the femur.
   (12) the inner ankle bone.
   (13) projection on the ilium.
   (14) a large cup-shaped articular cavity.

Questions Relating to the Patient Study

1. The nurse admitting Jane to the unit should place her in a

     a._____room alone.
     b._____cubicle with 3 infants.
     c._____cubicle with 1 other child of the same age.
     d._____cubicle with 3 other children of the same age.

2. Nursing care which should help Jane adjust to the hospital in the interval before Buck's extension was applied includes

     a._____hold her on your lap for feedings, pick her up frequently, give milk by bottle.
     b._____leave her in the crib at all times, change toys frequently, give milk by bottle.
     c._____hold her on your lap for feedings, give milk from a cup, add solid foods forcibly.
     d._____provide the toys she enjoys most, hold her on your lap for feedings, give milk from a cup.

3. The changes that should make you suspect that Jane's cast is too tight are

     a._____violent crying, elevation of temperature, abdominal distention.
     b._____bluish discoloration of the toes, swelling of the extremities outside the cast, abdominal distention.
     c._____refusal of food, elevation of temperature, vomiting.

4. As you are caring for Jane and believe the cast is too tight you should

     a._____provide diversional activities, place cotton padding under the edges of the cast, offer her a bottle of milk.
     b._____administer a sedative, elevate the extremities, discontinue play activities.
     c._____elevate the extremities, notify the nurse in charge, remove excessive padding from between the cast and the skin.
     d._____leave the child alone, notify the nurse in charge, record your observations on the patient's chart.

5. Reference is made to Jane's weak, fretful cry. This type of behavior might be explained on the basis of

     a._____malnutrition, strange surroundings, pain in the left hip.
     b._____emotional insecurity, malnutrition, fear of strangers.
     c._____fear of uniforms, pain in the left hip, hunger.
     d._____separation from her parents, hunger, fear of uniforms.

6. During the second hospitalization, a psychologist came to the unit to administer some tests to Jane. He reported that she was severely retarded mentally. Which of the phrases describing Jane's past development and adjustment do you associate with the mental retardation:

     a._____congenital dislocation of the hip, refusal of solid foods, frequent colds.

    b._____failure to sit alone, failure to talk, failure to stand or to pull
herself up.

    c._____fear of hospital personnel, malnutrition, mother's apparent lack
of interest in the child.

    d._____refusal of solid foods, frequent colds, fear of hospital personnel.

Questions for Discussion and Student Projects

1. Describe your plan of nursing care for Jane immediately after the first
admission, including

    a._____care of the skin to promote the healing of excoriations.

    b._____methods effective in removing fears and in demonstrating to the
child that she will be treated kindly.

    c._____technics of feeding liquids and solids.

    d._____toys suitable for Jane as determined by her interests and de-
velopment.

2. Discuss the mother's statement, "Keep her as long as you want to." Do
you think that this statement reflects an attitude which has contributed
to Jane's delayed development? If so, describe the type of care you
think Jane may have received at home.

3. Suppose you are a public health nurse going into the Kay home when
the mother is starting solid foods. How should you advise her to feed
Jane the first solid foods? What teaching should you give in relation to
Jane's refusal to accept orange juice? Is it common for infants to reject
orange juice at first?

4. Describe your plan for meeting the emotional needs of Jane Kay. Why
did she show signs of fear of the nurses and the doctors during the early
part of both admissions? How would you explain the change to a de-
manding behavior? How should these demands for attention be met?
Do you believe that nurses are justified in giving extra time and attention to one child in a pediatric unit, especially when it is felt that such
management will not be continued at home?

5. In the situation described, Jane's mother did not visit her during the
first month of hospitalization so it was necessary to teach all of the
home care at the time of dismissal. Prepare a plan of teaching showing
the material you would try to include in the short time allowed. What
demonstrations should be indicated? Do you think that written instructions should accompany those given verbally?

6. Do you believe that this family would derive benefit from public health
nursing visits? If so, what information should you include on the referral form?

Questions Relating to the Section in General

1. Congenital dislocation of the hip occurs most frequently in

    a._____white males.

    b._____Negro females.

    c._____Negro males.

    d._____white females.

2. The greatest number of dislocated hips in infancy
   a._____exist at birth.
   b._____develop at about 4 months.
   c._____develop gradually.
   d._____develop when the child begins to bear weight.

3. The cause of congenital dislocation is
   a._____malposition in utero.
   b._____not clearly understood.
   c._____based on hereditary factors.
   d._____inadequate diet of the mother during pregnancy.

4. Early symptoms of dislocation include
   a._____limited adduction of the affected side, widening of the perineum, stiffness of the joint on the affected side.
   b._____extreme mobility of the joint on the affected side, resistance to abduction on both sides, hyperextension of the hip on the affected side.
   c._____flexion of the hip on the affected side, elevation of the gluteal fold on the affected side, widening of the perineum.
   d._____limited abduction on the affected side, lordosis, stiffness of the joint on the affected side.

5. Symptoms observed after the child is walking include
   a._____waddling gait, lumbar lordosis, broad buttocks.
   b._____pain in the affected hip, widening of the perineum, waddling gait.
   c._____protuberant abdomen, shortening of the leg on the unaffected side, lumbar lordosis.
   d._____broad buttocks, widening of the perineum, stiffness of both hip joints.

6. The outstanding symptoms in cystic fibrosis of the pancreas are
   a._____vomiting, diarrhea, abdominal distention.
   b._____constipation, wasting of the gluteal muscles, decrease in appetite.
   c._____large frothy foul-smelling stools, wasting of the gluteal muscles, decrease in appetite.
   d._____fretfulness, decrease in appetite, failure to gain weight.

7. In cystic fibrosis of the pancreas the child's diet consists of foods
   a._____high in protein, low in fat, low in carbohydrate.
   b._____low in protein, sodium-free, high in carbohydrate.
   c._____low in fat, high in vitamins, high in carbohydrate.
   d._____high in protein, fat-free, low in carbohydrate.

8. The purpose of duodenal drainage in suspected cystic fibrosis of the pancreas is to determine the presence or absence of
   a._____trypsin.   c._____lipase.
   b._____amylase.   d._____sterase.

1. Plan a classroom demonstration to include
   a. the method of inspecting a young infant for all types of orthopedic deformities.
   b. the method of applying diapers to maintain proper body alinement in infants.
   c. the procedure for assisting the physician in measuring the length of the legs of infant and child.
2. What is the purpose of Buck's extension? Describe the responsibilities of the nurse who assists the physician in the application of Buck's extension. Would you lift the weights while caring for the patient? What measures should you take to prevent the child from being pulled toward the foot of the bed?
3. List the principles to be observed in caring for a small child with a newly applied cast. Describe your method of protection for a hip spica when the child has not developed bowel and bladder control.
4. What is the nurse's responsibility toward a 27-month-old child who has had no immunizations?
5. What are the facilities in your state and/or community for the care of mentally retarded children? Obtain information as to methods of making application for placement of a child in an institution for the mentally retarded, including the age at which a child will be accepted in your state.

Section 2. Nursing Care of Children
During the Pre-school Period

STUDY SUGGESTIONS: Before beginning the study of this Section, the student
will find it helpful to

A. Review

1. In anatomy and physiology texts: units on the circulatory, the genitourinary and the musculoskeletal systems.
2. In the medical-surgical part of this Guide, see the Sections on nursing
   disorders of the circulatory system, upper respiratory conditions (tuberculosis).
3. In nutrition texts: the nutritional needs of the preschool child, nutritional needs during lactation, low salt diets.
4. In pediatrics texts: immunization, child development (from 18 months
   to 6 years), nursing procedures, abdominal paracentesis, gavage, suction,
   spinal puncture, the administration of oxygen.
5. In public health nursing texts: pediatric clinics, the postpartum home
   visit.
6. In pharmacology texts: Chloromycetin, elixir phenobarbital, penicillin,
   para-amino-salicylic acid.
7. In microbiology texts: immunization, undulant fever, tuberculosis,
   tetanus.

B. Study

1. In pediatrics texts: the units relating to the nursing care of children
   with the specific disease condition under consideration.

C. Read the additional References listed before attempting to answer the questions relating to each patient study.

A VISIT TO THE CHILD HEALTH CONFERENCE—SITUATION STUDY

Mrs. Kramer took her 6-week-old son, Ralph, to the Child Health Conference at the suggestion of the visiting nurse. When the nurse had asked
Mrs. Kramer what plan the family had made for health supervision, the
mother replied that they were able to pay the family doctor for visits when
someone was sick but did not feel they could afford any "extras." Mrs.
Kramer was given the telephone number and location of the conference
and made an appointment for the baby.

On the day of the conference, Mrs. Kramer was greeted at the reception desk by a volunteer worker who showed her the waiting room and
explained where she might leave her wraps. The receptionist obtained the
identifying information needed to start Ralph's conference record and
gave it to the public health nurse, Miss Robinson.

The mother and baby were called into a small office where Miss Robinson introduced herself and explained the purpose and services of the

Child Health Conference. The nurse obtained and recorded information about the family's past health and the present plan for medical care during illness. Since this was Mrs. Kramer's first experience at the conference, additional time was allowed for questions and for Mrs. Kramer to recall the family medical history. The baby was then undressed and weighed, and, after a 10-minute wait, was taken by his mother and Miss Robinson into the doctor's office.

A complete physical examination was made, a few adjustments made in the baby's diet, and an explanation made of the plan for immunizations. Mrs. Kramer asked a few questions, the chief problem being whether or not to allow her 5-year-old son to spend a month at his grandmother's in the country. The doctor discussed the advantages and disadvantages of this proposed trip.

Miss Robinson spent a few minutes going over the doctor's instructions and making sure that the mother felt satisfied with the service. Mrs. Kramer was then instructed to stop at the receptionist's desk on her way out and to make an appointment for her next visit to the conference.

References

Jeans, Philip, Rand, Winifred, and Blake, Florence: Essentials of Pediatrics, ed. 4, pp. 100–105, Philadelphia, Lippincott, 1946.

Spock, Benjamin: The Pocket Book of Child Care, pp. 10–12, 181–184, New York, Pocket Books, 1946.

The Child Health Conference, Publication No. 261, Federal Security Agency, 1948. For sale by the Superintendent of Documents, Washington 25, D.C. Total pages 141, price 15 cents.

Questions Relating to the Situation Study

1. The visiting nurse planned for Mrs. Kramer to telephone for her own appointment because

   a._____mothers prefer making their own appointments.

   b._____the nurse did not have time.

   c._____mothers accept greater responsibility for attendance at conference when they make their own appointments.

2. The duties of a volunteer worker are usually to

   a._____make appointments, greet families, set up sterile supplies.

   b._____take the medical history, provide play materials for the children, set up exhibits.

   c._____greet families, make appointments, adjust the physical environment of the center.

   d._____advise mothers on child care, take medical histories, set up exhibits.

3. In case a child attending the conference shows signs of illness, Miss Robinson should

   a._____send him home immediately, make a future appointment.

   b._____call the family physician and report the symptoms, send the child home immediately.

c._____take the child's temperature, plan to make a home visit after the conference.

d._____isolate the child from others, ask the conference physician to advise the mother.

4. As the doctor explains the immunization program to Mrs. Kramer, he tells her that the baby will be inoculated against the following diseases before he is 1 year old:

a._____measles, whooping cough, scarlet fever, diphtheria.

b._____smallpox, whooping cough, diphtheria, tetanus.

c._____chicken pox, poliomyelitis, measles, smallpox.

d._____scarlet fever, tetanus, measles, typhoid.

5. Mrs. Kramer stated that her 5-year-old son had received immunizations for smallpox, diphtheria, tetanus and pertussis 2 years ago. The doctor told Mrs. Kramer that before the boy goes to the country for a month he should have

a._____a booster dose of tetanus toxoid, typhoid vaccine.

b._____re-vaccination for smallpox, typhus vaccine.

c._____typhoid vaccine, a booster dose for diphtheria, tetanus and pertussis.

d._____typhoid vaccine, anti-rabies serum.

6. Another question Mrs. Kramer asked related to the possibility of contracting undulant fever. The doctor should tell her that

a._____undulant fever is fairly rare.

b._____it would be safer to have pasteurized milk for the boy at all times.

c._____cows are all tested for possible infection.

d._____the risk of undulant fever is great enough to prohibit a month's stay in the country.

7. The purpose of a child health conference is to

a._____promote good health, prevent illness.

b._____provide immunizations, treat minor diseases.

c._____Adjust diets, prevent behavior problems.

d._____prevent illness, provide educational materials for mothers.

8. Children from one of the following age groups may attend child health conferences:

a._____birth to 2 years.

b._____birth to 10 years.

c._____6 weeks to 5 years.

d._____birth to 6 years.

9. During the first year of life, a baby should be checked by a doctor

a._____every 2 months.

b._____every 3 months.

c._____once monthly.

d._____twice yearly.

Questions for Discussion and Student Projects

1. Prepare a class report (suggested activity for one student) showing the duties or activities of the 3 public health nurses who served in the conference which Ralph attended.
2. Describe how Miss Robinson should instruct the mother when new foods are added, especially orange juice and cereal. Since Baby Kramer was breast fed and no formula is available, how should the mother moisten his cereal?
3. How should the visiting nurse respond to Mrs. Kramer when she refers to health supervision as "extras"? How can nurses teach the concept that preventive medicine is as essential as curative medicine?
4. Medical practice is known to vary in different areas. Prepare a list of foods usually given to babies in your community at the age of 6 weeks, 10 weeks and 6 months. At what age is orange juice started?
5. Suggestions are given below for group or class projects for student nurses having pediatric instruction and/or experience.

   a. Prepare an exhibit of toys for preschool children, emphasizing toys with educational value as well as specific safety features.
   b. Collect literature and posters suitable for teaching healthful practices. This material might be used in the outpatient department or pediatric clinic if no child health conference is available.
   c. Prepare a simple layette for a newborn infant. Designate articles for cold- and for hot-weather use.

6. Is there a child health conference in your community? If so, prepare answers to the following questions:

   a. Where does the conference meet?
   b. How often does it meet?
   c. Who are the individuals who provide the service, i.e. physician, nurse, etc.?
   d. How is the conference financed?
   e. How is eligibility for admission determined?

7. For a child health conference lasting 4 hours and giving service to 20 children, how many public health nurses would be needed, assuming 1 physician and 1 volunteer worker to be present?

A HOME VISIT BY A PUBLIC HEALTH NURSE—SITUATION STUDY

Miss Hopkins, a public health nurse, was making a visit in the home of Mrs. Long, who had returned the day before from the hospital with her 8-day-old baby girl. Mrs. Long was breast feeding the baby and reported that her milk supply seemed adequate. She asked Miss Hopkins to show her how to bathe and to weigh the baby. Following the bath demonstration, Mrs. Long sighed and said what really was bothering her was the behavior of her 2½-year-old son Danny. She told Miss Hopkins that he had been very good while she was in the hospital, but since her return he had been crying, wetting and soiling himself, and refusing to drink milk from a cup. Mrs. Long thought he might be jealous of his new baby sister but did not know how to handle the situation. She was quite annoyed at the regression in toilet habits because she had worked diligently to completely train him by the age of 18 months.

References

Spock, Benjamin: *The Pocketbook of Baby and Child Care,* pp. 184–193, 260–280, 290–296, New York, Pocket Books, 1946.
Strang, Ruth: An Introduction to Child Study, ed. 3, pp. 197–199, New York, Macmillan, 1951.

Questions Relating to the Situation Study

1. Mrs. Long asked the nurse how often she should feed the baby. Miss Hopkins' reply should be

   a._____every 4 hours.
   b._____every 3 hours.
   c._____every time he shows signs of hunger.
   d._____every time he cries.

2. The mother asked Miss Hopkins to explain to her the types of foods recommended during the period of lactation. The nurse should describe a

   a._____diet high in protein.
   b._____diet high in carbohydrates.
   c._____well-balanced diet with 1 quart of milk added.
   d._____diet low in fats and in roughage.

3. As Mrs. Long expressed her anxiety over Danny's behavior, the nurse should tell her that

   a._____it is natural for him to be jealous of the new baby.
   b._____he should be ignored as much as possible.
   c._____he will get over this behavior in a few days.
   d._____boys are more prone to show these signs than are girls.

4. Mrs. Long wanted to know what the nurse might suggest to get Danny to drink his milk again. She should be advised to

   a._____offer him rewards for each glass of milk taken.
   b._____ignore his refusals to take milk.
   c._____offer him the milk in a nursing bottle.
   d._____add chocolate and sugar to the milk.

5. Miss Hopkins should make the following suggestions for both parents to follow in their relationships with Danny:

   a._____try to get him to love the new baby.
   b._____show Danny that they love him as much as ever.
   c._____send him to his grandmother's for a week.
   d._____shame him for acting like a baby.

6. Since Mrs. Long is concerned over Danny's lapse in bowel and bladder control, the visiting nurse should tell her that
   a.____she trained him too early.
   b.____she did not train him early enough.
   c.____Danny is willfully annoying her.
   d.____as Danny feels less jealous, he will start using the toilet again.

Questions for Discussion and Student Projects

1. Assume you are Miss Hopkins, the public health nurse, going into the Long home. Describe the visit as it should be made, including how you should introduce yourself to the mother, the kinds of questions you should ask in order to learn as much as you can of the home situation, and the length of time you should remain in the home. Try to anticipate specific questions Mrs. Long might ask you concerning breast feeding, bathing the baby, and the baby's bowel movements.
2. Do you think it is common to hear descriptions of behavior similar to Danny's, especially that he was very good while the mother was away? Do you believe it was natural for Mrs. Long to be disturbed by his behavior following her return? What should you say or do to help her accept his actions and to see how she can relieve his anxieties.

Questions Relating to the Section in General

1. Jealousy occurs most commonly in the child who is
   a.____the only child, attending nursery school, has been sick frequently.
   b.____overly dependent upon his mother, around 2 to 2½ years old, unsure of his mother's love.
   c.____aggressive, around 5 years old, unsure of his mother's love.
   d.____undernourished, overly dependent, around 4 years old.

2. Entrance of a child into a nursery school should take place
   a.____after the new baby arrives.
   b.____2 or 3 weeks before the new baby arrives.
   c.____2 or 3 months before the new baby arrives.

3. The most suitable person to care for the 2½-year-old child while his mother is in the hospital is
   a.____the grandmother.
   b.____the aunt who is a graduate nurse.
   c.____a maid who has worked in the home.
   d.____a kind, mothering woman known by the child.

4. The mother of a child who is disturbed by a recent separation from her and who refuses to go to sleep at night should be told to
   a.____take him into bed with the parents.
   b.____sit by his crib until he goes to sleep.
   c.____lock him in his room.
   d.____let him cry it out.

5. Separation anxiety is most acute at the age of
  a._____1 year to 18 months.
  b._____2 to 2½ years.
  c._____3 to 4 years.
  d._____4 to 5 years.

6. The best advice to give parents on the subject of toilet training is
  a._____to wait until the baby shows he is ready.
  b._____to begin bowel training around 6 months of age.
  c._____to begin bladder training around 1 year of age.
  d._____to place the baby on the potty for 15 minutes at the same time each day.
  e._____that rectal suppositories are helpful in the establishment of bowel control.

7. The usual causes of regression in toilet habits are
  a._____drinking excessive amounts of water, malnutrition, resentment toward the mother.
  b._____too rigid controls set up by the mother, illness, loss of sleep.
  c._____illness, emotional stress, too rigid controls set up by the mother.
  d._____resentment toward the mother, malnutrition, loss of sleep.

8. The small child usually resists using a potty or toilet under the following conditions:
  a._____constipated stools, chronic fatigue of the child, a new baby in the home.
  b._____training started before the child was ready, child kept on the potty for too long at a time, child punished for accidents.
  c._____too many rewards offered, child does not understand what is expected of him, mother shows disapproval of the child's general behavior.
  d._____use of rectal suppositories, insufficient toys for the child, chronic fatigue of the child.

9. While there is variation in the growth rate of children in the United States, certain average figures have been determined for purposes of comparison:
  a. During the first year of life, the average infant
    (1)_____regains weight lost in the first few postnatal days by the end of the third week.
    (2)_____doubles his birth weight between the fourth and the sixth months.
    (3)_____tends to grow more rapidly when handled very little.
    (4)_____gains about 3 inches in length.
  b. During the second year of life, the average child
    (1)_____gains 6 to 8 pounds in weight.
    (2)_____gains about 6 inches in length.
    (3)_____trebles his birth weight.
    (4)_____doubles his birth weight.

10. The sleep habits of a 2 year old are most apt to be

    a._____resistance to going to bed at night, acceptance of the afternoon nap.

    b._____resistance to the afternoon nap, acceptance of going to bed at night.

    c._____resistance to going to bed at any time.

    d._____acceptance of going to bed at any time.

11. The average 2-year-old prefers

    a._____to feed himself, to help dress himself, action toys to picture books.

    b._____to be fed, to be dressed, picture books to action toys.

    c._____to feed himself, to help dress himself, picture books to action toys.

12. The toilet training of a 2 year old is usually

    a._____partial.   b._____complete.   c._____not started.

13. The average 2-year-old child's social development is best described by stating that he prefers to play

    a._____alone, but will share his toys and makes friends quickly with strangers.

    b._____alone, refuses to share his toys, tends to be shy with strangers.

    c._____with other children, usually shares his toys, makes friends quickly with strangers.

    d._____with other children, refuses to share toys, makes friends quickly with strangers.

14. The 2-year-old child's appetite is usually

    a._____increased for most foods.   c._____increased for new foods.

    b._____decreased for most foods.

15. The average 2-year-old child is able to use

    a._____sentences of 3 or more words, distinguish morning from afternoon.

    b._____single words or phrases only, distinguish morning from afternoon.

    c._____sentences of 3 or more words, but not distinguish morning from afternoon.

16. If a new baby arrives in the home, you would expect the 2 year old to be

    a._____very jealous.   b._____not at all jealous.   c._____indifferent.

Questions for Discussion and Student Projects—(*Continued*)

1. Describe how a mother should prepare a 2½-year-old child for the birth of a baby brother or sister. Include the following points:

    a. when he should be told.

    b. where the baby is coming from.

   c. changes to be made in the child's room, such as a room of his own
      or to a larger bed.

   d. entrance into nursery school.

2. How should the mother of a 2½-year-old child plan for his care during
the period of her hospitalization?
3. Describe various ways in which jealousy is manifested by the 2½-year-
old child and state how you think each of the symptoms should be
handled.
4. Make a list of fears which occur frequently between the ages of 2 and 4.
How should each one be explained to a mother who sees no reason for
her 3-year-old child to be fearful?
5. Describe ways in which a young child shows his readiness for toilet
training.
6. Write a short paragraph in your own words stating what you should
say to a young mother who asks your advice on methods most effective
in teaching her 18-month-old child to use the toilet.

THE DROWSY LITTLE BOY—PATIENT STUDY

Bobby, aged 2½ years, was admitted to the communicable disease unit
with a diagnosis of tuberculous meningitis. He was extremely drowsy,
convulsive and mildly cyanotic. Babinski's and Kernig's signs were
positive.

Orders on admission were:

   1. Prepare for lumbar puncture. Spinal fluid to laboratory for
      culture, cell count, protein and sugar.
   2. Infant soft diet as tolerated. Feed by gavage if necessary.
   3. Oxygen p.r.n.
   4. Urinalysis, CBC and differential.
   5. Routine investigation of contacts.
   6. Streptomycin 0.5 Gm. I.M. twice daily.
   7. P.A.S. Gm. 1 q.6 h. by mouth—gavage if necessary.
   8. Suction mucus from mouth and throat as necessary.
   9. Prepare for daily intrathecal streptomycin.

Bobby was placed in a single room. Oxygen was started immediately
after the lumbar puncture was completed. For the first few days Bobby
took small amounts of soft and liquid foods, but due to an inadequate
caloric intake it became necessary to feed him by gavage.

On the day following admission, the head nurse talked with the parents
to obtain information about all persons having close contact with Bobby
over the past few months. A list was prepared which included parents,
grandparents, aunts, uncles, close friends and baby sitters. The mother
assured the head nurse that she would urge all persons on the list to go at
once for a roentgenogram of the chest. At the end of a week, the hospital
physician was notified that Bobby's aunt, who had helped with his care,
was found to have active pulmonary tuberculosis. Her treatment was
carried out by her family physician.

Bobby remained in the hospital for several months.

References

Gesell, Arnold, and Ilg, Frances: The Infant and Child in the Culture of
    Today, pp. 177–201, New York, Harpers, 1943.
Siegel, Pearl T.: More about B.C.G., Am. J. Nursing, 49:753, 1949.

Questions Relating to the Patient Study

1. You would expect the laboratory results from an examination of the
   specimen of Bobby's cerebrospinal fluid to show

    a._____cell count 5, fluid slightly turbid, protein 100 mg. per 100 cc.
       of blood.
    b._____color clear, cell count 500, sugar 10 mg. per 100 cc. of blood.
    c._____tubercle bacilli present, fluid slightly turbid, protein 10 mg.
       per 100 cc. of blood.
    d._____tubercle bacilli present, fluid slightly turbid, cell count 500.

2. Bobby was placed in isolation because

    a._____personnel might become contaminated from the spinal fluid.
    b._____the patient may also have meningococcic meningitis.
    c._____the patient may have active pulmonary tuberculosis.
    d._____other children might contract tuberculous meningitis if in an
       open ward.

3. Signs of respiratory distress indicating that Bobby should receive an
   additional supply of oxygen are

    a._____cyanosis, rapid pulse, restlessness.
    b._____slow pulse, cyanosis, coma.
    c._____rapid respirations, perspiration, pallor.
    d._____cyanosis, coma, rapid respirations.

4. Gavage feedings for Bobby should be given

    a._____3 times daily.
    b._____every 2 hours.
    c._____every 6 hours.
    d._____every 4 hours.

5. The total amount given by gavage over a 24-hour period should be
   approximately

    a._____1200 cc.
    b._____5000 cc.
    c._____2500 cc.

6. The amount to be given at each feeding should be approximately

    a._____500 cc.
    b._____200 cc.
    c._____100 cc.
    d._____400 cc.

7. The ingredients in Bobby's **gavage** feedings over a 24-hour period should include

    a._____whole milk, orange juice, 1 egg.
    b._____orange juice, Karo syrup, water.
    c._____evaporated milk, egg, sugar.
    d._____thin cereal, skimmed milk, water.

8. Bobby's vomiting following a gavage feeding may be prevented by

    a._____removing the gavage tube rapidly.
    b._____removing the gavage tube slowly.
    c._____leaving the gavage tube in place over a 24-hour period.

9. Since Bobby was comatose for several weeks, special nursing care was needed to prevent the development of decubitus ulcers. The following type of care would be most effective in keeping his skin in good condition:

    a._____alcohol rubs, frequent changes of position, a rubber ring under the buttocks.
    b._____cool water sponges, oil rubs, restraint of the legs to prevent friction from the sheets.
    c._____frequent bathing, oil rubs, frequent changes of position.
    d._____alcohol rubs, restraint of the legs to prevent friction from the sheets, a rubber ring under the buttocks.

10. The nurse caring for Bobby during a convulsion should

    a._____restrain his arms and legs.
    b._____place a padded tongue blade between his teeth.
    c._____place him in a tub of water at a temperature of 105°F.
    d._____administer sedation as ordered.

11. Observations of the convulsion which should be included in the nurse's notes are the

    a._____areas of the body involved, the length of time of the convulsion, changes in color.
    b._____type of convulsion, changes in respirations, the length of time of the convulsion.
    c._____areas of the body involved, the behavior of the child following the convulsion, changes in color.
    d._____length of time of the convulsion, changes in pulse, the areas of the body involved.

Questions for Discussion and Student Projects

1. Describe your plan of nursing care for Bobby, including

    a. Observations:
    (1) the position the child assumes in bed.
    (2) the color of his skin, especially around the mouth and the nail beds.
    (3) signs to show the state of consciousness.

(4) sensory response and/or changes.

(5) muscular twitchings or convulsions.

(6) the character of the pulse and respirations.

b. Physical care:

(1) skin care to promote comfort and prevent excoriations.

(2) methods of feeding, as spoon, bottle or gavage.

(3) indications for the use of oral suction.

(4) the method of recording intake and output.

(5) the prevention of orthopedic deformities.

(6) the administration of medications.

c. Relationship with parents:

(1) precautions observed by the parents when visiting.

(2) the type of reassurance you can honestly give parents.

(3) suggestions for suitable toys parents may bring to hospital.

(4) provision for conference with the physician as desired.

(5) health teaching on the prevention of tuberculosis.

Questions Relating to the Section in General

1. Tuberculous meningitis occurs more frequently in:

a._____children under 3 years of age, the Negro race, both sexes equally.

b._____girls, the white race, children under 5 years of age.

c._____boys, the Negro race, children between the ages of 3 and 5 years.

d._____both sexes equally, the white race, children between the ages of 3 and 5 years.

2. Symptoms of tuberculous meningitis may be described according to three stages:

a. Prodromal stage:

(1)_____loss of appetite, vomiting, a fever of 103°.

(2)_____irritability, diarrhea, loss of appetite.

(3)_____constipation, convulsions, a fever of 104°.

(4)_____irritability, constipation, a fever of 100°.

b. Transitional stage:

(1)_____stupor, a fever of 105°, stiffness of the neck and the back.

(2)_____irritability, convulsions, a fever of 106°.

(3)_____stiffness of the neck, stupor, muscular twitching.

(4)_____bulging of the anterior fontanel, nystagmus, diarrhea.

c. Late stage:

(1)_____coma, a temperature of 97°, fixed pupils.

(2)_____convulsions, irregular pulse, diarrhea.

(3)_____paralysis, absence of reflexes, a fever of 100°.

(4)_____deep coma, a fever of 106°, fixed unresponsive pupils.

3. The tubercle bacillus enters the central nervous system as a result of

    a._____direct contact with persons having active pulmonary tuberculosis.
    b._____the use of unpasteurized milk.
    c._____tuberculous infection elsewhere in the child's body.

4. The chief action of streptomycin, an antibiotic, is

    a._____bacteriostatic.
    b._____bactericidal.
    c._____antiseptic.

5. Toxic symptoms noted during the use of streptomycin are

    a._____deafness, nausea, leukopenia.
    b._____coma, tinnitus, vomiting.
    c._____leukopenia, coma, diarrhea.
    d._____deafness, vomiting, constipation.

6. PAS (para-aminosalicylic acid) is given to

    a._____hasten the effectiveness of streptomycin.
    b._____delay the development of resistance to streptomycin.
    c._____prevent brain damage.
    d._____destroy tubercle bacilli.

7. BCG is indicated in persons who

    a._____have a positive tuberculin test, are under the age of 21 years.
    b._____are entering a school of nursing, have a positive tuberculin test.
    c._____are exposed to tuberculosis, are under 21 years of age.
    d._____have a negative tuberculin test, are exposed to tuberculosis.

8. Following the injection of BCG vaccine, the person develops a positive reaction to tuberculin at the end of

    a._____2 weeks.
    b._____4 months.
    c._____6 months.
    d._____1 year.

9. Match the following:

    a.__4__Opisthotonos.
    b.__3__Nystagmus.
    c.__1__Babinski's sign.
    d.__5__Intrathecal.
    e.__2__Kernig's sign.

(1) hypertension of the great toe when the bottom of the foot is stimulated with a sharp instrument.
(2) inability to extend the leg passively at the knee when the hip is flexed at a right angle.
(3) short, rapid, involuntary oscillation of the eyeball or eyeballs.
(4) arching of the back.
(5) into the spinal column.
(6) generalized muscular twitching.

10. At 2½ years the average child is said to be negativistic. From the list below check the methods mothers and nurses should use to lessen this type of behavior:
    a._____ignore the word "no" in his vocabulary.
    b._____insist upon the child carrying out all commands.
    c._____allow the child to make simple choices in matters which are not important.
    d._____teach the child that he must conform to household routines.
    e._____maintain some light humor toward his haughty behavior.

11. Feeding characteristics at this age are that the
    a._____child accepts new foods easily.
    b._____child shows definite food preferences.
    c._____appetite tends to be poor.
    d._____child enjoys green vegetables.
    e._____child shows little interest in between-meal snacks.

12. Suitable toys for the healthy child at 2½ years are
    a._____color books.
    b._____clay or Plasticine.
    c._____small plastic building blocks.
    d._____push-and-pull toys.
    e._____small cars.

13. True statements which describe the healthy average child of 2½ years are that
    a._____he is showing a strong urge for independence.
    b._____he plays well with children of his own age.
    c._____he goes to sleep readily at bedtime.
    d._____he is able to dress himself entirely.
    e._____he shows sudden shifts in behavior.
    f._____his speech is developing rapidly.
    g._____he is able to play alone for about an hour if his toys are interesting.
    h._____he resists all help with feeding.
    i._____he shows a frequent need to be dependent.
    j._____his growth is proceeding rapidly.
    k._____he is able to identify familiar animals in a picture book.
    l._____he expresses pleasure at hearing rhythmic music.
    m._____he pays little attention to books or magazines.
    n._____he prefers simple stories with no plot.
    o._____he has frequent temper tantrums.
    p._____he is in control of bowel and bladder function both day and night.
    q._____he enjoys performing simple household chores.

Questions for Discussion and Student Projects—(*Continued*)

1. Plan a classroom demonstration using a practice doll to show the method of holding a small child for a lumbar puncture.

2. Prepare a report (suggested assignment for one student) on the use of BCG and its effectiveness in the prevention of tuberculosis. What do the initials BCG represent?
3. In view of the emphasis which is placed upon the importance of mothers caring for their own babies, do you think that medical personnel are justified in removing a newborn infant from a mother who has active pulmonary tuberculosis?
4. What is the prognosis in tuberculous meningitis?
5. List other types of tuberculosis which affect young children and give the symptoms and medical treatment for each.
6. To obtain information on methods used to prevent tuberculosis, write to your State Health Department for printed material on tuberculosis control. Compare state and local activities and try to determine what the nurse's responsibility is in the total program. Is there compulsory inspection of milk and water in your community? What measures are taken to test milk cows for tuberculosis? Does your community have periodic campaigns to get chest roentgenograms of as many people as possible? Are preschool and school children tuberculin-tested at regular intervals? What provision is made for follow-up of those children with positive tests?

THE EDEMATOUS 3-YEAR-OLD CHILD—PATIENT STUDY

David Bromley, aged 3 years, was admitted to a large private room in a children's hospital with an admission diagnosis of nephrosis. His mother remained in the room during the entire hospital stay of 5 weeks. David brought a large collection of toys with him and received many more while there. He was an alert, active child with blond curly hair and soon became a favorite of all hospital personnel.

Mrs. Bromley told the nurses that David had had many colds during the past winter and that he had had pneumonia at the age of 2 years. He had been vaccinated for smallpox and immunized against diphtheria, pertussis and tetanus. During the previous week David began to have some swelling around his eyes and ankles, which progressed to the entire body. Mrs. Bromley was concerned chiefly with David's poor appetite and a fine, red rash over his lower abdomen.

Admission orders were as follows:

1. Bed rest.
2. Record intake and output.
3. High-protein, low-salt diet—substitute Lonolac for milk.
4. Record weight 3 times weekly.
5. Penicillin 50,000 units q. 4 h. for 3 days.
6. Elixir phenobarbital gr. ¼ at bedtime as necessary.
7. Laboratory examinations to include C.B.C., hemoglobin, sedimentation rate and daily urinalysis.
8. Blood pressure daily.

David's weight on admission was 40 pounds and there was generalized pitting edema of the face, abdomen, legs, feet and genitalia. On the second day, he developed diarrhea, for which Kaopectate was given. David's appetite remained poor in spite of all tempting foods offered him, and there was occasional vomiting. He was irritable at times during the hospital stay but after he became acquainted with a particular nurse he was friendly and happy with her.

At the time of discharge David had lost 8 pounds of weight. His eyes were still puffy and there was very slight edema of the hands and feet. Mrs. Bromley was told that he was not entirely well but that with the knowledge she had gained from the nurses, and with frequent visits by the physician, David could be cared for at home.

References

Jeans, Philip, Rand, Winifred, and Blake, Florence: Essentials of Pediatrics, ed. 4, p. 259 (abdominal paracentesis), 1946.

Heyman, Walter: Renal disorders in infants and children, Am. J. Nursing, 48:436, 1948.

Blumgarten, A. S.: Textbook of Materia Medica, Pharmacology, and Therapeutics, p. 238, (use of Kaopectate), New York, Macmillan, 1937.

Mitchell-Nelson: Textbook of Pediatrics, ed. 4, pp. 982–989, Philadelphia, Saunders, 1946.

Questions Relating to the Patient Study

1. Activities which should be most effective in securing bed rest for David are

   a._____change toys frequently, keep his skin clean and dry, permit unlimited visiting by his immediate relatives.

   b._____provide soft music, darken the room, remove all toys.

   c._____ask his mother to remain in the waiting room, offer the child rewards for resting, have the nurse remain with the child.

   d._____change toys as indicated by the child's interest, keep his skin clean and dry, maintain a comfortable position in bed.

2. David's skin needed special care because of excessive perspiration. The type of care which should be given is to

   a._____omit soap and water, use mineral oil for cleansing.

   b._____bathe twice daily with soap and water followed by a small amount of soothing powder.

   c._____bathe once daily followed by an alcohol rub.

   d._____bathe twice daily followed by an oil massage.

3. David's irritability most likely would be due to

   a._____irritation of the skin, being forced to remain in bed, being spoiled by too much attention.

   b._____abdominal discomfort, penicillin injections, strange surroundings.

   c._____generalized edema, skin irritation, abdominal discomfort.

   d._____being spoiled by too much attention, penicillin injections, skin irritation.

4. You would expect the laboratory report on the urinalysis to show
   a._____albumin 4+, many casts, lipoid bodies.
   b._____albumin 4+, many red cells, no casts.
   c._____albumin 1+, sugar negative, lipoid bodies.
   d._____albumin negative, specific gravity 1.001, many red cells.

5. You would expect the laboratory report of the blood examination to show
   a._____erythrocytes 4,500,000, leukocytes 6,000, normal sedimentation rate.
   b._____erythrocytes 4,800,000, leukocytes 20,000, elevated sedimentation rate.
   c._____hemoglobin 10 Gm. per 100 cc. of blood, elevated sedimentation rate, leukocytes 6,000.
   d._____erythrocytes 4,800,000, hemoglobin 10 Gm. per 100 cc. of blood, normal sedimentation rate.

6. You would expect David's daily average urinary output during the edematous phase to be approximately
   a._____500–600 cc.
   b._____50–150 cc.
   c._____300–400 cc.

7. Mrs. Bromley became upset because David wet the bed the first 2 nights they were in the hospital. In response to her anxiety you should tell her that the bedwetting
   a._____will be reported to her private physician.
   b._____is an indication of kidney disease.
   c._____probably results from drinking too much water at bedtime.
   d._____is to be expected during illness in a young child.

8. The purpose of the high-protein diet ordered for David was to
   a._____restore the albumin lost in the urine, maintain the nitrogen balance, raise the level of the serum protein in the blood.
   b._____restore the albumin lost in the urine, raise the level of the serum protein in the blood, prevent a loss of weight.
   c._____maintain the nitrogen balance, promote normal growth, prevent anemia.
   d._____raise the level of the serum protein in the blood, maintain the nitrogen balance, promote normal growth.

9. The purpose of a low salt diet was to
   a._____decrease thirst.
   b._____lessen perspiration.
   c._____prevent the retention of body fluids.
   d._____improve the appetite.

10. Lonolac was ordered for David as a milk substitute because it **is**
    a._____high in protein.   c._____low in fat.
    b._____low in sodium.   d._____high in carbohydrate.

11. David's weight showed a drop of 8 pounds as a result of

    a._____poor appetite.
    b._____an attack of diarrhea.
    c._____loss of fluids as edema disappeared.

12. The Kaopectate which was given to David is a preparation of kaolin with pectin added. This medication is classified as a (an)

    a._____carminative.
    b._____demulcent.
    c._____antiseptic.
    d._____sedative.

13. The expected action of Kaopectate is to

    a._____absorb moisture, coat the mucosal surfaces of the intestinal tract.
    b._____relieve intestinal cramps, improve the appetite.
    c._____reduce the rate of peristalsis, stimulate the flow of gastric juices.

14. Kaopectate usually is prepared for administration in a

    a._____capsule.
    b._____solution.
    c._____tablet.

15. Kaopectate usually is ordered

    a._____3 times daily.
    b._____every hour until diarrhea is controlled.
    c._____as 1 dose following each stool until the diarrhea is controlled.

Questions for Discussion and Student Projects

1. Describe your plan of nursing care for David, including

  a. Physical care:
    (1) position in bed.
    (2) skin care to promote comfort and prevent abrasions.
    (3) measures to relieve skin irritation due to rash.
    (4) prevention of exposure to infections.
    (5) provision for warmth and prevention of chilling.

  b. Feeding technics:
    (1) preparation of foods to provide interest.
    (2) methods to conserve energy at mealtime.
    (3) consistency of foods most acceptable to a 3-year-old child.
    (4) method of recording food and fluid intake.

  c. Emotional needs:
    (1) measures used to help the child feel accepted.
    (2) play materials suitable for the age and the type of illness.

(3) ways of establishing a wholesome relationship with the child's parents.

(4) recognition of signs of regression.

2. Prepare a plan for teaching Mrs. Bromley to care for David at home, including specific information on bathing, dressing, rest, toys, prevention of infection and care of the skin. How would teaching differ in this situation when the mother is present from that carried out only during visiting hours in wards? In which situation do you think teaching should be most beneficial? Give illustrations of desirable teaching which should take place through the mother's observation of the nurses giving care to David.

3. Describe your method of obtaining David's weight 3 times weekly. Is he permitted to stand on the scale? Does this procedure conflict with the order for bed rest?

Questions Relating to the Section in General

1. The cause of nephrosis is

a._____unknown.
b._____from bacterial infections.
c._____based on hereditary factors.

2. The outstanding features of nephrosis are

a._____recurrent edema, a fever of 103°F., albuminuria.
b._____poor appetite, an elevated blood pressure, recurrent edema.
c._____a fever of 101°F., albuminuria, normal blood pressure.
d._____recurrent edema, albuminuria, poor appetite.

3. In the following age groups, nephrosis occurs most frequently in

a._____6–9 years.
b._____4–7 years.
c._____under 3 years.
d._____over 8 years.

4. The onset in nephrosis is

a._____rapid with high fever and slight edema.
b._____rapid with severe edema and high fever.
c._____slow with slight edema and normal temperature.
d._____slow with severe edema and normal temperature.

5. The organism found most commonly in the respiratory tract during attacks of nephrosis is

a._____*Streptococcus hemolyticus.*
b._____*Pneumococcus.*
c._____*Staphylococcus.*
d._____*Streptococcus viridans.*

6. Complications which occur most frequently with nephrosis are

   a._____respiratory infections, rickets, decubitus ulcers.
   b._____anemia, respiratory infections, pneumococcic peritonitis.
   c._____malnutrition, meningitis, anemia.
   d._____anemia, rickets, pneumococcic peritonitis.

7. Check the statement below which describes the prognosis in nephrosis:

   a._____about 80 per cent of the children with nephrosis will recover
       completely.
   b._____about 50 per cent of the children with nephrosis will recover
       completely.
   c._____there is no hope for recovery.
   d._____there will be some residual kidney damage after the first attack
       of nephrosis.

8. The daily average output of urine for the child aged 1 to 3 years is

   a._____300–400 cc.
   b._____500–600 cc.
   c._____900–1,000 cc.

9. The daily average output of urine for the child aged 3 to 5 years is

   a._____900–1,000 cc.
   b._____300–400 cc.
   c._____600–700 cc.

10. The daily average output of urine for the child aged 5 to 8 years is

   a._____650–1,000 cc.
   b._____1,200–1,400 cc.
   c._____500–600 cc.

Questions for Discussion and Student Projects—(*Continued*)

1. Write to Mead Johnson Company, Evansville, Ind. (suggested project for one student) for information on Lonolac. Obtain samples of Lonolac from the hospital kitchen, if available. Prepare a report for the class giving the ingredients of Lonolac, showing how it is prepared and served, the reasons for giving and discussing some of the problems involved in the use of this substance.
2. Prepare a list of foods suitable for a 3-year-old child who is ordered a diet high in protein and low in salt. Plan sample menus for 3 days from your list.
3. At times an abdominal paracentesis becomes necessary for the child with nephrosis because of excessive pressure on the diaphragm. Describe the nursing care indicated by this treatment, including

   a. preparation of the child, both physically and emotionally.
   b. equipment needed.
   c. position of the child during the procedure.
   d. observations to be made during and after treatment.
   e. information to be recorded on the child's chart.
   f. care of the child and his bed as a result of seepage of fluid following the paracentesis.

4. Describe safety measures which are carried out in your hospital for the prevention of accidents. What is done to keep small children from falling out of beds or cribs? Make a tour of your pediatric unit for the purpose of detecting any physical hazards and report any found to the head nurse or the supervisor.

THE CHILD WHO WAS BURNT IN THE BRUSH FIRE—PATIENT STUDY

Four-year-old Donna Hawkins was admitted to the pediatric unit from the operating room where emergency treatment had been carried out for burns. Donna's clothing had caught fire while she was playing near a brush fire a few hours previously. She had second-degree burns over the left cheek, left forearm, anterior chest and legs, and third-degree burns over the lower back and abdomen. On admission to the ward a solution of 10 per cent dextrose in isotonic saline was being given intravenously at the rate of 40 drops per minute. Donna was quite drowsy.

Medical history showed that this child had received "triple shots" at the fourth, fifth and sixth months of life and a booster dose at 3 years. She had been vaccinated for smallpox at the age of 9 months.

Hemoglobin determination on admission was reported to be 100 per cent. Six hours later it was 110 per cent and blood plasma was given intravenously.

Donna remained in the hospital for a total of 5 months. During the first week intravenous fluids and plasma were given daily. Twice daily she received 300,000 units of fortified penicillin in aqueous solution intramusculary. Donna was kept in the dorsal position and every effort was made to maintain rest during this time. From the day of admission one of the major problems was Donna's nutrition. She refused both liquids and solids. The diet order was for protein Gm. 80, fat Gm. 50 and carbohydrate Gm. 150—total calories, 1,400. Penicillin was discontinued on the theory that this drug might be causing the poor appetite and Chloromycetin 250 mg. q. 3 h. was ordered orally. Phenobarbital elixir gr. ¼ was given as needed to produce relaxation.

Each week Donna was taken to the treatment room for a change of dressings. Healing was very slow. After 3 months the first of 4 skin grafts was done. Each time that preparations were made for skin grafting Donna cried and begged the nurses not to take her to the operating room. The child's appetite improved slightly after the first skin graft. The head of her crib was elevated, thus permitting her to feed herself and to use a bed tray for play.

Two weeks before discharge, Donna was allowed to be up walking. There was a flexion deformity of the hips of about 30° when the child was placed on her feet. Physiotherapy was ordered daily while in the hospital and Mrs. Hawkins was taught exercises and massage to be carried out at home. Below are the orders for Donna's continued care at home:

1. A diet high in protein, vitamins and iron.
2. Exercises and massage as taught by the physiotherapist.
3. Cod-liver-oil concentrate 10 drops daily.
4. At least 9 hours' sleep at night and a rest period each afternoon.
5. Return to the surgical clinic in 2 weeks.

References

Gesell, Arnold, and Ilg, Frances: The Infant and Child in the Culture of To-day, pp. 224–245, New York, Harpers, 1943.

Herschfield, John Winslow: The treatment of thermal burns, Am. J. Nursing 46:156, 1946.

Siler, Vinton E.: Burns and their treatment, Am. J. Nursing 42:994, 1942.

Spock, Benjamin: The Pocket Book of Child Care, pp. 280–286, 329–340, New York, Pocket Books, 1946.

Wallinger, Elsie: Burns and their nursing care, Am. J. Nursing 42:1000, 1942.

Questions Relating to the Patient Study

1. Symptoms of shock occurring soon after a severe burn include

   a._____pallor, rapid pulse, shallow respirations, elevated temperature.
   b._____slow pulse, rapid respirations, pallor, subnormal temperature.
   c._____low blood pressure, rapid pulse, elevated temperature, prostration.
   d._____pallor, subnormal temperature, weak rapid pulse, low blood pressure.
   e._____prostration, high blood pressure, rapid pulse, rapid respirations.

2. Symptoms of a toxic reaction occurring several hours after a severe burn include

   a._____flushed face, vomiting, slow pulse rate.
   b._____decreased urinary output, rapid pulse, flushed face.
   c._____dry mouth, slow pulse, decreased urinary output.
   d._____elevation of temperature, pallor, rapid pulse.
   e._____flushed face, slow pulse, coma.

3. The hemoglobin determination is higher than normal following a severe burn because of

   a._____shock caused by the burn.
   b._____loss of skin surface.
   c._____diminished fluid intake.
   d._____release of plasma into tissues at site of burn.

4. As Donna improves the mother and head nurse decide she no longer needs to be in a room alone. Of the possibilities below, it is best to place her in a

   a._____cubicle with another 4-year-old girl.
   b._____ward with 7 other small girls.
   c._____4-bed ward with 3 large girls.
   d._____ward with 3 girls and 4 boys.
   e._____4-bed ward with children aged 18 months to 3 years.

5. A diet high in protein is ordered to

   a._____aid in the repair of tissues.
   b._____promote growth.

    c._____help make up for the loss of nitrogen.

    d._____improve the appetite.

6. Methods which have been most effective in getting 4-year-old children to eat are to

    a._____serve small amounts, avoid all discussion of food, give a reward for food eaten at each meal.

    b._____serve small amounts, serve foods that are eaten with the fingers, avoid urging the child to eat.

    c._____serve dessert only when other foods have been taken, give daily rewards for foods eaten, stimulate competition with other children.

    d._____allow the mother to come in at mealtime and feed the child, prepare trays as attractively as possible, tell the child that if she eats well she will soon be well enough to go home.

7. Diversional activities for Donna during the time when she is in bed would include giving her

    a._____color books, picture magazines, small cuddly animals.

    b._____jigsaw puzzles, storybook dolls, a record player with records played by an adult.

    c._____modeling clay, finger painting, cut-out dolls.

    d._____small cuddly animals, finger painting, jigsaw puzzles.

8. Planned activities which might help correct the hip-flexion deformity when Donna is convalescing include

    a._____building with blocks while standing at a low table.

    b._____lying on her side in bed or on a table, keeping time to music, using both hands and feet.

    c._____reaching up on shelves to obtain play materials.

    d._____coloring in bed with her head elevated and with a bed tray across her lap.

9. The immunizing substance referred to as "triple shots" protects children against

    a._____pertussis, measles, diphtheria.

    b._____typhoid, pertussis, tetanus.

    c._____pertussis, tetanus, diphtheria.

    d._____measles, typhoid, diphtheria.

    e._____tetanus, diphtheria, pertussis.

10. Burns are often described as first-, second-, and third-degree in type. Match the following:

    a._____partial destruction of the skin.   (1) first degree.

    b._____full-thickness destruction of the skin.   (2) second degree.

    c._____erythema.   (3) third degree.

    d._____charring into muscle and/or bone.

    e._____erythema followed by vesicle formation.

11. Anemia is a frequent complication in patients suffering from burns. From the list below check the foods recommended in secondary anemia:

a._____milk.   f._____liver.
b._____eggs.   g._____cheese.
c._____vegetables, green.   h._____fruit.
d._____potatoes.   i._____pork.
e._____whole wheat cereal.   j._____navy beans.

Questions for Discussion and Student Projects

1. Prepare a list of various ways in which children usually become burned and present a method of prevention for each one.
2. What technics do you consider to be most effective in preparing a 4-year-old child to go to the operating room? What is the nurse's responsibility?
3. What methods would you use to lessen anxiety when taking a child to the treatment room for a painful procedure, during and after the procedure?
4. Plan a sample menu for a healthy 4-year-old child. Show modifications needed to adjust this menu to the diet ordered for Donna—protein 80 Gm., fat 50 Gm. and carbohydrate 150 Gm.
5. What measures do you believe could have been used to prevent the flexion deformity of Donna's hips?
6. Consider how parents may feel about an accident which could have been prevented. Prepare a list of possible responses the parents may make to the situation and give your reasons for including each one.
7. How do you think a student nurse feels toward a child who consistently refuses to eat? What should you have done if you had been responsible for Donna during the early phase of hospitalization when diet was a major problem?
8. From your own hospital situation, determine the approximate cost for maintaining a child in a pediatric unit for 5 months. In case the family cannot meet the expenses, what resources are available in your community?
9. Considering the immunizations that Donna had received in the past, do you think that additional tetanus toxoid should be given following the burns?
10. Describe your plan of nursing care for Donna, including

a. Physical care:

(1) position in bed for comfort and for prevention of deformities.
(2) administration of intramuscular injection—what areas of the body might be used when the lower back and buttocks have been burned?
(3) provision for warmth and the prevention of chilling.
(4) protection from infections.
(5) method of collecting the urine specimen.

(6) taking and recording blood pressure twice daily.

(7) recording intake and output.

b. Methods for meeting emotional needs:

(1) State how you would explain to Donna the need for remaining in the hospital; visiting regulations; the reason for restraints during the administration of intravenous fluids; the purpose of intramuscular injections. What would your response be if the child interpreted the needles as punishment?

(2) Describe the way in which home contacts might be maintained during a long period of hospitalization.

(3) Give some possible reasons for Donna's persistent refusal to eat.

c. Observations:

(1) character of pulse and respirations.

(2) color of skin.

(3) degree of responsiveness.

(4) changes in behavior during hospitalization.

CARDIAC SURGERY ON A 5-YEAR-OLD BOY—PATIENT STUDY

Joe Williams, aged 5 years, was admitted to the pediatric unit for cardiac surgery. The congenital defect, patent ductus arteriosus, was discovered by the family physician during a routine examination when Joe was 6 months old. Mrs. Williams stated that Joe had never been blue but had seemed short of breath if he ran fast or played too long. There had been episodes of coughing and difficult breathing when lying in a recumbent position. Now the family felt that some action should be taken to prepare Joe for entrance into school the following year.

Joe remained in the unit 5 days before surgery was done. During this time certain tests were carried out and Joe became acquainted with hospital personnel and routines. On the morning of the operation the nurse gave Joe his preoperative medication and took him to the operating room. Upon return he was placed in an oxygen tent and given continuous nursing care for the next 24 hours. Codeine gr. ¼ was given hypodermically for pain. Other orders included crystalline penicillin 400,000 units daily, fluids by mouth as tolerated and gradual return to full diet. On the third postoperative day Joe was up in a wheel chair, was walking on the fourth day, and went home on the eighth day following surgery.

Review Project

Prepare a drawing of the heart and the blood vessels showing circulation in the healthy individual. Include the following structures: Right auricle, right ventricle, left auricle, left ventricle, right lung, left lung, pulmonary artery, pulmonary veins, aorta, inferior and superior vena cava.

Using blue pencil to show areas of venous circulation and red pencil to show arterial circulation, draw small arrows to designate the direction of the blood flow. Using lead pencil and making dotted lines, show the location of the ductus arteriosus as it exists during fetal life.

References

Crystal, Dean K.: The operable cardiac anomalies, Am. J. Nursing 49:587, 1949.
Gesell, Arnold, and Ilg, Francis: The Infant and Child in the Culture of Today, pp. 246–251, New York, Harpers, 1943.
Potts, Willis J.: Tetralogy of Fallot, Am. J. Nursing 47:298, 1947; Pierson, D. Elizabeth: Nursing care of a child with tetralogy of Fallot, Am. J. Nursing 47:301, 1947.
Smith, Elizabeth M.: A nursing staff prepares for cardiac surgery, Am. J. Nursing 49:589, 1949.
Wallace, Mildred: Care of the child with tetralogy of Fallot, Am. J. Nursing 52:195, 1952.

Questions Relating to the Patient Study

1. In comparing Joe with a healthy 5-year-old boy, differences you would expect to see in Joe's growth are

   a._____shorter in stature, heavier in weight, delayed dentition.
   b._____taller in stature, lighter in weight, muscles less firm.
   c._____shorter in stature, muscles less firm, lighter in weight.
   d._____delayed dentition, muscles more firm, shorter in stature.

2. Personality characteristics for which to be alert as Joe is under your care include

   a._____dependence, stubbornness, lack of self-confidence.
   b._____fear of bodily damage, dependence, lack of self-confidence.
   c._____withdrawal from contacts with other children, fear of unfamiliar adults, dependence.
   d._____curiosity about new surroundings, friendliness, independence.

3. Recreational activities suitable for Joe in the period before surgery include

   a._____finger painting, color books, comic books.
   b._____push-and-pull toys, building blocks, color books.
   c._____trips around the hospital, record player, comic books.
   d._____jigsaw puzzles, building blocks, finger painting.

4. In order to help Joe in his adjustment to the hospital he should be admitted to a

   a._____single room.
   b._____cubicle with a 5-year-old boy who has had heart surgery.
   c._____large ward with 7 other children of various ages.
   d._____ward with 3 other children around 5 years of age.

5. In assigning someone to care for Joe in the preoperative period, the head nurse should choose a

   a._____senior student.
   b._____nursing aide.
   c._____different nurse each day.
   d._____nurse who will care for him following surgery.

6. Physical preparation indicated for Joe's surgery should include

    a._____taking his blood pressure twice daily, recording intake and output, keeping him in bed.

    b._____protecting him from infections, allowing him to be up and walking around the pediatric unit, giving him food and fluids as desired.

    c._____giving a daily enema, urging him to eat everything served to him, taking his blood pressure twice daily.

    d._____protecting him from infections, keeping him in bed, recording intake and output.

7. Methods you would expect to be effective in allaying Joe's anxiety about his operation are to

    a._____tell him as much about the operating room as he can understand, show him that you are going to take good care of him at all times, accompany Joe to the operating room.

    b._____provide suitable recreation, ignore questions about the operation, be very kind at all times.

    c._____tell Joe that lots of boys his age have operations, allow the parents to visit frequently, talk to Joe about his pets at home.

    d._____plan for Joe to get acquainted with the anesthetist, give him a sedative when he seems disturbed, ignore his questions about the operation.

8. The most desirable age for repair of Joe's defect is

    a._____in infancy.

    b._____between 5 and 12 years of age.

    c._____between 8 and 10 years of age.

    d._____after 13 years of age.

9. Joe's prognosis following successful surgery is for

    a._____life expectancy of about 25 years.

    b._____full life expectancy with normal activities.

    c._____life expectancy of about 10 years.

    d._____full life expectancy with limited activities.

10. Since tracheal irritation is a possible complication following endotracheal anesthesia, Joe should be observed for

    a._____cyanosis, increased pulse rate, labored respirations, restlessness.

    b._____cyanosis, coma, decreased pulse rate, Cheyne-Stokes respirations.

    c._____convulsions, elevated temperature, increased pulse rate, labored respirations.

    d._____pallor, subnormal temperature, Cheyne-Stokes respirations, weak pulse.

11. The nurse caring for Joe was instructed to encourage him to cough and to rotate him from side to back and to the other side every hour. The purpose of this activity is to:

a._____prevent hypostatic pneumonia.
b._____relieve pressure on the incision.
c._____prevent atelectasis.
d._____provide for the greater physical comfort of the child.

12. Unless specific orders are left you should regulate the oxygen concentration and the temperature in the oxygen tent as follows:

a._____oxygen concentration of at least 50 per cent, temperature 85°.
b._____oxygen concentration of at least 85 per cent, temperature 70°.
c._____oxygen concentration of at least 75 per cent, temperature 78°.
d._____oxygen concentration of at least 50 per cent, temperature 70°.

13. Joe's doctor wished him to have sufficient fluids by mouth in order to discontinue I.V. fluids as soon as possible. In case he resisted taking the liquids from the kitchen you should

a._____tell him the doctor will start intravenous fluids again.
b._____permit the mother to bring in his favorite beverages from outside the hospital.
c._____try a different kind of fluid every 15 minutes.
d._____record on the chart that he is un-co-operative.

14. Penicillin was ordered for Joe to

a._____promote healing of the chest wound.
b._____prevent pneumonia.
c._____prevent subacute bacterial endocarditis.
d._____prevent upper respiratory infection.

15. The defect in patent ductus arteriosus is caused by

a._____narrowing of the pulmonary artery.
b._____hypertrophy of the right ventricle.
c._____failure of a fetal blood vessel between the aorta and the pulmonary artery to close.
d._____failure of the valve between the right and the left auricles to close.

Questions for Discussion and Student Projects

1. Prepare a list of specific information you should obtain from Joe's mother in order to give him good nursing care while he is in the hospital.
2. Describe methods you should use to prepare Joe for the care he will receive at the time of surgery and immediately thereafter. Do you believe he should be taken on a trip to the operating room a day or two in advance where he is shown the rooms and is introduced to the personnel? Do you think he should see an oxygen tent before surgery? Should he be told that he will be in a single room on return from surgery, if such is in the plan?
3. How do you think Joe's parents feel before, during and after the operation? What is the nurse's responsibility toward them at these times?

4. What should you do if you are giving care to Joe and you are interrupted frequently by doctors and nurses from other wards coming in because they have never seen a patient with cardiac surgery? Is your first responsibility to care for the child or to help educate medical and nursing personnel?
5. As you are teaching Mr. and Mrs. Williams to care for Joe at home, what points do you believe should have the most emphasis? Prepare a list of the specific information to be given, including possible changes in Joe's behavior and personality characteristics. Do you think the parents need to be told that certain changes are to be expected?

Questions Relating to Congenital Heart Disease in General

[Questions 1 to 9 relate to the tetralogy of Fallot.]

1. Another congenital heart condition is known as the tetralogy of Fallot. The abnormal changes in heart structure are

   a._____stenosis of the pulmonary vein, hypertrophy of the right side of the heart, interventricular septal defect, dextroposition of the aorta.
   b._____hypertrophy of the left ventricle, stenosis of the pulmonary vein, interventricular septal defect, dextroposition of the aorta.
   c._____stenosis of the pulmonary artery, hypertrophy of the right side of the heart, interventricular septal defect, dextroposition of the aorta.
   d._____stenosis of the pulmonary artery, hypertrophy of the left ventricle, dilatation of the right auricle, interventricular septal defect.

2. Outstanding symptoms observed in the child with tetralogy of Fallot are

   a._____cyanosis, fatigue, clubbing of the ends of the fingers and the toes.
   b._____overweight, cyanosis, good appetite.
   c._____fatigue, cyanosis, hyperactivity.
   d._____cyanosis, poor appetite, restlessness.

3. Children with this congenital heart condition are extremely susceptible to

   a._____gastrointestinal disorders.
   b._____upper respiratory infections.
   c._____skin infections.
   d._____allergic conditions.

4. In tetralogy of Fallot the erythrocyte count is usually between

   a._____4 and 5 million per cubic millimeter.
   b._____2 and 3 million per cubic millimeter.
   c._____6 and 8 million per cubic millimeter.
   d._____7 and 9 million per cubic millimeter.

5. Reports of hemoglobin would be expected to show
   a._____10–12 Gm. per 100 cc. of blood.
   b._____16–24 Gm. per 100 cc. of blood.
   c._____25–30 Gm. per 100 cc. of blood.
   d._____8–10 Gm. per 100 cc. of blood.

6. The most suitable age for surgery for this type of heart condition is
   a._____in early infancy.
   b._____between the ages of 2 and 6 years.
   c._____between the ages of 7 and 14 years.
   d._____in early adolescence.

7. When parents talk to nurses about surgery for "blue babies," the nurse should tell them that
   a._____they should consult a surgeon competent in this field.
   b._____many heart conditions cannot be corrected by surgery.
   c._____all of the operations are successful.
   d._____very few of the operations are successful.

8. In tetralogy of Fallot, thrombosis in the cerebral vessels is one complication which may occur; it is caused by
   a._____elevation of the blood pressure.
   b._____infection in the blood stream.
   c._____an excessive number of red blood cells.
   d._____improper position in bed.

9. A measure usually successful in the prevention of thrombosis is
   a._____adequate hydration.
   b._____sedation.
   c._____elevation of the head of the bed.
   d._____administration of antibiotics.

10. A complication which may occur in any of the congenital heart conditions is subacute bacterial endocarditis. In order to assist the doctor in early recognition of this complication the nurse should be alert for
    a._____pallor, malaise, subnormal temperature.
    b._____convulsions, flushed face, a fever of 103°.
    c._____daily rise in temperature, irritability, thirst.
    d._____pallor, malaise, daily rise in temperature.

11. Symptoms expected in the later stages of subacute bacterial endocarditis include
    a._____small hemorrhagic areas in the skin and mucous membranes, diarrhea, fever.
    b._____raised nodules in the tissues or the ends of the fingers, subnormal temperature, coma.
    c._____small hemorrhagic areas in the skin and mucous membranes, abdominal pain, raised nodules in the tissues or the ends of the fingers.
    d._____abdominal pain, diarrhea, coma.

12. The causative organism in subacute bacterial endocarditis is most commonly

   a._____*Streptococcus viridans.*
   b._____*Staphylococcus aureus.*
   c._____*Streptococcus hemolyticus.*
   d._____*Staphylococcus albus.*

13. The most conclusive diagnostic finding is

   a._____elevation of the sedimentation rate.
   b._____positive blood culture.
   c._____changes in heart sounds.
   d._____the presence of anemia.

[The following questions relate to the development of the average 5-year-old child.]

1. The child is

   a._____able to print his own name, to write words legibly, to remember his home address.
   b._____able to print or write his own name, to write many words legibly, to remember his home address.
   c._____able to print his own name, to remember his home address, not able to write legibly.
   d._____unable to print or write, able to remember his name but not his home address.

2. This child is usually able to

   a._____dress and undress himself, enjoys "dressing up."
   b._____undress but not dress himself, resists "dressing up."
   c._____dress and undress himself, resists "dressing up."

3. He would be apt to

   a._____make friends easily with new adults.
   b._____be excessively shy with new adults.
   c._____show no interest in adults.

4. You would expect this child to

   a._____be very dependent upon his mother, dread going to school, be interested in the world outside his home.
   b._____be very dependent upon his mother, dread going to school, be interested only in his own home.
   c._____show increasing independence, be interested in the world outside his home, be eager to go to school.

5. In his play activities he shows

   a._____ability to share his toys, equal enjoyment of both boys and girls.
   b._____ability to share his toys, prefers to play with children of his own sex.

c.____inability to share his toys, prefers to play with children of the opposite sex.

d.____inability to share his toys or to play with other children.

6. You could expect this child to have temper tantrums.

a.____frequently.   b.____infrequently.   c.____never.

Questions for Discussion and Student Projects—(*Continued*)

1. Describe how nursing care differs in the pre- and postoperative periods in tetralogy of Fallot and in surgical repair of patent ductus arteriosus.
2. In the child with tetralogy of Fallot, why is it important for the nurse to know the type of operation performed in order to make accurate observations?
3. Prepare a list of equipment to be assembled in the room for use in the immediate postoperative period.
4. Describe activities which you believe a public health nurse should carry out while making periodic visits to a family whose child has a congenital heart condition. What is her responsibility in relation to continued medical care for the sick child, for prevention of illness in the entire family and for helping the family adjust to certain restrictions?

THE 6-YEAR-OLD HANDICAPPED CHILD—PATIENT STUDY

Julia Smith, aged 6 years, was seen in the out-patient department for a routine examination. Julia had been coming to the orthopedic clinic since the age of 1 year, when her condition was diagnosed as cerebral palsy, spastic paraplegia. On this visit, Mrs. Smith asked the doctor's advice about Julia entering public school and added that she hoped the special shoes might be unnecessary in the future.

The physician, nurse, mother and physiotherapist talked together following clinic in an effort to determine the best plan for Julia. A summary of the history follows:

Julia was born at full term following a long and difficult labor. The baby had difficulty swallowing at first but learned gradually to take an adequate diet. Her general development had always been slower than average, and medical aid was obtained because she was not sitting alone at 10 months. After the true nature of her difficulty was determined, physiotherapy was begun and continued once or twice weekly since that time. Night splints had been worn each night for the past 5 years and for 2 years long leg braces were used. At present Julia is able to walk unaided but her leg movements are jerky and special shoes are being used for daytime wear. This child's general health has been good. She has had chickenpox and a few colds. She has been immunized against diphtheria, whooping cough and tetanus, and vaccinated for smallpox. Julia has no brothers or sisters; the parents state that they wish to give all of their time to her.

During the conference with the doctor, nurse and physiotherapist, Mrs. Smith was chiefly concerned over how Julia would get along with other children since she had been with adults most of her life. A mutual decision was made to enroll her in public school and the nurse gave Mrs. Smith some guidance as to Julia's preparation for school. The doctor recommended that the special shoes be continued to be worn as additional support was needed for Julia's feet.

References

Jones, Margaret H.: The cerebral palsy child, Am. J. Nursing 46:465, 1946.
Kerr, Marion: Nursing responsibilities in cerebral palsy, Am. J. Nursing 46:469, 1946.
Abel, Marjorie: Feeding the child with cerebral palsy, Am. J. Nursing 50:558, 1950.
Film in sound and technicolor, "A Day in the Life of a Cerebral Palsy Patient," prepared at Phelps Clinic, Baltimore, Md. May be obtained through National Society for Crippled Children and Adults, Inc., Suite 1015, 11 S. LaSalle St., Chicago 3, Ill.

Background Review Questions

Match the following terms which are used in the study of cerebral palsy:

a._____motor cortex.
b._____hemiplegia.
c._____paraplegia.
d._____basal ganglia.
e._____pyramidal tract.
f._____monoplegia.
g._____extrapyramidal tract.
h._____tendon of Achilles.
i._____internal rotation.
j._____outward rotation.

(1) involvement of one side of the body.
(2) movement of a bone around a central axis, toward the midline of the body.
(3) an area in the cerebrum which controls voluntary planned movements.
(4) involvement of one extremity.
(5) paths from basal ganglia which promote purposeful co-ordinated movements.
(6) involvement of both lower extremities.
(7) an area in the cerebrum which controls associated movements.
(8) paths from the motor cortex which inhibit the action of muscles antagonistic to those attempting to contract.
(9) movement of a bone around a central axis, away from the midline of the body.
(10) involvement of both upper extremities.
(11) a band of tissue which connects the calf muscle to the heel bone.

Questions Relating to the Patient Study

1. From your knowledge of the effects of cerebral palsy you would expect Julia to show the following personality traits:

    a._____outgoing friendliness, seeking affection, inquisitiveness.
    b._____fear of unfamiliar situations, shyness, dependence.

   c._____aggressiveness, a tendency toward temper tantrums, destructive-
      ness.

   d._____emotional instability, lack of confidence, affectionate toward
      adults.

2. In order to evaluate Julia's mental status, she should be

   a._____given standardized intelligence tests to determine her I.Q.
   b._____gives tests prepared for cerebral palsy children only.
   c._____observed over long periods of time to determine the types of
      learning taking place in various areas.

3. Certain modifications of the daily diet for a 6-year-old child are indicated for Julia because of her difficulty:

   a._____increase in calories, protein and all vitamins.
   b._____increase in calcium and the vitamin-B group and decrease in
      calories.
   c._____increase in all vitamins and protein and decrease in calories.
   d._____increase in calories, protein and the vitamin-B group.

4. From the list of persons working together as a team to obtain the type
of care for Julia, check the one you consider to be the most vital
in attaining the care desired:

   a._____physiotherapist.
   b._____nurse.
   c._____mother.
   d._____physician.
   e._____social worker.

5. The nurse who works with Julia in the out-patient department
should be

   a._____friendly, calm, forceful.
   b._____kind, enthusiastic, affectionate.
   c._____calm, stern, exacting.
   d._____protective, affectionate, friendly.

6. The medical record showed that when Julia first began to walk she
used the "scissors-gait." This type of walking results from the following combination:

   a._____hip flexion, abduction of the thighs, outward rotation of the
      knees.
   b._____lordosis, outward rotation of the hips, knee flexion.
   c._____shortening of the tendon of Achilles, internal rotation of the
      knees, outward rotation of the hips.
   d._____hip and knee flexion, adduction of the thighs, shortening of the
      tendon of Achilles.

7. Leg braces were ordered for Julia to

   a._____assist her in walking.
   b._____prevent muscle contractures.

c._____prevent the development of bow legs.

d._____promote good posture.

Questions for Discussion and Student Projects

1. Assume you were the nurse in the out-patient department during the 5-year period of Julia's treatment. Outline a plan of health teaching for the parents including

   a. the nutrition of the family with emphasis on Julia's needs.

   b. physical care, such as bathing, dressing, toileting, sleep and rest, and improvised equipment for Julia.

   c. emotional aspects, such as development of independence, management of temper tantrums, suitable play materials, acceptance of the handicap by the parents, the child and other close relatives, and provision for contact with other children.

   d. the care of braces and night splints. How should the mother be taught to care for the skin? How would you encourage the mother to keep the braces and splints on when the child resists them?

   e. the health of Mrs. Smith. Make suggestions for recreation, measures for the simplification of housework and the possibility of having part of Julia's care given by the father or another person.

   f. methods to insure continued medical treatment for Julia. What should your response be to Mrs. Smith if she asked you about taking Julia to a clinic which advertises "quick cures" for cerebral palsy?

2. How do you think Mr. and Mrs. Smith felt when they were told that Julia had cerebral palsy? List a few possible attitudes and for each one state how nurses should be able to help parents accept the diagnosis.

3. Suppose you were the nurse who gave guidance to Mrs. Smith as to Julia's preparation for school. Prepare a list of points you should include to help this child and the mother in the adjustment to school.

4. What information do you think a school teacher should have about Julia? Who is the person responsible for giving this information to the teacher?

5. During the 5-year period of Julia's treatment, a public health nurse was visiting the Smith home periodically. What should her function be in the total plan of care? What kind of information should be exchanged between the hospital personnel and the public health nurse? What is the plan in your particular hospital for this type of co-ordinated care?

Questions Relating to the Section in General

1. Cerebral palsy may result from a variety of causes. From the items below, check the groups of most common causes:

   a._____faulty development of the brain in utero, injury at birth, postnatal brain damage.

   b._____injury at birth, feeblemindedness, postnatal brain damage.

   c._____faulty development of the brain in utero, injury at birth, mental retardation of the parents.

   d.____postnatal brain damage, psychosis of the mother, injury at
birth.

2. The number of cerebral palsy patients under the age of 21 years is
approximately

   a.____1 per 100,000 population.
   b.____500 per 100,000 population.
   c.____125 per 100,000 population.
   d.____220 per 100,000 population.

3. Cerebral palsy is classified into 3 main types. Check the frequency
with which each type occurs in the total number of cerebral palsy
patients, by encircling the appropriate figure:

   a.____Spastic: 25 per cent, 80 per cent, 45 per cent.
   b.____Athetoid: 10 per cent, 40 per cent, 60 per cent.
   c.____Ataxic: 15 per cent, 75 per cent, 50 per cent.

4. In the spastic type of cerebral palsy, brain damage is in the

   a.____motor cortex and pyramidal tract.
   b.____basal ganglia and extrapyramidal tracts.
   c.____cerebellum.

5. In the athetoid type of cerebral palsy brain damage is in the

   a.____motor cortex and pyramidal tract.
   b.____cerebellum.
   c.____basal ganglia and extrapyramidal tracts.

6. In the ataxic type of cerebral palsy brain damage is in the

   a.____basal ganglia and extrapyramidal tracts.
   b.____motor cortex and pyramidal tract.
   c.____cerebellum.

7. Physical manifestations seen frequently in the spastic type are

   a.____muscle spasm, imbalance, involuntary motion.
   b.____muscle spasm, strabismus, shortening of the tendons.
   c.____imbalance, nystagmus, involuntary motion.

8. Personality characteristics typical of the spastic type are that the
patient is

   a.____fearful, aggressive, affectionate.
   b.____friendly, loving, quick to anger.
   c.____fearful, introvertive, easily frustrated.

9. Physical manifestations seen frequently in the athetoid type are

   a.____muscle spasm, drooling, postural defects.
   b.____involuntary motion, facial grimacing, drooling.
   c.____muscle spasm, nystagmus, facial grimacing.

10. Personality characteristics typical of the athetoid type are that the patient is

    a._____friendly, affectionate, quick to anger.
    b._____fearful, introvertive, aggressive.
    c._____affectionate, friendly, slow to anger.

11. Physical manifestations seen frequently in the ataxic type are

    a._____muscle spasm, nystagmus, involuntary motion.
    b._____imbalance, strabismus, drooling.
    c._____imbalance, nystagmus, dizziness.

12. Personality characteristics typical of the ataxic type are that the patient is

    a._____friendly, aggressive, easily frustrated.
    b._____friendly, outgoing, quick to anger.
    c._____fearful, unhappy, slow to anger.

13. From your understanding of the area of the brain damaged in the 3 main types of cerebral palsy, check the type most often retarded mentally:

    a._____spastic.
    b._____athetoid.
    c._____ataxic.

14. When nerve cells of the brain and cord have been destroyed by disease or trauma, it is expected that

    a._____no regeneration will take place.
    b._____replacement by new cells will occur in about 2 years.
    c._____partial regeneration will take place with proper treatment.

15. Since at present there are not enough treatment centers to care for children with cerebral palsy, certain criteria have been set up for the selection of children for treatment. Check the factors which aid in this selection:

    a._____the financial status of the family, intelligence of the child, the severity of the handicap.
    b._____the intelligence of the child, the willingness of the parents to help with the treatment, the number of other children in the home.
    c._____the severity of the handicap, the willingness of the parents to help with the treatment, the mental ability of the child.
    d._____the age of the child, the financial status of the family, the severity of the handicap.

16. A large percentage of children with cerebral palsy have other physical difficulties. Those which occur most frequently are

    a._____speech defects, malnutrition, tuberculosis, visual disturbances.
    b._____hearing loss, diarrhea, rickets, sensory disorders.

    c._____visual disturbances, rickets, malnutrition, anemia.

    d._____speech defects, visual disturbances, hearing loss, sensory disorders.

17. From the following list of nursing observations, check those which are suggestive of cerebral palsy:

    a._____convulsions.
    b._____twitching of any muscles.
    c._____dilated pupils.
    d._____discoloration of the skin over the spine.
    e._____failure to raise the head by 6 months.
    f._____holding the head to one side at all times.
    g._____head banging.
    h._____involuntary or uncontrolled movements.
    i._____excessive tightness of the muscles.
    j._____crossed eyes.
    k._____difficulty in sucking.
    l._____stuttering when excited.
    m._____bedwetting.
    n._____grimacing.
    o._____drooling after 18 months.

Questions for Discussion and Student Projects—*(Continued)*

1. Study the list of causes given in Table 2 of the article by Dr. Jones in the *American Journal of Nursing*, pp. 465–468, July 1946. For each cause listed, state the nurse's responsibility, if any, in the prevention of cerebral palsy. Mention specific ways in which you should function to lessen the incidence of cerebral palsy.
2. Locate information on the costs of leg braces, night splints and orthopedic shoes for children. Estimate the cost of maintaining equipment of this type over a period of years for a growing child.
3. What facilities and services are available in your state and community for the care and treatment of cerebral palsy? Write to the Division of Services to Crippled Children in your state Health Department to learn the type of consultant service offered. What provision is made in your state for the education of handicapped children?

Section 3. Nursing Care of Children in the Early School Period

STUDY SUGGESTIONS: Before beginning the study of this Section, the student will find it helpful to

A. Review

1. In anatomy and physiology texts: the circulatory system and blood.
2. In medical nursing texts: rheumatic fever, leukemia.
3. In nutrition texts: nutritional needs of the child 6–12 years old, low-sodium diets.
4. In pediatrics texts: child development from 6–12 years, immunization.*
5. In pharmacology texts: atropine, ACTH, cortisone, penicillin, sodium salicylate.

B. Study

1. In communicable disease and pediatrics texts: the specific disease conditions under consideration.

C. Read the additional References listed before attempting to answer questions relating to each patient study.

JEAN HAS THE MEASLES AT HOME—PATIENT STUDY

A public health nurse went into the Patton home to care for 6-year-old Jean, who was ill with measles. Jean had been ill for 3 days, the rash having appeared on the morning of the nurse's home visit. The family physician had called and left the following orders:

> Remain in bed until the rash disappears.
> Diet as desired—encourage liquids.
> Keep children out of the patient's room.

The physician told Mrs. Patton that he would return later in the day to give gamma globulin to the 8-month-old baby and to the 3-year-old boy. Mrs. Patton asked the nurse to explain gamma globulin more fully, to teach her how to care for Jean, and to offer some suggestions for keeping Jean in bed. The public health nurse bathed Jean, changed the bed linens and demonstrated simple isolation technics to the mother. After the nurse had given Mrs. Patton the help she needed and had explained the purpose of gamma globulin, she left, saying that she would return the following day to give additional service to the family as needed.

References

Brackett, Arthur S.: The importance of vaccination and revaccination, Am. J. Nursing 52:847, 1952.

Kohn, Jerome, and Olson, Elsie: Whooping cough, Am. J. Nursing 50:723, 1950.

* Other questions on immunization are included in Section 2 of this Part.

Shetland, Margaret: Communicable disease nursing—1948, Publ. Health Nursing, 40:543, 1948.
The Control of Communicable Disease in Man, ed. 7, The American Public Health Association, 1790 Broadway, New York City 19, 1950. (Cost, $.40.)
Immunization against communicable diseases, Am. J. Nursing 52:844, 1952.

Background Review Question

Match the definition from the column on the right with its corresponding term in the column on the left.

a._____immunization.
b._____incubation period.
c._____concurrent disinfection.
d._____terminal disinfection.
e._____communicable period.
f._____carrier.
g._____contamination.

(1) rendering the personal clothing and physical environment free of infectious material at the time when the patient is no longer a source of infection.

(2) a person without apparent symptoms of a communicable disease, who harbors the specific agent and may serve as a source of infection.

(3) introduction of specific antibodies into a susceptible person.

(4) the presence of infectious material on surfaces, articles, clothing, water, milk, etc.

(5) the time between infection of a susceptible person and the appearance of signs or symptoms of the disease in question.

(6) the killing of pathogenic organisms as soon as possible after discharge of infectious materials from the body.

(7) the time during which the etiologic agent may be transferred directly or indirectly from the patient to another person.

Questions Relating to the Patient Study

1. As the public health nurse talked with Mrs. Patton about Jean's present illness, she learned that the early symptoms included
   a._____rash, fever, Koplick spots.
   b._____fever, redness of the eyes, watery drainage from the nose.
   c._____redness of the eyes, rash, diarrhea.
   d._____Koplick spots, lack of appetite, constipation.

2. Mrs. Patton asked the nurse to explain where the measles organism is located. The nurse should tell her that it is present in the
   a._____stools of infected persons.
   b._____air during an epidemic.
   c._____secretions of the nose and throat of infected persons.

3. The nurse should tell Jean's family that the disease is most readily transmitted to others

   a._____after the rash appears.
   b._____before the rash appears.
   c._____4–5 days before and 4–5 days after the rash appears.
   d._____during the period of desquamation.

4. The nurse should tell Mrs. Patton that symptoms which may be expected during the acute phase of measles are

   a._____hematuria, photophobia, cyanosis.
   b._____photophobia, itching of the skin, brassy cough.
   c._____diarrhea, cyanosis, profuse perspiration.
   d._____brassy cough, hematuria, malaise.

5. The temperature of Jean's room should be kept at approximately

   a._____90°.
   b._____68°.
   c._____80°.
   d._____72°.

6. In order to prevent eyestrain, the mother should

   a._____avoid letting Jean use her eyes, keep the room darkened.
   b._____keep Jean's eyes covered, remain in the room with the child at all times.
   c._____encourage Jean to play with large toys, prevent direct light toward Jean's eye.

7. Should Jean develop itching of the skin due to the measles rash, itching may be relieved by

   a._____bathing twice daily with soap and water.
   b._____adding bran or sodium bicarbonate to plain warm water for the daily bath.
   c._____omitting all bathing.
   d._____rubbing the skin twice daily with 70 per cent alcohol.

8. Mrs. Patton asked the nurse why the doctor seemed concerned about the two smaller children getting measles. The nurse should tell her that

   a._____growth is retarded by an attack of measles.
   b._____it is considered safer to have measles during the summer months than during the winter.
   c._____the doctor wants to spare the mother caring for two other sick children.
   d._____children under the age of 3 years are more prone to develop severe or dangerous complications.

9. In explaining gamma globulin the nurse should tell the mother that the material comes from

    a._____horse serum prepared in the state laboratory.
    b._____human blood serum obtained from persons who have had
          measles.
    c._____a synthetic preparation made by a chemical process.

10. Mrs. Patton asked the nurse how the material will be administered to
    the children. She should be told that it will be given
    a._____by mouth.
    b._____by needle intravenously.
    c._____hypodermically.
    d._____by needle into a large muscle.

11. In reply to a question as to how long the children would be protected
    from measles, the nurse should tell the mother that it will be for

    a._____2 years.
    b._____the rest of their lives.
    c._____about 4 weeks.
    d._____6 years.

12. The nurse explained to Mrs. Patton that the doctor planned to return
    the same day to give the gamma globulin because

    a._____prevention of the disease is possible only when gamma globulin
          is given within 3 or 4 days after exposure.
    b._____isolation of the patient, Jean, will not be indicated after the
          gamma globulin is given.
    c._____the family desires the 3-year-old boy to continue going to
          nursery school.

Questions for Discussion and Student Projects

1. Describe your plan for teaching Mrs. Patton to care for Jean in the
    home, including

    a. the preparation and serving of meals.
    b. bathing, changing bed linens, care of the hair, the eyes and the
       mouth.
    c. diversional activities suitable for Jean based on her interests, limita-
       tions to be observed because of illness and by isolation procedures.
    d. equipment needed, such as bedpan, food, tray, etc.
    e. isolation procedures which are safe and simple:

       (1) provisions for hand washing.
       (2) the use of an apron while giving care.
       (3) disposal of body secretions.
       (4) care of the dishes after use by the patient.
       (5) the method of handling contaminated linens and clothing.
       (6) concurrent and terminal disinfection as indicated by the nature
          of the disease.

    f. a daily schedule or plan for total care, allowing time for attention
       to other family members and for rest periods for Mrs. Patton.

2. Prepare a list of foods which would be suitable for Jean during the acute phase of measles. List a few points to be observed in planning a diet with Jean's mother, such as giving Jean a choice in the selection of foods, variety in preparing liquids, etc.

3. Describe how each of the following articles should be cleaned or disinfected at the time when Jean is considered to be no longer infectious:

   a. books and magazines.
   b. crayons.
   c. plastic toys.
   d. jigsaw puzzles.
   e. paper money.
   f. a wooly teddy bear.

Questions Relating to the Section in General

1. Measles is seen most frequently under one of the following conditions:

   a._____at age 1–10 years, in the winter months, in urban areas.
   b._____in rural areas, in the winter months, at age 6–12 years.
   c._____in the summer months, in all areas alike, at age 1–10 years.
   d._____in urban areas, at age 6–12 years in the summer months.

2. Complications of measles most commonly seen are

   a._____nephritis, otitis media, lobar pneumonia.
   b._____heart disease, tuberculosis, bronchopneumonia.
   c._____otitis media, bronchopneumonia, corneal ulcers.
   d._____nephritis, heart disease, bronchopneumonia.

3. Of the following organisms, scarlet fever is caused by

   a._____*Streptococcus viridans.*
   b._____*Streptococcus hemolyticus,* group A.
   c._____*Staphylococcus aureus.*
   d._____*Streptococcus hemolyticus,* group B.

4. Scarlet fever may be prevented by

   a._____immunization.
   b._____vaccination.
   c._____avoidance of contact with infected individuals.
   d._____quarantine of active cases.

5. The complication most dreaded in scarlet fever is

   a._____nephritis.
   b._____deafness.
   c._____heart disease.
   d._____adenitis.

6. Infants should be vaccinated against smallpox at the age of

   a._____1 year.
   b._____6 months.

c.____18 months.
d.____2 years.

7. Smallpox vaccinations should be repeated every
 a.____10 years.
 b.____7 years.
 c.____5 years.
 d.____2 years.

8. Smallpox vaccination is contraindicated in
 a.____malnutrition.
 b.____eczema.
 c.____congenital heart disease.
 d.____tuberculosis of the spine.

9. Of the following age groups, the highest mortality in whooping cough occurs in
 a.____2–6 years.
 b.____13–16 years.
 c.____birth–1 year.
 d.____6–10 years.

10. The most frequent serious complication of whooping cough is
 a.____otitis media.
 b.____bronchopneumonia.
 c.____nephritis.
 d.____encephalitis.

11. The communicable period in whooping cough is from
 a.____the onset of catarrhal symptoms through about 3 weeks of spasmodic coughing.
 b.____3 days before the onset of the first cough through 6 weeks of coughing.
 c.____6 weeks after the onset of paroxysms or whoop.
 d.____10 weeks after the onset of the first cough.

12. In caring for a child with whooping cough, the air in the room or ward should be
 a.____moist, of a temperature of about 72°, dust free.
 b.____of a temperature of 72°, dry, well ventilated.
 c.____of a temperature of 85°, moist, dust free.
 d.____dry, of a temperature of 80°, well ventilated.

13. Should a mother ask regarding natural immunity to whooping cough, the nurse should tell her that
 a.____natural immunity exists during the first 4 months of life.
 b.____newborn babies have little or no immunity to whooping cough.
 c.____newborn babies have natural immunity to whooping cough if the mother has had the disease.
 d.____natural immunity exists during the first 2 months of life.

14. The Schick test is used to determine a person's susceptibility to

    a._____scarlet fever.
    b._____tuberculosis.
    c._____diphtheria.
    d._____typhoid fever.

15. The function of all nurses in the *control* of communicable disease should be to

    a._____give bedside care to patients.
    b._____stress the need for and value of immunizations.
    c._____teach mothers to give care to children ill in homes.
    d._____teach community groups the dangers of communicable disease.

16. Teaching prevention of communicable disease is most effective before illness occurs. Preventive teaching should include

    a._____personal cleanliness, early isolation in suspected illness, immunization whenever possible.
    b._____adequate nutrition, avoidance of public gatherings, personal cleanliness.
    c._____daily inspection for sore throats, early isolation in suspected illness, adequate nutrition.
    d._____periodic medical supervision, daily school attendance, avoidance of public gatherings.

17. Match the incubation period from the column on the right with its corresponding communicable disease in the column on the left:

    a.___3___chickenpox (varicella).   (1) 10–15 days.
    b.___6___diphtheria.   (2) 7–16 days.
    c.___7___German measles (ru-   (3) 2–3 weeks.
          bella).   (4) 3–38 days.
    d.___8___influenza.   (5) 2–5 days.
    e.___1___measles (rubeola).   (6) 2–5 days.
    f.___9___mumps (infectious par-   (7) 14–21 days.
          otitis).   (8) 24–72 hours.
    g.__10___whooping cough (pertus-   (9) 12–26 days.
          sis).   (10) 7–21 days.
    h.___2___smallpox.
    i.___5___scarlet fever.
    j.___4___typhoid fever.

18. From the following list of communicable diseases, check those which are preventable by the development of artificial active immunity:

    a._____chickenpox.   f._____mumps.
    b._____smallpox.   g._____undulant fever.
    c._____poliomyelitis.   h._____scarlet fever.
    d._____pertussis.   i._____typhoid fever.
    e._____diphtheria.   j._____tetanus.

Questions for Discussion and Student Projects—(*Continued*)

1. Describe your plan of nursing care for a 10-month-old infant hospitalized for whooping cough, including

   a. feeding—amounts, frequency, technics, foods recommended and foods to be avoided.
   b. emergency care during severe paroxysms.
   c. measures to promote sleep and rest.
   d. isolation procedures as determined by the nature of the organism.
   e. parent teaching.

2. Prepare a report for class (suggested project for one student) explaining the meaning of two terms: (1) placarding and (2) quarantine. State the advantages and disadvantages to the public and to the health department of these two control measures. Describe current practices used in your community for the control of communicable disease.

KENNETH HAS HIS TONSILS OUT—PATIENT STUDY

Kenneth White, aged 7 years, came into the hospital to have his tonsils and adenoids removed. He was admitted one afternoon, went to the operating room the following morning, and was discharged to his home the next day. Kenneth had been told by his parents that he would be put to sleep for the operation and that his throat would be sore when he awakened. A preoperative medication of codeine gr. ¼ and atropine ⅟₃₀₀ was given hypodermically on call to surgery. Kenneth complained of being very thirsty and somewhat hungry while waiting to go to the operating room, but asked little about the actual procedure. Mr. and Mrs. White spent an hour with Kenneth before he went to surgery and were waiting in his room when he returned.

Vomiting was moderate in the early postoperative period and there was an occasional streak of bright red blood in the mucus from Kenneth's throat. By noon he was awake asking for ice cream and water.

References

Bellam, Gwendoline: Tonsillectomy without fear, Am. J. Nursing 51:244, 1950.
Benz, Gladys: Pediatric Nursing, pp. 278–284, St. Louis, Mosby, 1948.
Gesell, Arnold, and Ilg, Frances: The Child from Five to Ten, pp. 131–138, New York, Harpers, 1946.
Spock, Benjamin: Baby and Child Care, pp. 358–361, 380–382, New York, Pocket Books, Inc., 1946.

Questions Relating to the Patient Study

1. The nurse admitting Kenneth to the ward should place him in a

   a._____double room with another boy who has just had a T & A.
   b._____room alone.
   c._____cubicle with 3 other boys near his age.
   d._____ward with 7 other children older than Kenneth.

2. If Kenneth should ask the nurse why he has to have his tonsils and adenoids removed, she should tell him that

    a._____the doctor will answer his questions later.
    b._____it will help him to grow faster.
    c._____almost all children have their tonsils and adenoids removed.
    d._____it is done to prevent frequent colds and sore throats.

3. In order to help Kenneth feel comfortable as he is admitted to the unit, the nurse should

    a._____introduce him to the other children and to the nurses, provide diversional activity, explain all procedures before they are carried out.
    b._____tell him he is to remain in bed, send all his personal articles home, provide comic books.
    c._____explain all procedures before they are carried out, tell him he is to remain in bed, give him a bedside radio.
    d._____introduce him to the other children and to the nurses, send his parents home, give him something to eat.

4. You would expect Kenneth's anxiety during his hospital stay to be a result of

    a._____separation from his parents.
    b._____fear of strange places.
    c._____fear of bodily pain.
    d._____fear of unfamiliar adults.

5. On the morning of the operation, which of the following symptoms would be of most concern to the physician?

    a._____nasal discharge, nausea, thirst.
    b._____skin rash, nasal discharge, elevated temperature.
    c._____elevated blood pressure, hunger, skin rash.
    d._____constipation, headache, thirst.

6. While waiting for Kenneth to be called to the operating room, suitable activities are

    a._____looking at picture books, having the mother read to the child, playing a record player with an adult changing the records.
    b._____playing checkers with another boy, reading comic books, listening to the radio.
    c._____working puzzles, reading children's magazines, observing other patients.

7. When called to the operating room, which of the following hospital people should accompany him?

    a._____an orderly from the operating room.
    b._____a nursing aide from the pediatric unit.
    c._____the nurse who has been assigned to him.
    d._____a nurse from the operating room.

8. In the immediate postoperative period, you would expect Kenneth's pulse to be

    a._____weak and thready.
    b._____rapid and bounding.
    c._____slow and irregular.
    d._____soft and intermittent.

9. You would expect Kenneth's skin upon return from surgery to be

    a_____cold and clammy.
    b._____dry and flushed.
    c._____mottled and moist.
    d._____moist and flushed.

Questions for Discussion and Student Projects

1. Describe the preparations you should make for Kenneth's postoperative care. Prepare a list of articles which should be in his room.
2. How do you think the parents need to be prepared for Kenneth's appearance upon his return from the operating room? Plan a short classroom discussion on the possible reactions of the parents when seeing their child anesthetized, vomiting, and with the possibility of bleeding. Do you think parents are disturbed at the sight of a few streaks of bright red blood in the oral excretions following a tonsillectomy?
3. In your hospital, how soon following surgery would you be permitted to give water or ice cream to Kenneth? Why do children frequently ask for ice cream following a T & A?
4. How long should a nurse remain at Kenneth's bedside after the operation? Why is it important to make careful and almost continuous observations of the child in the postoperative period?
5. Describe the nursing care you should give to make Kenneth comfortable after he reacts from the anesthetic. Is it usual for children to be restless at this time? Should he be encouraged to talk or to keep quiet? Do you think there would be an indication for sedation?
6. Do you expect Kenneth to behave as an average 7-year-old boy would in a play or school situation? If any changes are expected, state what they might be and describe how you as a nurse should respond to these changes in behavior.
7. What preparation do you think Mrs. White needs to give care to Kenneth at home? What type of rest should be continued at home? What foods are permitted the post-T & A patient and what foods are discouraged?

Questions Relating to the Section in General

1. Unless there is some urgent reason for taking out tonsils and adenoids at a particular time, the most suitable age for this operation is around

    a._____4 years.
    b._____7 years.
    c._____10 years.
    d._____14 years.

2. Tonsils and adenoids are made up of

    a._____lymphoid tissue.
    b._____connective tissue.
    c._____mucous membranes.
    d._____scar tissue.

3. Tonsils are removed most frequently to correct

    a._____swollen cervical glands, nervousness, feeding difficulties.
    b._____stuttering, malnutrition, chronic fever.
    c._____tonsillitis, swollen cervical glands, chronic fever.
    d._____nervousness, chronic fever, feeding difficulties.

4. Adenoids are removed most frequently to correct

    a._____mouth breathing, poor school performance, restlessness.
    b._____repeated upper respiratory infections, poor appetite, night-mares.
    c._____recurrent attacks of otitis media, restlessness, poor school performance.
    d._____repeated upper respiratory infections, mouth breathing, recurrent attacks of otitis media.

5. Laboratory procedures generally carried out before a T & A are

    a._____urinalysis, sedimentation rate, hemoglobin.
    b._____complete blood count, serology, platelet count.
    c._____urinalysis, complete blood count, bleeding and clotting time.
    d._____serology, sedimentation rate, complete blood count.

6. Of the following properties, codeine is classified as being

    a._____analgesic.
    b._____hypnotic.
    c._____sedative.

7. The average dose of codeine for a 7-year-old child is

    a._____1 gr.
    b._____½ gr.
    c._____⅛ gr.
    d._____¼ gr.

8. Symptoms of an overdose of codeine are

    a._____perspiration, rapid pulse, lowered rate of respiration.
    b._____itching of the skin, coma, slow respirations.
    c._____perspiration, constipation, delirium.
    d._____restlessness, contracted pupils, slow pulse.

9. The average dose of atropine for a 7-year-old child is

    a._____$\frac{1}{100}$ gr.
    b._____$\frac{1}{600}$ gr.
    c._____$\frac{1}{450}$ gr.
    d._____$\frac{1}{300}$ gr.

10. Of the following plants, atropine is obtained from

a.____foxglove.   c.____belladonna.
b.____hemp.   d.____poppy.

11. Early symptoms of atropine poisoning include

a.____dry red skin, contracted pupils, rapid pulse, slow respirations.
b.____dilated pupils, dry red skin, rapid pulse, rapid respirations.
c.____coma, contracted pupils, perspiration, slow pulse.
d.____dilated pupils, rapid pulse, perspiration, confusion.

12. Late symptoms of atropine poisoning include

a.____restlessness, subnormal temperature, delirium.
b.____pallor, strong bounding pulse, confusion.
c.____stupor, confusion, rapid weak pulse.
d.____coma, convulsions, wet clammy skin.

13. Aside from the presence of bright red blood, symptoms of bleeding following a T & A are

a.____pallor, weak thready pulse, cold clammy skin.
b.____rapid bounding pulse, Cheyne-Stokes respirations, loss of consciousness.
c.____restlessness, rapid shallow respirations, flushed face.
d.____slow respirations, pallor, dry flushed skin.

14. The nurse's responsibilities in event of bleeding following a T & A are to

a.____notify the physician, give a stimulant, elevate the head of the bed.
b.____supply additional warmth, prepare for a blood transfusion, elevate the foot of the bed.
c.____notify the physician, supply additional warmth, keep the child as quiet as possible.
d.____give a sedative, ask the parents to leave the room, notify the head nurse.

Questions for Discussion and Student Projects—(*Continued*)

1. What are the policies in your hospital in regard to parents visiting children who are having their tonsils and adenoids removed? In case visiting is permitted only once on the morning of operation, which time do you think is most beneficial to the child— immediately before he is taken to surgery or immediately after his return?

2. Assuming you are assigned to care for a 6- or 7-year-old child who has come into the hospital for a T & A, and who has had no previous preparation for the experience, describe how you should explain to the child what is to happen, trying to anticipate some specific questions the patient may ask.

3. What should you do when a child complains of being thirsty and

hungry as fluids and food are withheld for operative procedures? Is there a playroom in your pediatric unit where the child could be placed while other children are having breakfast?

[Questions 1–6 refer to the development of the average 7-year-old child]

1. He is usually able to

    a_____tell the time of day by the clock, accept responsibility for being "on time," observe respect for the property of others.

    b._____tell the time of day by the clock, but be unable to accept responsibility for being on time or for observing respect for the property of others.

    c._____tell morning from afternoon, but be unable to tell the time of day by the clock.

2. This child usually enjoys

    a._____radio and television programs, reading more than active games.

    b._____radio and television programs, active games more than reading.

    c._____active games more than reading, spends little time with radio or television.

3. He is apt to

    a._____indulge in fanciful daydreams, cry frequently, have frequent temper tantrums.

    b._____indulge in fanciful daydreams, try very hard not to cry, have no temper tantrums.

    c._____not indulge in fanciful daydreams, try very hard not to cry, have frequent temper tantrums.

4. His relationships with adults show

    a._____a need for approval, an acceptance of physical demonstration of affection, a liking for his school teacher, attempts to please adults.

    b._____little need for approval, a dislike for physical demonstration of affection, dislike for all school teachers, little effort to please adults.

    c._____a need for approval, rejection of physical demonstration of affection, a liking for his school teacher, attempts to please adults.

5. His activities demonstrate an ability to

    a._____adjust to competitive sports, accept losing at games, adjust to interruptions of activities, show perseverance in most activities.

    b._____show perseverance in most activities, but adjusts poorly to competitive games, is a poor loser, and resents interruptions of his activities.

    c._____accept interruptions of activities, show perseverance in activities, but unable to adjust to competitive games and is a poor loser.

6. He prefers to be dressed

    a._____neatly at all times.

    b._____untidily.

    c._____neatly when going to school, untidily at play.

THE CARE OF A CHILD WITH A FATAL ILLNESS—PATIENT STUDY

Elaine Dixon, aged 9 years, was admitted to the pediatric unit with a diagnosis of acute lymphatic leukemia. Her chief complaints were weakness, abdominal pain and ulcerations in the mouth. Mrs. Dixon reported that Elaine had been well until about 10 days ago when she lost interest in her school work, cried frequently and refused to eat solid foods. The family physician was consulted. He referred Elaine to a local pediatrician for diagnosis and treatment.

Admission orders were as follows:

    1. Bed rest.

    2. Diet as tolerated, using as little salt as possible.

    3. C.B.C. and differential.

    4. Urinalysis daily.

    5. Phenobarbital gr. ½ at bedtime as necessary.

A senior nursing student admitted Elaine to a single room and explained various activities of the ward to the child and to her mother. On the third day of hospitalization an order was left for Elaine to receive ACTH 25 mg. q. 6 hours. Blood transfusions of 500 cc. of whole blood were given weekly. Mr. and Mrs. Dixon were permitted to visit their daughter as often as they wished. Elaine seemed to show improvement after the first week, but later failed to respond to any form of treatment and died 1 month after admission to the hospital.

Reference

Cooke, Jean V.: Leukemia in children, Am. J. Nursing 50:353, 1950.

Background Review Questions

1. Erythrocytes are formed in the

    a._____liver.

    b._____bone marrow.

    c._____spleen.

    d._____spinal cord.

2. Erythrocytes are destroyed in the

    a._____blood stream.

    b._____liver.

    c._____spleen.

    d._____lymph glands.

3. The normal blood platelet count is

    a._____10,000 to 15,000 per cubic millimeter.

    b._____100,000 to 150,000 per cubic millimeter.

    c._____250,000 to 600,000 per cubic millimeter.

4. In leukemia the platelet count is

    a._____increased.
    b._____decreased.
    c._____not changed.

5. Match the following:

    a._____hyperplasia.   (1) periods of general improvement of symp-
    b._____petechiae.   toms.
    c._____ecchymosis.   (2) decrease of the leukocyte count.
    d._____remission.   (3) formation of blood.
    e._____exacerbation.   (4) increase in severity of disease.
    f._____neoplasm.   (5) formation of red cells.
    g._____leukopenia.   (6) small spots caused by bleeding into the
    h._____stomatitis.   skin or the mucous membrane.
    i._____erythropoietic. (7) abnormal multiplication of tissue cells.
    j._____hematopoietic. (8) new and abnormal growths.
                             (9) hemorrhages into the skin or the mucous
                                membranes.
                    (10) enlargement of the lymph nodes.
                    (11) inflammation of the mouth.

Questions Relating to the Patient Study

1. From the list below check the activities which the nurse should carry out to help Elaine in her adjustment to the hospital:

    a._____Introduce herself by name.
    b._____Show Elaine how to call the nurses.
    c._____Send all personal articles home with the mother.
    d._____Tell Elaine to ask for anything she wants to eat.
    e._____Tell the mother not to bring in any food.
    f._____Explain the use of the bedpan.
    g._____Tell Elaine to ask for toys anytime she wishes to play.
    h._____Refer all questions to the head nurse.
    i._____Remain with the child while blood is drawn for tests.
    j._____Tell Elaine she is too big to cry.
    k._____Assure the mother that Elaine will be well enough to go home soon.
    l._____Explain what is meant by bed rest.

2. Bleeding from mucous membranes occurred during the latter phase of hospitalization and was due to

    a._____a decrease in the platelets in the blood.
    b._____vitamin-C deficiency.
    c._____an increase in leukocytes.
    d._____a decrease in lymphocytes.
    e._____general malnutrition.

3. Since Elaine had little interest in food, the nurse was trying at all times to get her to eat. The activities which should be most effective are to

a._____serve foods only as requested, decorate the tray for each meal, have the child keep a record of the food eaten.

b._____prepare surprises often, serve liquids only, remain with the child while she eats.

c._____permit the mother to bring food from home, prepare surprises often, serve soft and liquid foods.

d._____serve foods only as requested, remain with the child while she eats, have the child keep a record of the food eaten.

Questions for Discussion and Student Projects

1. Describe your technics for giving an individualized type of nursing care to Elaine as indicated by certain symptoms, such as bleeding and ulcerations of the mouth, extreme tenderness of the skin (especially over the joints and the abdomen), poor appetite, excessive weakness, and bleeding from the mucous membranes of the rectum.
2. Prepare a summary of information you think the parents should be given as to Elaine's disease and the outlook for recovery. Include suggestions for the parents concerning their actions and attitudes while visiting Elaine which should lessen her anxiety.
3. At the time ACTH is begun as treatment, what do you think the parents should be told concerning changes to be expected in Elaine's appearance and behavior?
4. About 1 week before Elaine died, the priest came to her room to administer the last rites of the Catholic Church. What is the nurse's responsibility in preparation for this religious service? What would your response be to the child should she question you about the possibility of her death?
5. Plan a classroom discussion on ways in which nurses should express sympathy to the parents when a child dies. Do you consider it unprofessional to let the parents see that you are upset or grieved by a death?
6. What should you do in case Elaine's parents asked you to recommend an undertaker for them?

Questions Relating to the Section in General

1. ACTH is a substance obtained from the

a._____anterior lobe of the pituitary gland of animals.

b._____adrenal cortex of hogs.

c._____posterior lobe of the pituitary gland of cattle.

2. Certain changes in the child usually observed a few days after treatment with ACTH has begun are

a._____a moon-shaped face, dry skin, increased appetite.

b._____decreased appetite, diarrhea, acne.

c._____increased appetite, acne, a moon-shaped face.

d._____acne, fever, lassitude.

3. A low-sodium diet is ordered with ACTH to

a._____improve the appetite.

b._____decrease the urinary output.

    c._____lessen thirst.

    d._____prevent the retention of body fluids.

4. The type of leukemia seen most frequently in children is

    a._____chronic monocytic.

    b._____acute lymphatic.

    c._____acute myelogenous.

    d._____chronic lymphatic.

    e._____aleukemic.

Questions for Discussion and Student Projects—(*Continued*)

1. Occasionally a specimen of bone marrow is obtained from the child to aid in the diagnosis of leukemia. Describe the procedure used in your hospital. Is the child taken to the operating room or is the procedure carried out in the ward? What is the responsibility of the nurse in preparing the child both physically and emotionally?
2. Suggested report for one student: Determine the cost of ACTH per dose, and for treatment over a period of 3 weeks. Why is this drug expensive? When was ACTH first used? For what conditions has it proved to be most beneficial?
3. What is the policy in your hospital regarding replacement of blood used for transfusions? What requirements must be met by a donor who offers blood for transfusions?
4. What facilities are available in your hospital or community to pay for ACTH in instances where the family cannot meet this expense?

DIANA MUST REST—PATIENT STUDY

Diana Hill, a 10-year-old girl, was convalescing from an attack of acute rheumatic fever which had left moderately severe heart damage. Diana had been in the hospital for 5 months when orders were written for preparation for discharge. The nursing student responsible for Diana summarized her illness as follows:

> Diana has had frequent colds and sore throats since the age of 3 years and had a T & A at the age of 8. Mrs. Hill stated that Diana's appetite had always been poor although she was described by the admitting physician as being well nourished. On admission Mrs. Hill told the doctor that 2 weeks ago Diana had a swollen right ankle, cried easily and was very irritable. She gave Diana an aspirin tablet and in a short time the ankle no longer bothered her. The day before admission, both knees and both elbows became swollen, stiff and painful and Diana had a nose bleed lasting about 5 minutes. Her appetite was described as increasingly poorer. Temperature on admission was 100.2°, pulse 88, respirations 24. During the past month, Diana had lost 6 pounds in weight.
>
> Laboratory findings at the time of admission were reported as follows: RBC 4,100,000, WBC 15,250, hemoglobin 11 Gm. per 100 cc. of blood, urinalysis negative, throat culture positive for *Streptococcus hemolyticus*, sedimentation rate 60.

Diana remained in bed during the entire hospital stay but was permitted a high back rest during the day. Penicillin 400,000 units was given daily for the first week. Sodium salicylate gr. 10 and sodium bicarbonate gr. 5 were given 4 times daily for 3 weeks.

Two heart lesions developed soon after admission—mitral stenosis and aortic insufficiency. Although Diana's general condition seemed to improve and her joint pains decreased, the heart lesions grew more pronounced. At the end of 6 weeks new orders were written for (1) ACTH 25 mg. every 6 hours, (2) low-sodium diet (not more than 2 Gm. of sodium per day), (3) blood pressure daily, (4) daily record of weight and (5) record of intake and output. Later the ACTH was discontinued and cortisone 50 mg. was given 3 times daily, which was to be continued at home. Diana's heart sounds were much better but she was ordered to remain in bed at home until further improvement occurred.

References

Blecha, Elmira: Low sodium diets, Am. J. Nursing **51**:464, 1951.

Gesell, Arnold, and Ilg, Frances: The Child from Five to Ten, pp. 212–217, New York, Harpers, 1946.

Sadler, Sabra: Rheumatic Fever Nursing Care in Pictures, Philadelphia, Lippincott, 1949.

———, and Seibel, Elizabeth: The child with active rheumatic fever and her nursing care, Am. J. Nursing **46**:170, 1946.

Strang, Ruth: Development in the Preadolescent Years, *in* An Introduction to Child Study, pp. 487–539, New York, Macmillan, 1951.

Wilson, D. Laurence: ACTH and cortisone in clinical practice, Am. J. Nursing **50**:649, 1950.

Diversions for the Sick, John Hancock Mutual Life Insurance Co., Boston, Mass. 22 pages. Free on request.

Questions Relating to the Patient Study

1. As the nurse talks with Diana about her care at home, she should give the following reason for continuing bed rest:

   a._____the doctor has ordered bed rest.
   b._____being up may cause a recurrence of the joint pain.
   c._____the heart trouble may get worse.
   d._____rest helps her to get entirely well again.

2. The nurse should suggest several possible types of diversional activity for Diana. From those listed below, check the ones most suitable:

   a._____continuing school work, learning to knit, water coloring.
   b._____reading, coloring with crayons, listening to quiet radio programs.
   c._____watching television, writing letters for other family members, sewing.
   d._____continuing school work, talking to friends on the telephone, planning the family menus.

3. In the conference with Mrs. Hill, the nurse should instruct her to

    a._____prepare a strict schedule, permit no exceptions in the routine.

    b._____remain within calling distance at all times, plan an occasional treat for Diana.

    c._____allow Diana to help plan her own schedule, plan for an occasional treat.

    d._____prepare family meals around Diana's wishes, permit no visitors in the child's room.

4. Assume that a public health nurse has made a home visit to help Mrs. Hill prepare for bringing Diana home. The nurse makes a report to the hospital physician describing the home. From the list below, check conditions most essential to safe care at home:

    a._____absence of infection, a warm dry house, a bed alone and if possible a room alone for the child.

    b._____no other children in the home, the mother willing to give proper care, a warm dry house.

    c._____absence of infection, no other children in the home, a bathroom near the patient's room.

    d._____adequate nutrition assured, the mother willing to give proper care, the family able to buy necessary medications.

5. During the time in which Diana received sodium salicylate, the nurses should be alert for the following toxic effects:

    a._____nausea, diarrhea, edema of the extremities, headache.

    b._____gastric distress, nausea, ringing in the ears, vomiting.

    c._____constipation, deafness, nausea, headache.

    d._____gastric distress, diarrhea, rash, edema of the face.

6. Sodium bicarbonate was given with sodium salicylate to reduce one of these undesirable side effects:

    a._____ringing in the ears.

    b._____headache.

    c._____rash.

    d._____gastric distress.

7. Sodium salicylate is classified as

    a._____antibiotic and antipyretic.

    b._____analgesic and antipyretic.

    c._____sedative and analgesic.

    d._____hypnotic and antipyretic.

8. Sodium salicylate and sodium bicarbonate were discontinued before ACTH was administered to Diana because

    a._____expected benefits were not being produced.

    b._____low sodium intake is indicated in ACTH therapy.

    c._____beneficial effects of ACTH are reduced in the presence of any other drug.

9. Following the administration of ACTH to Diana some of the changes listed below may be observed:

   a.____appetite is decreased, weight is gained, joint pain is diminished.
   b.____weight is lost, appetite is improved, the sedimentation rate is lowered.
   c.____appetite is increased, joint pain is decreased, the sedimentation rate is lowered.
   d.____joint swelling is decreased, appetite is decreased, the sedimentation rate is elevated.

10. You would expect these changes in Diana's appearance during the first few days of ACTH therapy:

   a.____purplish discoloration of the fingertips, acne, loss of hair, pallor.
   b.____rounding of facial contours, pallor, clubbing of the ends of the fingers and the toes, acne.
   c.____acne, loss of hair, purplish striae over the abdomen and the thighs, rounding of facial contours.
   d.____pallor, dilated pupils, acne, loss of hair.

11. Laboratory reports would show the following changes in Diana's blood cells after ACTH was started:

   a.____increase in red cells, increase in white cells, decrease in eosinophils.
   b.____decrease in red cells, decrease in white cells, increase in eosinophils.
   c.____increase in red cells, decrease in white cells, decrease in eosinophils.

12. Blood chemistry examinations from Diana during treatment with ACTH would show

   a.____elevation of potassium, calcium and phosphorus, elevation of blood sugar, lowering of sodium and chlorides.
   b.____lowering of potassium, calcium and phosphorus, lowering of blood sugar, elevation of sodium and chlorides.
   c.____elevation of blood sugar, lowering of potassium, calcium and phosphorus, elevation of sodium and chlorides.

13. The low-sodium diet was ordered for Diana to

   a.____prevent excessive urinary activity.
   b.____prevent retention of body fluids.
   c.____decrease thirst.
   d.____decrease appetite.

Questions for Discussion and Student Projects

1. Do you believe that nurses in hospitals are able to give better care to children as information is available about home conditions? List certain facts you would like to have concerning the Hill family as you are giving care to Diana.

2. Describe your plan for teaching Mrs. Hill to provide for Diana's needs at home following discharge from the hospital, including

   a. bathing, changing bed linens and bed positions.
   b. clothing for Diana to wear during the day.
   c. preparation and serving of meals.
   d. elimination.
   e. protection from infections.
   f. sleep and rest.
   g. recreation.

3. Suggested class report for one student: Ascertain the total cost of the penicillin, ACTH, cortisone, sodium salicylate and sodium bicarbonate given to Diana during her 5-month stay in the hospital. What provisions are made in your community to assist a family unable to pay for medications?

4. Do you think that Diana's parents should be told that certain physical changes are to be expected during ACTH therapy? If so, describe how you should prepare them for these changes.

5. Prepare a list of foods which Diana would be permitted on a low-sodium diet, including items essential for a growing 10-year-old girl. Plan a few sample menus, trying to make allowances for the likes and dislikes of any 10-year-old child with whom you are acquainted.

Questions Relating to the Section in General

1. The symptoms most typical of rheumatic fever are

   a._____pain in the joints, loss of weight, a fever of around 102°.
   b._____epistaxis, a fever of around 100°, dry skin.
   c._____swelling in the joints, a fever of around 103°, damp skin.
   d._____skin nodules, painful swollen joints, elevated sedimentation rate.
   e._____elevated sedimentation rate, damp skin, poor appetite.

2. Rheumatic fever occurs most frequently in:

   a._____school age children (7–14 years), poor housing, the temperate zone.
   b._____a cold damp climate, all economic groups, school children.
   c._____poor nutritional status, a dry climate, poor housing.
   d._____the temperate zone, wealthy families, families with a history of rheumatic fever.
   e._____school children, well-nourished children, a cold damp climate.

3. Recurrences of rheumatic fever may be prevented by

   a._____avoidance of upper respiratory infections, a high-protein diet, immunization programs.
   b._____limited activity, a high-vitamin diet, sodium salicylate.
   c._____general adequate nutrition, wholesome living conditions, avoidance of upper respiratory infections.
   d._____immunization programs, limited activity, plenty of sunshine.

4. The presence of rheumatic nodules is an indication that

    a._____carditis is developing.
    b._____rheumatic fever is in an active phase.
    c._____the prognosis is unfavorable.
    d._____rheumatic fever is in a quiescent phase.

5. The arthritis of rheumatic fever

    a._____results in permanent stiffness of the joints.
    b._____produces atrophy of the muscles around the affected joints.
    c._____recovers completely.
    d._____returns as rheumatoid arthritis in adult life.

6. Nursing care during the active phase of rheumatic fever should be directed toward the attainment of physical rest. Under the general headings below are listed certain methods of providing the desired rest. Check those which you believe to be most effective:

  a. Position in bed:

     (1)_____elevate the head of the bed, place personal articles nearby, allow the child to face interesting activities.
     (2)_____change the position every hour, maintain a recumbent position, allow one pillow under the head.
     (3)_____allow the child to sit on the edge of the bed for 15 minutes daily, place personal articles near, allow one pillow under the head.

  b. Care of the skin:

     (1)_____bathe twice daily with soap and water, allow the child to assist with the bath, dust folds of the skin freely with bath powder.
     (2)_____bathe daily with soap and water, give an alcohol back rub twice daily, give partial baths in addition as needed.
     (3)_____give oil baths only, allow the child to assist with the application of oil, use olive oil.

  c. Elimination:

     (1)_____carry the child to the bathroom, give enemas as needed, measure all urinary output.
     (2)_____allow the child to get the bedpan from the stand, nurse removes child from bedpan, measure all urinary output.
     (3)_____bedpan to be warmed, nurse lifts child to bedpan, small pillow to be placed as support under the child's back.

  d. Placement in the pediatric unit:

     (1)_____in room alone.
     (2)_____in room with one other child of about the same age.
     (3)_____in a 6-bed ward.
     (4)_____in a 4-bed ward with a screen around the patient's bed.

e. Care of the hair:

(1)____shampoo each week with water.
(2)____shampoo as needed with a dry shampoo.
(3)____brush vigorously each day.
(4)____allow the child to comb his own hair daily.

f. Clothing while in bed:

(1)____loose-fitting hospital pajamas.
(2)____hospital gown only.
(3)____child's own favorite pajamas.
(4)____nightgown and bed jacket.

g. Feeding:

(1)____child to be fed entirely by a nurse.
(2)____child may assist by feeding self part of each meal.
(3)____emphasis placed on importance of eating all of food served.
(4)____parents should take turns coming in to feed the child.

h. Emotional security or contentment is increased by

(1)____changing play materials frequently, unlimited visitors, maintaining contacts with the family.
(2)____attendance at weekly movies, assurance that the nurses are concerned with the welfare of all children in the unit, unlimited visitors.
(3)____the nurse's acceptance of any regressive tendencies, faith in the doctors, having one's own money to spend.
(4)____maintaining contacts with the family, assurance that the nurses are concerned with the welfare of all children in the unit, the nurse's acceptance of any regressive tendencies.

7. Chorea is described as one of the rheumatic diseases. It occurs most frequently in

a.____boys, summer months, age 6 to 15 years.
b.____girls, spring months, age 6 to 15 years.
c.____boys and girls alike, spring months, age 10 to 14 years.
d.____girls, winter months, age 10 to 14 years.

8. In chorea the onset is

a.____rapid with involuntary movements.
b.____rapid with chills and fever.
c.____slow with a low-grade fever.
d.____slow with a history of clumsiness.

9. The outstanding symptoms in chorea are

a.____involuntary muscular movements, emotional instability, indistinct speech.
b.____fever, an elevated sedimentation rate, involuntary muscular movements.

    c._____swollen joints, fever, emotional instability.

    d._____joint pain, indistinct speech, fever.

10. The prognosis in chorea is for

    a._____complete recovery in about 1 year.

    b._____residual heart damage.

    c._____complete recovery in 1 to 4 months.

    d._____the condition to become chronic.

11. The child with active chorea should be placed in one of the following locations in the unit:

    a._____in a cubicle with one other girl.

    b._____in a 4-bed ward.

    c._____in a room alone.

    d._____in a 6-bed ward.

12. The 10-year-old girl prefers social contacts with

    a._____teen-age girls.

    b._____other ten-year-old girls.

    c._____teen-age boys.

    d._____adults.

13. Favorite books read by 10-year-old girls deal with subjects such as

    a._____adventure and mystery.

    b._____religion and philosophy.

    c._____love and romance.

    d._____family life and biographies.

14. Ten-year-old boys enjoy reading books on the following subjects:

    a._____adventure and mystery.

    b._____love and romance.

    c._____family life and biographies.

    d._____religion and philosophy.

15. The years between 8 and 12 are described in terms of health as being

    a._____dangerous because of accidents.

    b._____the healthiest years of a child's life.

    c._____hazardous because of communicable disease.

    d._____the years in which mental illness has its beginning.

16. The leading cause of death in children between the ages of 8 and 12 is

    a._____rheumatic fever.

    b._____communicable diseases including tuberculosis.

    c._____accidents.

    d._____poliomyelitis.

17. While 10-year-old children develop interests in a variety of hobbies, the one that is a universal favorite is

    a._____learning to play a musical instrument.

    b._____carpentering.

c.___collecting things.

d.___reading.

18. One of the statements below is most descriptive of the 10-year-old child's relationships with others:

a.___he is selfish and lacking in sensitivity to the welfare of other people.

b.___he is un-co-operative in play and in school.

c.___he has a tendency toward temper tantrums.

d.___he has a strong sense of justice and fair play.

Questions for Discussion and Student Projects—(*Continued*)

1. In your hospital, what plans are made to investigate home conditions before a convalescent patient is dismissed? How is the report submitted to hospital personnel?

2 Suggested report for one student: Prepare a nursing care plan for a 10-year-old girl with chorea including

a. suitable play equipment.

b. feeding technics.

c. care of the skin.

d. placement in a pediatric unit.

e. prevention of bodily injury.

3. Plan a classroom discussion around characteristics in a nurse which are particularly desirable when giving care to a chorea patient. Are these same qualities suitable for the nurse caring for other types of pediatric conditions? Do you think that, with conscious effort, nurses are able to develop characteristics known to be desirable in certain fields of nursing?

4. What are the facilities in your community for the recreation and the guidance of school children? Prepare a list of clubs which 10-year-old boys and girls may join. What are the objectives or purposes of these clubs?

5. What should your response be to the parents of a 10-year-old child who are distressed at the persistent reading of comic books? Part of the mother's concern is that the child will develop criminal tendencies and another expressed fear is that the child will never appreciate more desirable literature. (See the Strang reference, pp. 515–516.)

Section 4. Nursing Care During the Adolescent Period

Study Suggestions: Before beginning the study of this Section, the student will find it helpful to

A. Review

1. In anatomy and physiology texts: the units on the female reproductive system, the central nervous system, the musculoskeletal system.
2. In nutrition texts: nutritional needs in the adolescent period.

B. Study

1. In pediatrics, medical nursing and/or communicable disease nursing texts: the specific disease conditions under consideration.*

C. Read the additional References listed before attempting to answer the questions relating to each patient study.

THE SCHOOL HEALTH PROGRAM—SITUATION STUDY

Miss Carr, the nurse assigned to school No. 88, had spent most of one morning assisting the school physician with physical examinations. Pupils scheduled were high school freshman girls and 10 had been examined. Before the doctor arrived, Miss Carr spent about 15 minutes with the entire group of girls talking about healthful living and answering questions. During the examinations, one 14-year-old girl was discovered to have scabies. Miss Carr arranged to visit the home later that day to determine whether or not other members of the family were so affected and what provisions were made by the family for medical care.

At the end of the physical examinations, Anna, a 13-year-old girl, asked Miss Carr for a few minutes of her time. When the nurse and Anna were alone, Anna stated that she needed to know more about her monthly periods. She added that she had known for a long time from observing an older sister that such a condition is to be expected, but no one had really explained it. Miss Carr drew a few simple diagrams on the blackboard to illustrate certain parts of the female anatomy, and after some general discussion, Anna said she understood it.

As Miss Carr was leaving the school building, she stopped at the principal's office to discuss a meeting which had been held the previous evening. The principal had asked Miss Carr to represent nursing at a PTA meeting where the problem of drug addiction was discussed. One of the parents had become alarmed because recently she had heard that some kind of "dope" was being sold to the high school students and she

* Narcotic addiction and emotional disturbances are also considered in the section on psychiatric nursing.

wanted an investigation made. The meeting had been attended by school personnel, parents, the school physician, Miss Carr, and others interested in community welfare. A plan had been agreed upon to attempt to prevent the use of narcotics by high school students.

References

Hoffman, H., Sherman, Irene, Krevitsky, F., and Williams, F.: Teen-age drug addicts arraigned in the narcotic court of Chicago, J.A.M.A. 149:655, 1952.

Ratcliff, J. D.: A sane look at teen-age drug addiction, Parents Magazine pp. 41, 76, November 1951.

Reilly, Margaret, G.: Juvenile acne, Am. J. Nursing 50:269, 1950.

Sellew, Gladys: Health supervision of the school child, pp. 176–191, and Diseases and conditions of the skin and hair, pp. 391–399, *both in* Nursing of Children, Philadelphia, Saunders, 1948.

Spock, Benjamin: Puberty development, in Baby and Child Care, New York, Pocket Books, Inc.

The control of communicable disease in man, 7th ed., Am. Pub. Health Assoc. 1790 Broadway, New York City 19, 1950.

Guiding the adolescent, Fed. Sec. Agency Publication No. 225, pp. 5–10, Rev. 1946.

Questions Relating to the Situation Study

1. One of the questions asked by a pupil was, "What is the physical examination like?" Miss Carr should tell them

   a._____to wait and see.
   b._____that it will last about 15 minutes.
   c._____that each girl is partially undressed and wears a white robe over her underclothing.
   d._____that they should not waste the doctor's time with idle questions.

2. Another pupil asked Miss Carr to explain to them why the physical examinations were done. She told them that

   a._____the purpose is to keep school children in the best possible health.
   b._____parents demand this service.
   c._____it is required by state law.
   d._____many children who cannot afford private medical care are thus assured of periodic physical examinations.

3. As the diagnosis of scabies was made by the school physician, you would expect to see the following symptoms:

   a._____itching of the entire body, vesicles in the palms of the hands, a fever of 100°F.
   b._____itching of the skin between the fingers, small dark spots over the fingers, dermatitis of the hands.
   c._____a red raised rash over the neck and the chest, enlarged cervical lymph glands, itching of the neck and the chest.
   d._____loss of hair over the top of the head, crusty formations back of the ears, itching of the scalp.

4. After the condition of scabies is discovered, the procedure which is most appropriate in a school health program is to

   a._____send a note to the family, give the child a prescription for an ointment, send a note to the principal's office.

   b._____send the child home at once, warn all others in the class to watch for signs of scabies, send a note to the family.

   c._____send a nurse to visit the home, refer the child to his family physician, report the condition to the principal's office.

   d._____send the child home at once, give the child a prescription for an ointment, report the condition to the home room teacher.

5. Suppose you are the nurse making the home visit and the mother asks you what caused scabies. You should tell her

   a._____it is associated with uncleanliness.

   b._____it is caused by a very small parasite, called a mite.

   c._____it is a fungus infection.

   d._____the cause is not clearly understood.

6. In case you are asked how the disease is spread, you should explain that it is usually spread by

   a._____drinking from the same glass.

   b._____using another person's comb.

   c._____eating from another person's plate.

   d._____intimate association with an infected person.

7. In general, scabies may be prevented by

   a._____frequent hand washing, general cleanliness, use of one's own personal toilet articles.

   b._____use of medicated soaps, immunization, a daily bath.

   c._____frequent change of bed linens, use of one's own personal toilet articles, alcohol rubs.

   d._____immunization, alcohol rubs, a daily bath.

8. Suppose the mother you are visiting asks you how she can keep the two preschool children from getting scabies from the older girl. You should tell her to

   a._____boil all dishes used by the patient, soak all of her linens in a weak Lysol solution before placing them with the family wash, keep the children separated.

   b._____prevent close contact between preschool children and the patient, wash her hands thoroughly after giving care, use hot water and soap in washing the patient's clothing and bedding.

   c._____destroy all books and papers used by the patient, burn sulfur candles in the patient's room when treatment is completed, keep other children out of the patient's room.

9. In talking with Anna about menstruation, Miss Carr should tell her that

a._____she should expect to have painful cramps, she should spend the first day in bed, all physical exercise should be abandoned.

b._____delayed menstruation is a sign of tuberculosis, she should avoid dancing during a period, she should eat lightly during a period.

c._____menstruation is a normal process, daily bathing should be continued, periods may be irregular during early adolescence.

d._____a physician should be consulted if cramps are severe, she should avoid baths, she should eat lightly during a period.

Questions for Discussion and Student Projects

1. Prepare a list of suitable activities of a school nurse. Do you think she should spend the major portion of her time and efforts working toward the prevention of illness or working with children who have physical handicaps?

2. What are some of the common physical defects you would expect Miss Carr to encounter among school children?

3. Assume you are this school nurse and have 10 high school freshman girl students waiting 15 minutes for physician. What would you do with this period? Do you believe the girls would be interested in health teaching? What questions do you think they might ask the nurse? What points should you include?

4. Describe how you think the menstrual function should be explained to Anna. Prepare a simple drawing of the anatomic parts you believe should be included in the explanation. What terms do you think should be used to give her an adequate understanding of the process?

5. State how you would answer each of the following questions should Anna ask them:

   a. Why does a period occur every month?
   b. Do boys have menstrual periods? Why not?
   c. Over how many years do menstrual periods continue?
   d. Do you consider it fair for women to have this inconvenience?
   e. Is it desirable to use vaginal tampons?
   f. May I take aspirin tablets for cramps?

Questions Relating to the Section in General

1. During early adolescence physical growth shows a

   a._____slow increase in height.
   b._____rapid increase in weight.
   c._____slow increase in both height and weight.
   d._____rapid increase in both height and weight.

2. Comparison of the physical growth of boys and girls in early adolescence shows that

   a._____boys grow more rapidly than girls.
   b._____girls grow more rapidly than boys.
   c._____growth proceeds at the same rate in both sexes.

3. In late adolescence, comparison of growth for boys and girls shows that

   a._____boys grow more rapidly than girls.
   b._____girls grow more rapidly than boys.
   c._____growth proceeds at the same rate in both sexes.

4. The child who is in a rapid growth spurt is prone to be

   a._____restless.
   b._____tired.
   c._____overactive.
   d._____aggressive.

5. Adolescent children are often troubled by the skin condition called acne. The usual causes of acne are

   a._____overexposure to the sun's rays, constipation, overweight.
   b._____emotional tensions, underweight, lack of sunshine.
   c._____excessive oil in the skin, constipation, dietary indiscretions.
   d._____menstrual disturbances, excessive oil in the skin, lack of sunshine.

6. The average age at which puberty development starts in girls is

   a._____10 years.
   b._____13 years.
   c._____9 years.
   d._____11 years.

7. The average age at which menstruations starts is

   a._____13 years.
   b._____10 years.
   c._____12 years.
   d._____11 years.

8. The average age at which puberty development starts in boys is

   a._____10 years.
   b._____13 years.
   c._____9 years.
   d._____11 years.

9. Children who have not started developments expected for their particular age should be

   a._____examined by a physician.
   b._____given a high-protein, high-vitamin diet.
   c._____given additional rest periods.
   d._____assured that the expected developments will start since individual children mature at different rates.

10. Measures effective in the prevention of acne are

   a._____a low-calorie diet, daily cleansing of the skin with soap and water, outdoor exercise.

b._____daily cleansing of the skin with soap and water, regular bowel habits, a well-balanced diet.

c._____a high-vitamin diet, cleansing the skin with cold cream only, regular bowel habits.

d._____a high-calorie diet, daily cleansing of the skin with cold cream, outdoor exercise.

11. Ringworm is occasionally a problem among school children. Skin eruptions are caused by

a._____a fungus growth.

b._____bacterial infection.

c._____a sensitivity to certain contacted objects.

d._____virus organisms.

12. The school nurse should explain to pupils that ringworm is

a._____not contagious.

b._____expected to recover spontaneously.

c._____frequently accompanied by secondary infections.

d._____spread by both direct and indirect contact.

13. Ringworm of the scalp usually results in the loss of patches of hair. Mothers of children so affected should be told that

a._____the hair will grow again in a few weeks.

b._____the bald spots will be permanent.

c._____the hair will grow again at puberty.

d._____scars will be left on the areas of the scalp affected by ringworm.

14. Another condition occurring among school children is the presence of head lice. Which of the following terms refers to head lice?

a._____Pediculosis corporis.

b._____Pediculosis capitis.

c._____Pediculosis pubis.

15. Symptoms of head lice are

a._____itching of the scalp, enlarged lymph glands at the base of the scalp, restlessness.

b._____a fever of 100°F., itching of the scalp, fatigue.

c._____loss of appetite, lethargy, itching of the scalp.

16. Head lice may be prevented in school children by

a._____daily inspection of all heads, weekly shampoos at home, separate hand towels for all children.

b._____the use of separate toilet articles by all children, no exchange of head gear among children, a minimum amount of close contact between children.

c._____frequent handwashing, daily inspection of all heads, clean toilet facilities.

17. In general, pediculosis of any type is associated with

a._____poor housing.

b._____low economic status.

c.____a lack of personal cleanliness.
d.____delinquent behavior.

18. From the following list of observations check those which could cause you to suspect that a high school student might be using a habit-forming drug:

    a.____excessive day dreaming.
    b.____an increase in appetite.
    c.____loss of interest in school work.
    d.____loss of weight.
    e.____restlessness.
    f.____withdrawal from social contacts with school mates.
    g.____aggressiveness.
    h.____contracted pupils in eyes.
    i.____loss of appetite.
    j.____secretive behavior.
    k.____gain in weight.
    l.____depression.
    m.____increased interest in competitive sports.

19. A teacher asks the school nurse to see a high school student who is having abdominal cramps, nausea and vomiting. The nurse should

    a.____call the school physician, send the student home, notify the mother by telephone.
    b.____take the student home, notify the mother by telephone, notify the principal's office.
    c.____ask the mother to come to the school, place the child on a bed or table, call the school physician.
    d.____keep the student quiet, ask the mother to come for the child, advise the mother to call the family physician.

Questions for Discussion and Student Projects—(*Continued*)

1. Prepare a sample diet which would provide for the total nutritional needs of a high school freshman. Divide the foods into 3 separate meals and explain why each item is included for the particular meal.
2. Describe what you should say to help a young girl recognize the value of eating a satisfactory breakfast.
3. From your knowledge of subjects taught in high schools, list specific areas in which health teaching could be included. Do you think health should be taught as a separate course or included in a variety of subjects?
4. At what age in a girl's life should menstruation be explained? Who do you think should be responsible for giving this information?
5. Suppose you were called upon to meet with parents and school personnel to help prepare a program for the prevention of narcotic addiction in your community. What information do you think you would need about drug addiction and about your particular school program?

6. When you were in high school, what plan was in effect to prevent the spread of communicable skin diseases? Who assumed responsibility for the maintenance of a sanitary environment?
7. Describe how you should inspect a child's head for pediculosis as she is being admitted to the hospital. Do you think this part of the admission procedure should be carried out while the mother is present?
8. What is the treatment for head lice in your hospital, and what are the precautions to be observed in carrying out the treatment?
9. Describe how you should explain to an older child that she has pediculosis, including possible methods of contracting the condition and measures for prevention.

THE BOY WITH POLIO—PATIENT STUDY

Jeffry Taylor, aged 12 years, was admitted in July to the communicable disease unit of a general hospital. His chief complaints were stiff neck and inability to use his right arm. Jeffry had gone swimming at a nearby pool and 2 days later began to complain of soreness and swelling of his cervical glands. He did not feel able to carry out his usual activities and did not wish to eat. The parents took Jeffry to the family physician who gave him a prescription for some white tablets. The day prior to admission, Jeffry complained of pain in his right shoulder and back, and of a slight discomfort in both legs. On the morning of admission, he could not raise his right arm above his head. Backache was severe and his temperature was 100°F. by mouth.

Neuromuscular examination revealed the following:

1. Marked nuchal rigidity.
2. Abdominals equal in all 4 quadrants.
3. Kernig's and Babinski signs negative.
4. Knee jerks hyperactive but equal.
5. Ankle jerks hyperactive but equal.
6. Biceps reflexes weak on the left and absent on the right.
7. Inability to elevate the right arm and shoulder.
8. No weakness of the hands, the forearms or the lower extremities.
9. Poker spine.

Spinal fluid examination revealed the following:

Cell count, 75 lymphocytes.
Protein, 46 mg.
Sugar, 58 mg.
Pandy, trace.
Chlorides, 123.6.

Jeffry was placed in a specially prepared bed and warm moist packs were applied 3 times daily to his right shoulder, upper arm, back and cervical spine. His position was changed every 2 hours from prone to back-lying alternately. After 5 days Jeffry's temperature was normal and he was taking a general diet. At the end of 2 weeks he was allowed up in a chair for his meals and 3 days later was discharged to a convalescent home.

Background Review Questions

1. Match the following muscles with the correct function:

a.____deltoid.
b.____erector spinae (sacrospinalis).
c.____gastrocnemius.
d.____trapezius.
e.____rhomboids.
f.____hamstrings.
g.____latissimus dorsi.
h.____sternocleidomastoid.
i.____diaphragm.
j.____pectorals.
k.____quadriceps femoris

(1) flexes knee.
(2) flexes head laterally on neck.
(3) extends forearm.
(4) draws arm downward and forward across chest and aids in chest expansion.
(5) draws arm downward and backward and rotates it.
(6) extends foot, flexes lower leg.
(7) extends spine.
(8) elevates arm, aids in backward and forward motions of arm.
(9) rotates scapula, draws head backward.
(10) extends knee.
(11) retracts and elevates scapulae.
(12) contracts chest.
(13) flexes forearm.

2. Match the following related terms:

a.____nucha.
b.____cervical.
c.____prone.
d.____calcaneus.
e.____plantarflexion.
f.____anterior horn cells.
g.____peripheral.

(1) heel bone.
(2) in the spinal cord.
(3) away from the center.
(4) nape of the neck.
(5) back lying.
(6) ankle bone.
(7) region of the neck.
(8) extension of the foot.
(9) face lying.

3. Prepare 2 drawings to illustrate the parts of the body which are affected by the polio virus:

a. a cross-section of the spinal cord showing the location of the anterior horn cells.
b. a vertical drawing of the spinal cord showing pathways of the peripheral nerves which supply impulses to the muscles of the upper and the lower extremities.

References

Anderson, Gaylord W., and Arnstein, Margaret G.: Communicable Disease Control, ed. 2, pp. 280–293, New York, Macmillan, 1949.
Funsten, Robert V., and Calderwood, Carmelita: Orthopedic Nursing, ed. 1, pp. 410–466, St. Louis, Mosby, 1943; ed. 2, pp. 474–544, 1949.
Knocke, Frederick J., and Knocke, Lazelle: Rehabilitation, pp. 115–132, and Surgery, pp. 168–174, in Orthopedic Nursing, Philadelphia, Davis, 1951.

Nursing for the Poliomyelitis Patient, prepared and published by the Joint Orthopedic Nursing Advisory Service of the National Organization for Public Health Nursing and the National League of Nursing Education, 2 Park Avenue, New York City 6. 88 pages, price $.35.

Siedenfeld, Morton A.: Psychological considerations in poliomyelitis care, Am. J. Nursing 47:369, 1947.

Questions Relating to the Patient Study

1. As Jeffry is being admitted to the unit, certain observations are helpful to the physician in planning treatment and in appraising the immediate degree of illness. Those which are most significant at this time are

   a._____type of respirations, signs of urinary retention, muscular weakness.

   b._____signs of muscle spasm, lacerations of the skin, position the child assumes in bed.

   c._____evidence of malnutrition, position the child assumes in bed, signs of urinary retention.

   d._____type of pulse, signs of emotional anxiety, orthopedic deformities.

   e._____type of respirations, muscular weakness, evidence of malnutrition.

2. In regard to the care of Jeffry's skin on admission, the nurse should

   a._____give him a soap and water bath.

   b._____give him a brisk alcohol rub.

   c._____oil the entire body with warm olive oil.

   d._____omit all skin stimulation during the acute phase of the disease.

3. The purpose of the moist packs ordered for Jeffry was to

   a._____prevent stiffening of the joints.

   b._____relieve muscle spasm.

   c._____improve circulation to the muscles.

   d._____prevent the progression of muscular weakness.

4. The warm moist packs are contraindicated for Jeffry in the following circumstances

   a._____a temperature of 100°F. or over, skin rash, extremely hot weather.

   b._____objections made by the patient, insufficient nursing personnel, skin rash.

   c._____extremely hot weather, objections made by the parents, a temperature of 100°F. or over.

   d._____upper respiratory infection, insufficient nursing personnel, objections made by the patient.

5. During the first few days, Jeffry's right arm should be

   a._____held close to his body.

   b._____elevated on a pillow.

    c._____maintained at a right angle to his body.

    d._____kept in a position most comfortable for Jeffry.

6. Jeffry was turned every 2 hours in order to

    a._____prevent hypostatic pneumonia, improve the circulation, provide interest for the child.

    b._____promote rest, allow for frequent observations of the skin, prevent orthopedic deformities.

    c._____improve the circulation, promote rest, prevent hypostatic pneumonia.

    d._____prevent decubitus ulcers, promote rest, prevent hypostatic pneumonia.

7. As the nurses change Jeffry's position in bed, of the following methods they should

    a._____turn Jeffry's entire body as a unit, supporting the extremities only at the joints.

    b._____ask the child to help move himself by placing one arm around the nurse's shoulders.

    c._____wrap the child in a sheet and turn him by a rolling motion.

8. In case Jeffry's parents told you they were concerned that 2 younger children in the family might develop polio, you should tell them that

    a._____there is no reason to fear this possibility.

    b._____the other children should be observed for symptoms and early medical care obtained if symptoms develop.

    c._____they should consult their family physician about giving penicillin to the other children as a preventive measure.

    d._____the children should be kept in bed most of the time.

9. The parents might ask you whether or not Jeffry may have been exposed to polio while in swimming 2 days before the onset. You should tell them that

    a._____studies have shown that the incubation period is between 3 and 35 days.

    b._____it is unwise for any child to go swimming in a public pool during the polio season.

    c._____studies have shown swimming pools and bathing beaches to be a common source of polio infection.

Questions for Discussion and Student Projects—(*Continued*)

1. Plan a classroom demonstration of the preparation of the bed currently recommended for Jeffry.
2. Using a student nurse or an ambulatory patient, show how pillows and pads should be used to relieve muscle spasm in the parts so affected in Jeffry.
3. Describe your plan of nursing care for Jeffry while he is a patient in the communicable disease unit, including

a. Bed rest:

  (1) position in bed to promote comfort and to prevent deformities.
  (2) care of the skin, mouth, hair and nails.
  (3) methods for changing the position in bed.
  (4) measures to promote adequate rest and sleep.

b. Dietary factors:

  (1) nutritional needs as determined by illness.
  (2) methods of feeding.
  (3) method of keeping record of intake.
  (4) addition of salt when excessive amounts of body fluids are lost.

c. Elimination:

  (1) signs of urinary and/or fecal retention.
  (2) methods of keeping record of output.
  (3) precautions to be observed when placing Jeffry on the bedpan.

d. Charting:

  (1) notations regarding muscle spasm, tightness around specific joints, and signs of paralysis of muscles.
  (2) complaints made by Jeffry.
  (3) appetite, including food and fluids taken.
  (4) observations regarding elimination.
  (5) Jeffry's emotional reaction to his illness.

e. Visitors:

  (1) explanation of isolation precautions to parents.
  (2) teaching general communicable disease prevention to Jeffry's parents.
  (3) recommendation of suitable gifts for Jeffry.

f. Psychologic considerations:

  (1) explanation of all procedures to Jeffry.
  (2) plan for spending time with Jeffry listening to him and talking as needed.
  (3) response to questions regarding fears of being crippled.
  (4) recommended activities appropriate for Jeffry according to his age, interests and illness.
  (5) methods used to maintain interest in Jeffry's previous activities.

4. Describe how Jeffry and his parents should be prepared for care in the convalescent hospital. What should your response be to the parents if they insist that they are able to give the necessary care at home?

5. Jeffry's chief weakness was in his right deltoid. Prepare a plan of appropriate recreational activities for Jeffry based on his age, his interests and the limited use of his right arm. What suggestions should you make to prevent overuse, with resulting overdevelopment, of the left arm?

Questions Relating to the Section in General

1. Poliomyelitis occurs most commonly in

    a._____the late summer months, adults, eastern United States.
    b._____children under 10 years, the middle summer months, western United States.
    c._____southern United States, adults, the early fall months.
    d._____children under 10 years, the later summer months, in any part of the United States.

2. In poliomyelitis, the virus attacks the anterior horn cells in the spinal cord. The function of the anterior horn cells is to

    a._____transmit motor impulses to the muscles.
    b._____transmit sensory impulses to the brain.
    c._____co-ordinate motions of the trunk and the lower extremities.
    d._____transmit sensory impulses to the muscles.

3. Damage to the anterior horn cells is done during

    a._____the period of isolation.
    b._____the acute stage.
    c._____any relapse caused by improper treatment.

4. In the light of present knowledge of poliomyelitis, the most effective control measures during an epidemic are to

    a._____keep children indoors, close the schools, avoid contact with new groups of people.
    b._____avoid crowds, close swimming pools and beaches, encourage outdoor play.
    c._____encourage outdoor play except in the hot sun, avoid contact with new groups of people, promote environmental sanitation.
    d._____continue with children's usual activities, encourage well-balanced meals, inspect children daily for early symptoms.

5. In poliomyelitis, changes in spinal fluid to be expected are

    a._____pressure normal, cell count increased, sugar increased.
    b._____pressure increased, cell count increased, protein elevated.
    c._____sugar increased, cell count normal, chlorides increased.
    d._____pressure normal, fluid cloudy, chlorides increased.

6. In the bulbar type of poliomyelitis, pathologic changes are in the

    a._____cerebrum.
    b._____cervical region of the spinal cord.
    c._____medulla oblongata.
    d._____cerebellum.

7. Symptoms of bulbar polio are

    a._____nasal quality of the voice, irregular respirations, difficulty in swallowing.

b.____paralysis of the respiratory muscles, cyanosis, coma.

c.____excessive mucus in the throat, convulsions, slow pulse.

d.____difficulty in swallowing, paralysis of the respiratory muscles, urinary retention.

8. Signs of involvement of the muscles of the upper thorax are

   a.____flushing of the face, rapid shallow respirations, flat rigid abdomen.

   b.____cyanosis, rapid shallow respirations, flat rigid chest on the affected side.

   c.____retraction of the intercostal muscles, deep regular respirations, cyanosis.

   d.____pallor, slow shallow respirations, expanded chest wall.

9. Signs of involvement of the diaphragm are

   a.____expanded chest, urinary retention, irregular respirations.

   b.____cyanosis, flat rigid chest, ballooned abdomen on exhalation.

   c.____prominent eyeballs, cyanosis, flat rigid chest.

   d.____expanded chest, prominent eyeballs, ballooned abdomen on exhalation.

10. In case packs are ordered for the patient who has muscle spasm of the upper thorax or diaphragm, the nurse should

    a.____use only light-weight lay-on packs, apply packs every few minutes until respirations are improved.

    b.____apply packs every 2 hours, pin packs on loosely.

    c.____apply packs every few minutes, fasten packs securely with safety pins.

    d.____use only light-weight lay-on packs, apply packs every 4 hours.

11. Occasionally braces are ordered for polio patients during the convalescent stage. The purpose of the brace or braces is to

    a.____provide additional support to the involved part, prevent muscular atrophy, assist the child in walking.

    b.____assist the child in walking, prevent deformities, prevent muscular atrophy.

    c.____maintain the involved part in the desired position, prevent deformities, prevent stretching of the affected muscles.

12. Arthrodesis is the surgical procedure which

    a.____retards growth of an extremity.

    b.____stabilizes a joint.

    c.____provides for greater movement of a joint.

13. The purpose of a tenotomy is to

    a.____prevent further deformity.

    b.____stabilize a joint.

    c.____lengthen a muscle.

14. An osteotomy is done to

    a._____change the alignment of a bone.
    b._____provide for free movement of a joint.
    c._____retard growth of an extremity.

15. Epiphyseal arrest is a surgical procedure which

    a._____stabilizes a joint.
    b._____retards growth of the unaffected extremity.
    c._____lengthens a muscle.

Questions for Discussion and Student Projects— *(Continued)*

1. Describe how you should explain to parents that a lumbar puncture is a necessary part of the diagnostic procedures. What should your response be to parents who say they believe a lumbar puncture to be a dangerous procedure?

2. Suppose you are a public health nurse working in a rural area and become responsible for supervising the transportation of an acutely ill polio patient to a nearby hospital. Describe ways in which you should plan for the trip with the least discomfort or damage to the patient.

3. What are the regulations of your state and local health departments for the control of poliomyelitis? Are all patients isolated? If so, for how long? Are families quarantined after a patient has been diagnosed as polio? If so, for how long? What activities may be continued by individuals exposed to the disease? Is there a health department regulation which affects the disinfection of excreta? Is there a definite procedure for concurrent and terminal disinfection of articles used in the care of the patient?

4. Make a list of professional workers who are concerned with the care of polio patients. State the function of each person and show how the efforts of all workers should be co-ordinated to obtain the best care for the patients.

5. Plan an observation, if possible, in the physical therapy department to observe (a) a patient having a muscle examination and (b) muscle re-education technics as carried out by the physical therapist.

6. Plan a demonstration of the nursing care indicated for the patient in a respirator.

7. How should nurses prepare the patient psychologically for being placed in the respirator? What do you think the parents should be told about the purpose of a respirator? Try to anticipate specific questions parents might ask you about this type of care and prepare an answer for the possible questions.

8. Assume you are the nurse caring for a child during the convalescent stage of polio, and long leg braces are being used. Describe how you should teach the mother to care for the child and the braces at home, including prevention of pressure areas, care of the appliance, knowledge of proper fitting and the importance of wearing the brace.

9. What is meant by the term "physiologic rest position"? Plan a class-

room demonstration using an ambulatory patient or a student nurse to show positions of good body alignment in back, face and side lying.

10. Describe methods used in your hospital to prepare the operative site for orthopedic surgery. Why is it desirable to provide extra care of the skin when surgery is to be performed on a bone or joint?
11. Write your State Vocational Rehabilitation Service to learn what your state offers to disabled persons. Prepare a report for class (suggested project for one student) to explain the rehabilitation program as it operates in your state, including

   a. eligibility of the person needing assistance.
   b. vocational and educational counseling available.
   c. training facilities available for applicants.
   d. sources of funds for support of the program.
   e. job placement following training.
   f. follow-up of the disabled person.

12. Prepare a list of crippling conditions which usually result in some degree of disability. What is the nurse's responsibility toward patients who are temporarily or permanently disabled?
13. Describe how you should explain the services of your state rehabilitation program to a 16-year-old boy in your community who is confined to a wheel chair as a result of poliomyelitis.
14. What are the functions of the National Foundation for Infantile Paralysis? How does this organization secure financial support?
15. Investigate current research in the development of a "preventive vaccine" for poliomyelitis. What are some of the difficulties encountered in the prevention and control of this disease?

THE TRUANT—PATIENT STUDY

Charles Braddock was a 14-year-old boy from juvenile court who had been admitted to the pediatric unit for a physical examination. He got along fairly well with the 3 other boys in his ward where he had spent the previous week. Various tests and procedures, including electroencephalogram, roentgenograms of the skull, the chest and the long bones, and laboratory examinations were all reported to be within normal limits. Charles was 5 feet, 11 inches tall, and weighed 155 pounds. He had been in good health all of his life.

Charles was brought to the hospital by a probation officer from juvenile court. In a conference with the social worker the officer explained that Charles had been in trouble several times in the past 4 years due to stealing and truancy. There was also a history of enuresis over the past 6 years. Charles had been apprehended by a local policeman for stealing cigarettes from a grocery store, and, since this was his third offense, the policeman notified the family and Charles was admitted to juvenile court. The probation officer described the home as follows:

The parents had separated twice, but live together at present. The father works most of time and the family live in moderate circumstances. Siblings consist of an older sister aged 17 and two brothers aged 11 and 8. The

420   *Nursing Care of Children*

older sister is said to be superior in school work, in music and in relationships with people.

Charles told the student nurse assigned to his ward that he was in the eighth grade but hated school and planned to leave as soon as he was old enough. He was polite, obedient and co-operative in his relationships with hospital personnel. The night nurse reported that he masturbated rather frequently, and was restless in his sleep.

Charles remained in the hospital for a few more days when he was referred to Child Guidance Clinic for treatment. He returned to juvenile court for a hearing and was dismissed to his parents.

References

Beverly, Bert I.: A Psychology of Growth, pp. 119–146, 186–197, New York, McGraw-Hill, 1947.
Mitchell-Nelson: Psychologic Disorders, *in* Textbook of Pediatrics, ed. 4, pp. 1008–1023, Philadelphia, Saunders, 1945; ed. 5, pp. 1252–1272, 1950.
Oed, Minnie K.: Helping the bewildered adolescent, Am. J. Nursing 50:298–301, 1950.
Spock, Benjamin: Baby and Child Care, pp. 325–326, New York, Pocket Books, (Available at most drug stores—$.35.)
Strang, Ruth: Development and Guidance of Adolescents, *in* An Introduction to Child Care, ed. 3, pp. 647–675, New York Macmillan, 1951.
Whitman, Samuel: Child guidance clinic, Hygeia, The Health Magazine September, 1945.
Guiding the Adolescent, Federal Security Agency Publication 225, pp. 55–68. For sale by the Superintendent of Documents, U.S. Government Printing Office, Washington 25, D.C. 83 pages, price $.25. (Free copies available to health workers.)

Questions Relating to the Patient Study

1. In studying Charles' past history, you would suspect that his undesirable behavior was caused by

   a._____the separations of his parents, insufficient money, jealousy of his younger brothers.

   b._____mental retardation, jealousy of his older sister, rejection by his mother.

   c._____unstable family life, jealousy of his older sister, lack of personal satisfactions.

   d._____rejection by his mother, the separations of his parents, rapid gain in height and weight.

2. The night nurse who discovered Charles masturbating should

   a._____ignore the activity.

   b._____place a screen around his bed.

   c._____ask him to stop.

   d._____give him something else to do.

3. You would suspect that Charles' enuresis was associated with

   a._____excessive masturbation.

   b._____hostility toward his parents.

   c._____lack of success in school.
   d._____early sexual maturation.

4. In case Charles wet the bed while in the hospital, the nurse caring for him at the time should

   a._____insist that he change the bed linens.
   b._____shame him for his babyish behavior.
   c._____change the bed making no comments.
   d._____let him remain indefinitely in the wet bed.

5. The head nurse in the unit where Charles was placed should

   a._____assign someone to watch him at all times to prevent escape.
   b._____encourage personnel to treat him in the same manner as other patients.
   c._____restrict visitors to the mother only.
   d._____censor all of his outgoing mail.

6. While Charles was in the hospital, one of the boys in the ward accused him of stealing some stamps from his collection. The student nurse assigned to the boys should

   a._____report the episode to the head nurse.
   b._____tell the boy to let Charles keep the stamps.
   c._____search through Charles' personal articles to see if he has the stamps.
   d._____tell Charles it is a sin to steal.

7. Nurses' notes during Charles hospitalization should have emphasis on the following points:

   a._____reaction to physical examination, attitude toward parents at visiting hour, appetite.
   b._____description of specific types of behavior, complaints of physical discomfort, sleep habits.
   c._____remarks about home situation, attitudes toward authority, relationships with other boys.
   d._____responsiveness toward friendly adults, description of specific types of behavior, attitude toward parents at visiting hour.

Questions for Discussion and Student Projects

1. What provisions should a student nurse make for Charles' recreation while he is in the hospital? From your knowledge of the interests of a 14-year-old boy, prepare a plan of activities for Charles, making adjustments as indicated by his present situation. Do you think nurses should purchase special materials for recreation for Charles?
2. Describe how you should explain to Charles the services of a Child Guidance Clinic. How should you respond to Charles if he stated that he refused to attend the clinic?
3. Suppose one day the boys in the ward teased Charles about being so tall and heavy for 14 years. Describe how you should explain to them

differences in rates of growth. Do you think boys are more disturbed at unusually slow or at unusually rapid growth?

Questions Relating to the Section in General

1. Measures designed to prevent juvenile delinquency should be practiced

   a._____from the birth of a child.
   b._____at the time of entrance into school.
   c._____during the preadolescent period.
   d._____from the beginning of the adolescent period.

2. Certain basic emotional needs are present in all individuals. Check those below which must be met in the development of a healthy personality:

   a._____to be financially secure, to be loved, to have freedom to play.
   b._____to be healthy, to have spending money, to belong to a family.
   c._____to be loved, to belong to a family, to be recognized as a worthwhile person.
   d._____to achieve success in school, to belong to a group or gang, to be recognized as a person.

3. Worry or anxiety over physical appearance at adolescence is observed most frequently in

   a._____boys, children from wealthy families, children showing superior intelligence.
   b._____girls, children from economically deprived families, children of average intelligence.
   c._____boys and girls alike, children in moderate financial circumstances, children who fail in school.
   d._____boys and girls alike, children from all economic levels, children except those severely retarded mentally.

4. Instruction regarding sex tends to

   a._____cause adolescents to indulge in sexual relations.
   b._____reduce tension in social activities.
   c._____produce a greater incidence of asocial behavior.
   d._____increase the incidence of masturbation.

5. Children who begin maturation early may be expected to

   a._____become larger than the average child.
   b._____develop undesirable modes of behavior.
   c._____attain full growth earlier than the average child.
   d._____attain full growth later than the average child.

6. Truancy from school should be viewed as an

   a._____early symptom of delinquency.
   b._____indication that the child is undergoing some type of conflict.
   c._____evidence of failure in school.
   d._____indication that school work is insufficient challenge.

7. During adolescence special nutritional needs are for

   a._____high protein, high vitamin, high fat.
   b._____low fat, high carbohydrate, vitamin D.
   c._____low carbohydrate, low fat, vitamin B.
   d._____high protein, low fat, vitamin D.

8. One of the most vital needs of the adolescent is to

   a._____be in the company of friendly adults.
   b._____belong to a group near his own age and with similar interests.
   c._____experience romantic relationships with members of the opposite sex.
   d._____help people or groups who are in need.

Questions for Discussion and Student Projects—(*Continued*)

1. Suggested classroom report for one student—Obtain information, by personal interview if possible or by correspondence, describing facilities for the care of juvenile delinquency in your community. Include the following points:

   a. Ages of children receiving care. At what age is a young person who breaks the law handled by a juvenile court rather than by a civil court maintained for adults?
   b. Incidence of offenders by age and by sex.
   c. Types of offenses occurring most frequently.
   d. Relationship of delinquency to housing, geographic areas and economic status of parents.
   e. Personnel reponsible for services of juvenile court, including qualifications and functions of each.
   f. Procedures used. What is the difference between a hearing and a trial? How are decisions reached as to disposition of the offenders?
   g. Plans for the follow-up or the supervision of children known to juvenile court.

2. What recreational facilities are available in your community for teen age youngsters? From your readings and observations, prepare a list of activities most popular for boys and girls between the ages of 13 and 18 years.

3. In your state, what is the minimum age for leaving school? What are the usual reasons for high school students leaving before graduation?

4. Certain types of behavior which may occur during adolescence are cheating, running away from home, eating excessively, withdrawal from social contacts and speech disorders. Describe how you should advise parents who express anxiety to you because of any of the above symptoms.

Section 5. Planning for the Nursing Care of Hospitalized Children

In the previous Sections, certain conditions have been described which required hospitalization of the child. In this last Section, you are to consider facilities and methods recommended to provide the type of nursing care which promotes recovery of the child with the least amount of emotional trauma and with the greatest amount of physical comfort. Under facilities will be included the ward and its equipment; under methods, the planning and execution of all activities which provide safe, individual nursing care for children in the unit.

STUDY SUGGESTIONS: Before beginning the study of this Section, the student will find it helpful to review:

1. The nursing care needs of the children listed as hospitalized patients.
2. The summary Section in Part One, Nursing Care of Adult Patients with Medical and Surgical Disorders.
   The references listed in this Section supplement those listed in the Section cited above.

Listed are the name, age and diagnosis of each patient admitted:

Dickie Harrison	aged 3½ weeks	Pyloric stenosis
Susie	" 3 months	Cleft lip repair
Johnnie Keller	" 4 "	Intussusception
Margaret Green	" 5 "	Infantile eczema
Shirley Mae	" 9 "	Infantile diarrhea
Jane Kay	" 18 to 27 "	Congenital dislocation of the hip
David Bromley	" 3 years	Nephrosis
Donna Hawkins	" 4 "	Burns
Joe Williams	" 5 "	Congenital heart disease
Kenneth White	" 7 "	Tonsillectomy
Elaine Dixon	" 9 "	Leukemia
Diana Hill	" 10 "	Rheumatic fever
Charles Braddock	" 14 "	Emotional disorder

References

Frank, Ruth: Parents and the pediatric nurse, Am. J. Nursing 52:76, 1952.
Latham, Helen: Safe care for hospitalized children, Am. J. Nursing 51:403, 1951.
Leino, Amelia: Organizing the nursing team, Am. J. Nursing 51:665, 1951.
————: Planning patient-centered care, Am. J. Nursing 52:324, 1952.
McClure, Catherine T: Guest in the house, Am. J. Nursing 49:775, 1949.
Randall, Margaret: The assignment of patients and duties, in Ward Administration, pp. 156–174, Philadelphia, Saunders 1949.
Smith, Anne Marie: Play for Convalescent Children, New York, Barnes, 1941.

Spock, Benjamin: Baby and Child Care, p. 360, New York, Pocket Books.
Stevens, Marian: Visitors are welcome on a pediatric ward, Am. J. Nursing **49**:233, 1949.
Wilkins, Gladys: The role of the nurse in the admission of children to hospitals, Nursing Research **1**:36, 1952.

Questions and Student Projects

1. The drawing on this page shows a suggested plan for a pediatric unit with facilities for 17 patients. Reproduce this drawing on paper, and, using the children's names, show where you should place each one in the unit. Be able to explain your reasons for placing them as you do.
2. Prepare one or more drawings of pediatric units which you believe would provide for the total needs of the patients described and which would eliminate unnecessary steps for personnel.

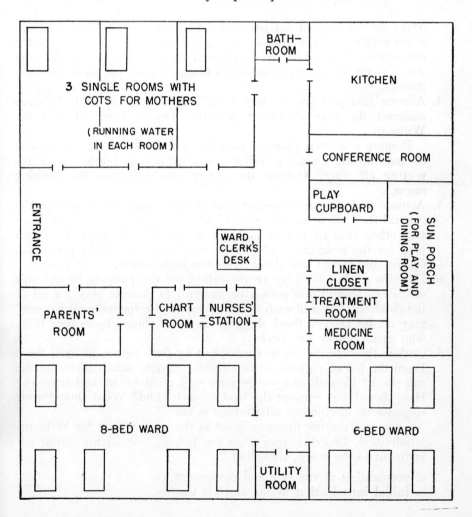

3. Personnel assigned to the pediatric unit consist of the following:

7 A.M. to 3:30 P.M.	3 to 11 P.M.	11 to 7 A.M.
Head nurse	General staff	General staff
Assistant head nurse	nurse____1	nurse____1
General staff nurse____1	Student	Student
Student nurses____4	nurses____3	nurse____2
Practical nurse____1	Nursing	Nursing
Nursing aide____1	aide____1	aide____1
Ward clerk____1		
(hours 8–4:30)		
Volunteer____1		
(hours 9–4)		
Kitchen maid____1		
(on ward at meal time only)		

Make an assignment for one day when all personnel are present. Since a 40-hour week is observed, each person will be off duty for 2 consecutive days. Make an assignment sheet for one week, showing the days off for each person and 5 hours of class per week for each student.

4. Assume that you are on duty from 7 A.M. to 3:30 P.M. You are assigned the care of David Bromley, Donna Hawkins and Joe Williams.

    Prepare a written plan for your day's activities to meet the needs of each of the children. What are your responsibilities when reporting off duty? Outline the report you will give the evening nurse.

5. Assume that you are a senior student nurse assigned to relieve the general staff nurse on her evening off duty. To assist you, you have two other student nurses and a nursing aide. Prepare a written plan for the assignment of patients and duties to all the personnel. Outline the report you should give the night nurse.

6. Describe a plan for play or recreation for the patients in the unit described. Should one person be assigned to provide play for all of the children or should each nurse be responsible for her own patients' play needs? Do you think the play cupboard should be locked? If so, who should carry the key?

7. Outline the activities to be carried out by each person at meal time. From the list of patients, which children might eat at tables on the sun porch? How should you prepare each child for his or her meals? How should you present the food to each child? What should your response be to children who refuse to eat?

8. Assume you are the nurse assigned to the room where Joe Williams is admitted. Describe your plan for helping Joe in his initial adjustment to the ward, including

    a. preparation of the crib and equipment.
    b. initial introduction to Joe and his mother.

   c. explanations of his immediate surroundings to Joe.

   d. information about Joe to be obtained from his mother.

   e. explanations of visiting rules to Joe and to his mother.

   f. answers to questions concerning the operation to be done.

   g. observations and recording of Joe's behavior in relation to signs of fears or evidence of anxiety.

   h. your response toward Joe when he cries at the time his mother leaves.

9. Describe the two methods of assignment of duties known as the case method and the functional method. Explain the advantages and the disadvantages of both methods in the care of children in the hospital.

10. Plan a classroom discussion (perhaps a report from one student showing the policies followed in other hospitals) relating to visiting hours in the pediatric department of your hospital. What are some of the problems associated with visiting hours? Do you believe that children are benefited or harmed by daily visiting by parents? Describe ways in which nurses may use the visiting hour for health teaching to the parents.

11. Suppose you were given a sum of money considered adequate for setting up an organized play program for a 30-bed pediatric unit with patients of all ages. Assuming that you are able to pay the salary of a qualified director for the program, prepare a suggested plan including

   a. educational requirements and personal characteristics of the director.

   b. types and number of various toys, books and magazines, crafts, construction materials, etc., to be purchased.

   c. provision for group activities in the unit, such as singing, playing games, having parties, showing movies, etc.

   d. storage space for play materials.

   e. play space for ambulatory patients or for those in wheel chairs and carts.

12. In recent years several states have provided for the preparation and licensure of practical nurses. Write to your State Nurses Association or to the State Board of Nurse Examiners for information on recent or proposed legislation affecting practical nurses in your state. Do you think prepared practical nurses should be assigned to pediatric units? If not, state your reasons. If so, what specific duties do you approve assigning to these nurses?

Part Three
Nursing Care of the Psychiatric Patient

Section 1. Nursing Care of Neurotic People

THE "PERFECT LADY"—PATIENT STUDY

Mrs. Young, aged 27 years, was admitted to the hospital 2 weeks ago. For the past 5 months, according to her story, she has been becoming increasingly "tense and jittery" and has often had the feeling that she might hurt people, especially her husband. It has been taking her longer and longer to get her usual household tasks completed and lately she has had to repeat many of the activities several times before being able to go on with something else. While working about the house she often feels compelled to throw whatever she has in her hand and then feels that she might "just take off and run." She has many somatic manifestations accompanying these periods of tenseness.

Since entering the hospital, Mrs. Young has been rather restless and frequently comments on her periods of dizziness and her headache. She is always very neatly dressed, takes an hour each morning to apply her cosmetics and then requires the same amount of time to touch them up before she leaves the ward. In the evening she takes 2 hours to get ready for bed, folding each article of clothing neatly, straightening the contents of the dresser drawers, realigning the shoes on the floor of her closet, and applying various creams and lotions to her face and arms.

Last week when she had an appointment for a psychologic examination the nurse told her about it on the evening before. She became increasingly restless, took 4 hours to get ready for bed and then paced the floor for the rest of the night. The appointment for the examination was canceled and a second one was arranged for yesterday. This time the nurse informed Mrs. Young of her appointment 10 minutes before she was to leave. Her immediate reaction was "Oh! How can I get ready?" as she began to rearrange her dress and apply her make-up. She was 10 minutes late for the appointment and told the psychologist she had a terrific headache and couldn't think and finally burst into tears.

She is very slow and precise in the routine ward activities and usually completes her meal one-half hour after all the other patients have finished eating. She often repeats, "It's torture—you don't know how it is—yet it's so silly but I have to do it. Is it my mind? Am I going crazy?"

Mrs. Young's mother provided the following information: her daughter had had the usual childhood illnesses although she was never seriously ill; she was toilet trained at 1 year and except for an occasional accident "didn't give me any trouble from then on." She was really "Mother's little helper" and always seemed much older than she really was; she practically took over the management of the household when she was 9 years old, at which time her father died and her mother had to go to work. She was a good housekeeper even at that age and kept everything neat and clean but "that is the way I trained her." During childhood she had frequent headaches but the doctor said that nothing was wrong and she

431

would probably outgrow them; "I had to caution her all the time about playing too hard because she always was a tomboy. I would make her come in and sit on a chair and when I'd remind her that she might get sick and then wouldn't be able to help mother she'd behave. We also found that it helped to tease her about playing with the boys." During the time she was in high school, she would come right home after school, straighten the house and then prepare the evening meal; she never wanted to run around like the rest of the girls except to go to some church function with mother; she had a job in a grocery store on the week-ends and learned to save her money just like mother had so she was able to pay for her own education.

References

Cottrell L.: Understanding the adolescent, Am. J. Nursing **46**:181, 1946.

Kalkman, Marion: Introduction to Psychiatric Nursing, pp. 296–313, New York, McGraw-Hill, 1940.

Lourdes, Sr. Mary: Understanding children, Am. J. Nursing **46**:770, 1946.

Maslow, A., and Mittleman, B.: Principles of Abnormal Psychology, pp. 417–453, New York, Harpers, 1951.

Peplau, Hildegard: Interpersonal Relations in Nursing, pp. 17–309, New York, Putnam, 1952.

Preston, George: The Substance of Mental Health, New York, Rinehart, 1943.

Waters, Jane: Achieving Maturity, pp. 56–77, 131–151, 167–224, New York, McGraw-Hill, 1949.

Weiss, M.: Nursing care of a psychoneurotic patient, Am. J. Nursing **46**:41, 1946.

Whittenberg, Rudolph M.: So You Want to Help People, New York, Association, 1947.

Questions Relating to the Patient Study

1. When Mrs. Young asks, "Am I going crazy?", the nurse should respond

   a._____"It bothers you, doesn't it?"
   b._____"It's silly to think about such things."
   c._____"We don't use the word 'crazy' in psychiatry."
   d._____"Why, no! What makes you think that?"

2. Mrs. Young's intense feelings about wanting to throw things is usually referred to as a (an)

   a._____compulsion.
   b._____delusion.
   c._____fantasy.
   d._____obsession.

3. Mrs. Young's handwashing indicates that she probably has some fixation at which of the following levels?

   a._____oral.
   b._____anal.
   c._____oedipal.
   d._____latent.

4. When Mrs. Young complains of a headache, the nurse should respond

    a._____"I'll ask your doctor for some medication for relief."
    b._____"You'll feel better after a while."
    c._____"You're feeling a little more tense today?"
    d._____"Why don't you lie down in your room for a while?"

5. The nurse should inform Mrs. Young before a routine nursing procedure is carried out

    a._____just as she goes into Mrs. Young's room with the equipment.
    b._____just prior to going into her room with the equipment.
    c._____about 10 minutes before getting the equipment ready.
    d._____about 2 hours in advance of the time for the procedure.

6. The most probable reason for Mrs. Young's anxiety is

    a._____fear that she has a brain tumor.
    b._____fear that others will harm her.
    c._____a feeling that she will lose control of herself.
    d._____worry about paying for the high cost of hospitalization.

7. In relation to Mrs. Young taking so long to eat, the action which would be appropriate for the nurse is to

    a._____insist that she eat alone in her room.
    b._____insist that she return her tray at the same time as the others.
    c._____arrange for her tray to be served first.
    d._____tell her that she will have to try to eat faster.

8. Mrs. Young's compulsions serve best as a release for her

    a._____antisocial tendencies.
    b._____feelings of anxiety.
    c._____asocial traits.
    d._____intellectual ability.

9. The nurse should explain the ward routines in detail to Mrs. Young because it is

    a._____difficult for Mrs. Young to comprehend hospital routine.
    b._____essential that unanticipated experiences be minimized for her at this time.
    c._____important that she learn to appreciate what is to be done for her.
    d._____necessary that she comply with all hospital regulations.

10. The pattern of Mrs. Young straightening her dresser drawers so frequently is an example of

    a._____athetoid movements.
    b._____compulsive acts.

    c._____"normal" hehavior.
    d._____obsessive tendencies.

Questions for Discussion and Student Projects

1. Mrs. Young apparently has many dependent longings. Why, then, was she able to assume so much responsibility as a child in caring for the house?
2. Outline the characteristics of each phase of psychosexual development. Compare these with the characteristics of Mrs. Young's development. In phases in which Mrs. Young's psychosexual development is not described, hypothesize as to what you think happened to her during that period.
3. During Mrs. Young's childhood, a physician told her that she would probably outgrow her headaches. How do you think doctors and nurses should handle such a problem today? Support your statements.
4. What are some of the probable reasons why, as a child, Mrs. Young seemed older than she really was?
5. What situations during Mrs. Young's childhood might have contributed to her feelings of rejection?
6. What could the nurse do to decrease the time Mrs. Young takes to carry out her routine personal hygiene?
7. When Mrs. Young has feelings that she might hurt someone, do you think she really would? Why?
8. Assume that you are planning a party for a group of patients which includes Mrs. Young. How might you bring Mrs. Young into the plans so that the experience would be of therapeutic value? Support your decisions.
9. What incidents in Mrs. Young's pattern of everyday living are probably a reflection of her repressed hostility? What would be the nurse's rôle in relation to these aspects of her behavior?
10. What would you anticipate as being characteristic of Mrs. Young's pattern of interpersonal relations? What needs does this pattern reflect? How might the nurse provide care which fulfills these needs?
11. What would you hypothesize about Mrs. Young's true feelings about her mother? What experiences in her childhood were significant in influencing these feelings?

Questions Relating to the Section in General

1. The estimated percentage of the untreated individuals with psychoneuroses who are thought to recover spontaneously through healthy interpersonal experiences is

    a._____5 per cent.
    b._____10 per cent.
    c._____15 per cent.
    d._____20 per cent.

2. Factors which are important in determining an individual's response to frustration are

    a._____availability of substitutes.
    b._____personality structure.
    c._____strength of the drive.
    d._____strength of the barrier.

3. Anxiety may be described as

    a._____anticipation of danger.
    b._____a feeling of helplessness.
    c._____increased muscular tension.
    d._____related to specific objects.

4. Characteristics which are typical of the individual with a psycho-neurosis are that he

    a._____displays marked anxiety.
    b._____expresses impulses directly.
    c._____rigidly controls social behavior.
    d._____seeks dependent relationships.

5. The individual who feels that he can be successful only through a favorable stroke of luck is most apt to reveal a predominant trend in his interpersonal relations of

    a._____dependence.
    b._____detachment.
    c._____domination.
    d._____mistrust.

6. The immediate reactions which might be anticipated if an individual was prevented from performing an intense compulsion are

    a._____agitation.
    b._____apprehension.
    c._____calmness.
    d._____resignation.

7. The areas in which obsessions may be manifested are the

    a._____affective.
    b._____ideational.
    c._____motor.
    d._____sensory.

8. Tendencies which are characteristic of the individual with a de-pendent-submissive attitude in his interpersonal relations are that he

    a._____has a constant dread of loneliness.
    b._____has difficulty assuming responsibility.
    c._____has difficulty making independent decisions.
    d._____reveals the need for authoritative support in most situations.

9. The pattern of reaction formation is most typical in symptom neuroses of

    a._____anxiety states.
    b._____conversion hysteria.

    c._____neurasthenia.
    d._____obsessive-compulsive state.

10. Behavior patterns which are characteristic of the individual with an obsessive compulsive reaction are

    a._____lack of anxiety.
    b._____marked indecision.
    c._____repetitious behavior.
    d._____social withdrawal.

11. The term which best describes an individual's behavior when he has a conflict is

    a._____adaptive.
    b._____hesitant.
    c._____tense.
    d._____vacillating.

12. According to Kalkman, the characteristics which are typical of the individual in an anxiety state are

    a._____a feeling of impending doom.
    b._____inability to relax.
    c._____restlessness.
    d._____somatic complaints.

13. The methods which are acceptable as a means of studying personality are

    a._____controlled laboratory situations.
    b._____objective observations.
    c._____pain-stimulus experiments.
    d._____word-association tests.

14. Patterns which are general methods of coping with frustration are

    a._____abandoning the goal.
    b._____accepting a substitute goal.
    c._____getting around the barrier.
    d._____removing the barrier.

15. The characteristics which you would expect in a girl during the oedipal phase of development are

    a._____curiosity about sex differences.
    b._____identification with her mother.
    c._____intense admiration of both parents.
    d._____interest in "gangs" with girls her age.

16. The age at which frustration would be the most detrimental to the child is

    a._____1 month.
    b._____6 months.

    c._____12 months.
    d._____18 months.

17. Of the following periods, in the Freudian concept of personality development, the age span including 4 to 6 years is known as

    a._____anal.
    b._____latent.
    c._____oedipal.
    d._____oral.

18. The term which best describes the nurse's action if she could recognize and identify feelings and emotions of another person without ever having personally experienced these feelings and emotions is

    a._____empathy.
    b._____identification.
    c._____projection.
    d._____sympathy.

19. Miss Albert is very neat, meticulous, stingy and unresponsive. The age when one would hypothesize that she had probably been overly frustrated is

    a._____birth to 1 year.   c._____2 to 3 years.
    b._____1 to 2 years.   d._____4 to 5 years.

20. Suggestibility is most characteristic of the individual with

    a._____anxiety state.   c._____conversion hysteria.
    b._____anxiety hysteria.   d._____obsessive-compulsion state.

21. The pattern which is most characteristic of the individual with a traumatic neurosis is

    a._____dizziness.   c._____nightmares.
    b._____irritability.   d._____paralysis.

22. A 24-year-old woman is extremely punctual, scrupulously neat and clean and strongly disapproving of those who do not possess these qualities. She is also stingy with both money and affection. The childhood background would be expected to reveal that she

    a._____received little real affection.
    b._____received parental interest on the basis of strict obedience.
    c._____was subjected to strong disciplinary measures.
    d._____was toilet trained very early.

23. When Jack discovered he could not make the highest grades in his class, he concentrated on becoming the best at basketball. This is an example of

    a._____compensation.   c._____displacement.
    b._____conversion.   d._____idealization.

24. The term which best describes an individual who makes an emotional response to an organic illness is

    a.____neurotic reaction.   c.____psychosomatic reaction.
    b.____organic reaction.   d.____psychotic reaction.

25. The factors which are apt to motivate the individual who has a tendency to dominate in his interpersonal relations are

    a.____fear of being deprived.   c.____fear of being rejected.
    b.____fear of being dominated.   d.____feelings of self doubt.

26. In contrast to the behavior of the "mature" individual, the behavior of the neurotic individual is more

    a.____compulsive.   c.____intense.
    b.____exaggerated.   d.____rational.

27. *Directions:*
    Place the number of the definition (from the right-hand column) which most accurately defines the pattern of behavior in the left-hand column in the space to the left of the word to be defined.

    Definitions   *Patterns of Adjustment*

    a.__4__identification.   (1) the satisfaction of desires in day
    b.____insulation.   dreaming.
    c.____fixation.   (2) a return to patterns of behavior
    d.__1__phantasy.   which were useful earlier.
    e.__9__projection.   (3) camouflage of motives unacceptable
    f.__3__rationalization.   to one's self.
    g.__5__reaction formation.   (4) experiencing the same feelings and
    h.__2__regression.   actions of another person simul-
    i.__8__repression.   taneously.
    j.__7__sublimation.   (5) development of overt behavior the
    k.__6__none of these.   direct opposite of unconscious de-
                                        sires.
                                    (6) development of logic-tight compart-
                                        ments.
                                    (7) redirection of desires from socially
                                        unobtainable goals into acceptable
                                        activities.
                                    (8) subconscious "forgetting."
                                    (9) transfer of unacceptable actions or
                                        attributes to others.

Questions for Discussion and Student Projects—(*Continued*)

1. Differentiate between a neurosis and a psychosis.
2. Describe Freud's concept of the reality principle.
3. What are the main characteristics and functions of the id, the ego and the super ego?
4. Differentiate between the following phases in child development: oral, anal, oedipal, latent.

5. What implications does Gesell's theory of progression-regression have for the understanding of psychiatric patients?
6. How does the convulsive seizure differ in a patient with conversion hysteria from that in a patient with epilepsy?
7. What is the estimated percentage of patients in the general hospital with serious psychiatric disorders? How does this figure compare with the number of beds for psychiatric patients?
8. How many nurses are employed in caring for psychiatric patients? What is the estimated number needed? What provisions are made in the National Health Act to help remedy this situation?
9. How does the number of psychiatrists compare with the number of physicians who specialize in other fields?
10. Describe the development of the mental hygiene movement in the United States.

Section 2. Nursing Care of Patients with Cerebral Incompetence

THE YEARS AFTER FORTY—PATIENT STUDY

Mr. Greene, a 50-year-old school teacher, was admitted to the hospital 3 months ago. Mr. Greene is now on the geriatric unit in a State Hospital and has a partial paralysis of his right arm. Upon admission he complained of dizziness, headache and fatigue and stated that something had happened to his memory. There was a slight slurring of speech and he cried frequently. His wife stated that he had apparently been in good health until one morning recently he complained of a severe headache. At school he slumped in his chair and was exceedingly weak. He was first taken to a general local hospital but was transferred to the State Hospital after he attempted to jump out the window. His comment at that time was that he was trying to get away from the snakes that were all over his bed and on the floor of his room.

Since his admission to the State Hospital, his speech has cleared up and there has been no recent evidence of hallucinations. His dizziness and headaches have disappeared, but in addition to not being able to use his right arm, he shuffles his feet when he walks and occasionally pitches forward. On some days he cries for long periods of time, is irritable and states that his mind is gone. At other times he is a pleasant person and has a fairly good memory for both recent and remote events.

Mr. Greene is a Catholic; he taught history in the local high school. He has a bachelor's degree from the State Teachers College and was well thought of by his colleagues, his students and their parents.

References

Burton, Arthur, and Harris, Robert E., Editors: Case Histories in Clinical and Abnormal Psychology, pp. 346–380, New York, Harpers, 1947.

Cameron, Norman: The Psychology of Behavior Disorders, pp. 141–186, 338–426, 540–575, Boston, Houghton Mifflin, 1947.

Ingram, Madeline: Principles of Psychiatric Nursing, pp. 281–304, Philadelphia, Saunders, 1949.

Kalkman, Marion E.: Introduction to Psychiatric Nursing, pp. 125–166, New York, McGraw-Hill, 1950.

Muller, Theresa: The Nature and Direction of Psychiatric Nursing, pp. 138–153, 212–226, Philadelphia, Lippincott, 1950.

Orgel, Samuel: Psychiatry Today and Tomorrow, pp. 81–142, 177–194, New York, International Universities Press, 1946.

Mental Hygiene in Old Age, Family Welfare Association of America, 1937. (Pamphlet.)

Questions Relating to the Patient Study

1. The physician probably would diagnose Mr. Greene's condition as

    a._____cerebral arteriosclerosis.
    b._____involutional melancholia.
    c._____manic-depressive, depressed phase.
    d._____senile psychosis.

2. Providing that Mr. Greene has no further complications, the nurse would anticipate that his illness would be characterized by

    a._____increased paralysis of muscles.
    b._____an increased number of headaches.
    c._____short periods of remission.
    d._____decreased use of his right arm.

3. The factors which are most influential in determining the degree of personality change in Mr. Greene are the

    a._____current family relationships.
    b._____degree of economic independence.
    c._____rapidity of degenerative changes.
    d._____strength of personality integration.

4. The primary aim of the nursing care plan for Mr. Greene should be to

    a._____encourage a minimum level of performance.
    b._____encourage an optimum level of performance.
    c._____enforce a strict habit-training program.
    d._____keep him as quiet as possible.

5. The diversional activity which would be most suitable for Mr. Greene is

    a._____playing pingpong.
    b._____reading historical documents.
    c._____singing old-time songs with others.
    d._____watching television.

6. The typical onset for an individual with Mr. Greene's illness is between the ages of

    a._____40 and 50.   b._____50 and 60.   c._____60 and 70.
    d._____70 and 80.

7. In regard to Mr. Greene's total behavior, the most important aspect that the nurse should observe in order to carry out an optimum nursing care plan is

    a._____food and fluid intake.   c._____periods of accessibility.
    b._____degree of emotional labil-   d._____bowel and bladder control.
    ity.

8. The nurse caring for Mr. Greene in the general hospital should arrange his room so that it would have

a.＿＿dim lighting during the   c.＿＿good lighting during the
    night.   night.
b.＿＿good lighting during the   d.＿＿subdued lighting during
    day.   the day.

9. The symptom typical of Mr. Greene's illness is

    a.＿＿emotional lability.   c.＿＿paranoid tendencies.
    b.＿＿ideas of reference.   d.＿＿sadistic tendencies.

10. When Mr. Greene becomes restless at night and cannot sleep, the
    nurse should first

    a.＿＿ask the doctor to order a sedative.
    b.＿＿give him a wet sheet pack.
    c.＿＿give him warm milk.
    d.＿＿let him sleep more during the day.

11. Mr. Greene wanders up and down the hall; on several occasions he
    came to the nurse's station and began examining the contents of the
    waste basket for a letter which he accused the nurse of discarding.
    The nurse should

    a.＿＿ask the attendant to insist that he remain in the day room.
    b.＿＿restrain him in a chair.
    c.＿＿tell him to go back to the day room.
    d.＿＿suggest that she help him write another letter.

Questions for Discussion and Student Projects

1. Outline a plan for the nurse

    a. when Mr. Greene's wife visits him.
    b. when Mr. Greene is discharged.

2. What occupational therapy activities would be suitable for Mr. Greene?
3. What complications would the nurse anticipate when caring for Mr.
   Greene? What are the symptoms of the complications?
4. Would Mr. Greene be likely to be given electroshock therapy? Why?
5. Why do patients like Mr. Greene sometimes injure themselves when
   they have hallucinations?
6. Why would nurses who resent authority be apt to dislike caring for
   Mr. Greene?
7. Why is Mr. Greene's performance likely to vary from time to time?
8. What foods should be included in Mr. Greene's diet? Why?
9. Will Mr. Greene be likely to conform to hospital routines? Support
   your decision.

Questions Relating to the Section in General

1. The increase in the older population is the result of

    a.＿＿increased birth rate.   c.＿＿control of communicable dis-
    b.＿＿curtailed immigration.   eases.
                                        d.＿＿higher living standards.

2. The increasing number of aged in the United States may result in

   a._____conservative government budgets.
   b._____diminished demands for luxuries.
   c._____fewer changes in laws.
   d._____liberal political policies.

3. The ratio of elderly people in State hospitals is

   a._____decreasing steadily.   c._____increasing in isolated instances.
   b._____increasing steadily.   d._____remaining about the same.

4. In generations to come the characteristic which will be most probable in regard to population trends is a

   a._____decreased number of women of all age groups.
   b._____decreased number of elderly women.
   c._____surplus number of elderly women.
   d._____surplus number of men of all age groups.

5. The population trend which is expected to occur by 1990 is that 1 person in

   a._____8 will be 65 or older.
   b._____18 will be 65 or older.
   c._____28 will be 65 or older.
   d._____38 will be 65 or older.

6. Simple deterioration is characterized by

   a._____increased impressionability. c._____nocturnal restlessness.
   b._____progressive memory defect.   d._____increased irritability.

7. The major health hazards in older people are characterized by

   a._____multiple causation.   c._____prominent symptoms.
   b._____progressive course.   d._____sudden onset.

8. The most appropriate action of the nurse in caring for the senile individual is to

   a._____encourage him to do as much as possible for himself.
   b._____encourage activities that require fine detailed movement.
   c._____terminate activities before he becomes fatigued.
   d._____vary his daily routine of activities frequently.

9. Confabulation refers to

   a._____circumstantiality in regard to recent events.
   b._____fabrications invented to fill memory gaps.
   c._____facts in regard to remote events.
   d._____none of the above.

10. When young nurses give specific directions to elderly patients they are apt to respond

   a._____co-operatively.   c._____resentfully.
   b._____pleasantly.   d._____none of the above.

11. In old age, most commonly memory

    a._____for recent events is lost first.
    b._____for remote events is lost first.
    c._____loss for both recent and remote events occur simultaneously.
    d._____is not usually impaired.

12. Structural changes which occur in old age are

    a._____dry thick skin.   c._____increased body weight.
    b._____hypertrophied heart.   d._____thickened arterial walls.

13. An hallucination is a disorder of

    a._____affectivity.   c._____orientation.
    b._____memory.   d._____perception.

14. The symptom which would be classified as a disorder in progression of thought is

    a._____circumstantiality.   c._____ideas of reference.
    b._____flight of ideas.   d._____perseveration.

15. The term which is classified as a disorder of thinking is

    a._____delusion.   c._____hallucination.
    b._____dementia.   d._____illusion.

16. The terms which are classified as disorders of thought are

    a._____delusion.   c._____idea of reference.
    b._____hallucination.   d._____obsession.

17. The term which is not a disorder of the content of thought is

    a._____delusion.   c._____idea of reference.
    b._____flight of ideas.   d._____obsession.

18. The term which would describe the experience of an individual who thought he heard a machine gun while his neighbor was mowing the lawn is

    a._____delusion.   c._____identification.
    b._____hallucination.   d._____illusion.

19. An illusion is a disorder of

    a._____affect.   c._____perception.
    b._____consciousness.   d._____thinking.

20. Of the following disturbances of consciousness, the patient is completely inaccessible in

    a._____confusion.   c._____stupor.
    b._____clouding of the sensorium.   d._____coma.

21. The term which would best describe the experience of an individual who complained of a lack of sensation is

    a._____depersonalization.   c._____isolation.
    b._____displacement.   d._____rationalization.

22. The phrase which defines a hallucination is

    a._____an idea, contrary to fact, that cannot be changed by reasoning.
    b._____a loss of memory pertaining to time, place and person.
    c._____a sensory perception without an external stimulus.
    d._____a state of bewilderment, embarrassment and perplexity.

23. The term which would describe the experience of an individual who "recognized" his dead child's voice in the clatter of the lawn mower is

    a._____delusion.   c._____identification.
    b._____hallucination.   d._____illusion.

Questions for Discussion and Student Projects—(*Continued*)

1. Differentiate between the symptoms of senile psychosis and cerebral arteriosclerosis.
2. In our culture, why do elderly men have more difficulty in adjusting to life situations than elderly women?
3. How does our culture compare with others in the treatment of the aged individual?
4. What are some of our cultural lags in the treatment of the aged?
5. In what conditions other than those discussed will cerebral incompetence be found?

Section 3. Nursing Care of Autistic and Suspicious People

"WHY DON'T PEOPLE LIKE ME?"—PATIENT STUDY

Mr. Ryan, admitted to the hospital 2 weeks ago, is a 24-year-old bank clerk who left college after the second year. He often speaks of "not having enough schooling" and of "feeling different on the ward because others there seemed more educated." Mr. Ryan lives with his family who say that he has always been a "most obedient child who never required harsh discipline." Nevertheless, he was also described as being stubborn, moody, sulky, brooding and very sensitive as a child. He had never displayed much initiative except in keeping his toys very neatly arranged and would then have a temper tantrum if anyone accidentally disarranged them. He usually played with other children but would often say "they didn't want me to play." Many times he would come home from school and tell about a new toy or gadget that some other boy had, and how much better it was than any he had. He had not enjoyed the usual roughhouse activities of boys but preferred to keep his clothes clean and to associate more with adults. This his mother had seemed to encourage as she related this information very proudly.

During the few months previous to admission, he had become progressively more irritable and "imagined things like people following him." He had become critical of his mother, "picked on her all the time," continually finding fault with everything she did and then becoming very angry, swearing, and occasionally breaking a piece of furniture during these periods.

On the ward he has been heard to comment, "I can take orders O.K. but I don't like being pushed around." He usually sits and watches the other patients in their activities and often tells them what they should have done in certain instances. He has played ping-pong a couple of times with the nurse and always strikes the ball so hard that it goes out of bounds. Even when participating in some activity his attention is frequently distracted from what he is doing as he looks about the room taking in the telephone, the doorways, the nurse, the radio and the movements of the other patients.

Yesterday when he was playing "Rummy" with the nurse he recounted the cards repeatedly before dealing them. During the game he suddenly said, "What's going on around here, anyway?" Then as the doctors walked by the room he said in an undertone, "They're looking at me like I'm a gambler." His intake of nourishment is adequate although he spends much time looking over his tray each time before eating and throughout the meal continually makes derogatory remarks about the food.

446

References

Biddle, W. E.: The Nurse and "spontaneous" recovery in schizophrenia, Am. J. Nursing 49:371, 1949.

Clawson, G.: Nursing care of psychiatric patients receiving insulin therapy, Am. J. Nursing 49:621, 1949.

Kalinowsky, Lothar B., and Hoch, Paul: Shock Treatment, 16–23, 40–55, 92–101, 228, New York, Grune and Stratton, 1950.

Kalkman, Marion: Introduction to Psychiatric Nursing, pp. 129–131, 279–285, 293–296, New York, McGraw-Hill, 1950.

Matheny, R., and Tepolis, M.: Nursing care for the acutely ill psychotic patient, Am. J. Nursing 50:27, 1950.

Render, Helena Willis: Nurse Patient Relationships in Psychiatry, pp. 140–153, New York, McGraw-Hill, 1947.

Renee (Pseud): Autobiography of a Schizophrenic Girl, New York, Grune and Stratton, 1951.

Thorner, Melvin W.: Psychiatry in General Practice, pp. 250–290, Philadelphia, Saunders, 1949.

Questions Relating to the Patient Study

1. In general, Mr. Ryan's prognosis is probably not so good as that of patients with

   a.____catatonic schizophrenia.   c.____simple schizophrenia.
   b.____schizo-affective disorder. d.____all of the above.

2. In hypothesizing about Mr. Ryan's early behavior, of the following periods of development the nurse would anticipate that he experienced the most trauma or deprivation during the

   a.____anal period.   c.____oedipal period.
   b.____latent period. d.____oral period.

3. Mr. Ryan's super ego can best be described as being

   a.____absent.   c.____weak.
   b.____intense. d.____none of these.

4. The activity which the nurse should encourage Mr. Ryan to pursue in his present state is

   a.____assisting the occupational therapist put away the tools.
   b.____playing with the punching bag.
   c.____watching mystery stories on television.
   d.____wrestling with other male patients.

5. Therapeutically, the nurse can help Mr. Ryan most by serving as support for his

   a.____ego. c.____super ego.
   b.____id.   d.____none of the above.

6. In dealing with Mr. Ryan's general behavior the principle(s) which would be most helpful to the nurse in understanding him is (are)

a.____behavior is purposeful.   c.____behavior has a cause.
b.____behavior evolves from needs.   d.____all of the above.

7. When Mr. Ryan bats the pingpong ball out of bounds, he is most likely expressing his

a.____disinterest in the game.   c.____hostility toward others.
b.____feelings of depression.   d.____inability to play the game.

8. The symptom which is most characteristic of Mr. Ryan's behavior is

a.____depressive tendencies.   c.____masochistic traits.
b.____grandiose ideas.   d.____paranoid ideas.

9. Mr. Ryan's illness is most typical of

a.____involutional melancholia with paranoid tendencies.
b.____catatonic schizophrenia.
c.____paranoia.
d.____paranoid schizophrenia.

10. A nurse was supervising a group of patients on the sun porch while they were listening to a radio program. Suddenly Mr. Ryan jumped up, began pounding on the window pane, and shouted, "I have to get out of here, my children are on fire."
Of the following emergency responses the nurse should

a.____try to divert Mr. Ryan's attention by talking to him.
b.____instruct a reliable patient to seek other personnel for additional help.
c.____make a physical approach from behind by grasping Mr. Ryan's wrists.
d.____call loudly for the assistance of other members of the personnel.

Questions for Discussion and Student Projects

1. What are some of the factors which probably increase Mr. Ryan's feeling of insecurity? How can the nurse help him feel more secure?
2. Describe how the nurse should respond to Mr. Ryan in the following situations:

a.____Mr. Ryan criticizes her while she is attempting to carry out a nursing procedure for another patient.
b.____Mr. Ryan asks, "What's going on around here, anyway?"
c.____Mr. Ryan repeatedly refuses to drink fluid of any type.
d.____Mr. Ryan becomes sarcastic with other patients.

3. Why might Mr. Ryan become hesitant to carry out even little requests made by the nurses?
4. What changes in Mr. Ryan's behavior should make the nurse most alert? Why?
5. What factors in Mr. Ryan's childhood may have contributed to his present illness?

6. Hypothesize in regard to the type of person you think Mr. Ryan's mother was.
7. What additional information should the nurse collect by the technics of observation in order to make a more complete nursing care plan for Mr. Ryan?
8. Contrast the behavior of Mr. Ryan with that of a patient diagnosed as catatonic schizophrenia.
9. If Mr. Ryan receives deep insulin therapy, describe the type of relationship the nurse will try to develop just prior to his going into coma and immediately after awakening from coma.
10. If Mr. Ryan becomes drowsy in the afternoon after he has received an insulin treatment, describe the nurse's immediate action.

"JUST LEAVE ME ALONE"—PATIENT STUDY

This is Miss Lillianthal's second admission to the hospital. She is 25 years old and for the past few months has been working as a record clerk in a nearby metropolitan area. She is the youngest child and the only girl in a family of 6 children. During her early school years she was described as a lovable child who was well liked—rather shy, and seeming to become frightened any time there was any dissention. Her mother described her as a "strong-willed" child who required very strict discipline to get her to conform and proudly said, "Sometimes I had to spank her a dozen times a day but it finally made an impression." As a child she frequently ran away from home saying that she was going to find her father whose work kept him away from home most of the time. She seldom played with the girls in the neighborhood but would tag after her brothers, who constantly ridiculed her about being a "tomboy."

Miss Lillianthal was a brilliant student in school and she began to spend more and more of her time browsing in books.

She got her first job when 21 years old, and one evening when the family was away moved all of her belongings into a rooming house on the other side of town. Her mother would call her a dozen times a day and ask her to come back home. The mother could not understand it because Miss Lillianthal had never had to take any responsibility.

Since entering the hospital Miss Lillianthal's behavior has been very inconsistent. At meal time she would sometimes sit alone and nibble at her food. She'd eat for a few minutes and then stop and stare straight ahead. At other times, she would devour her food very rapidly, eating everything that was placed before her and even snatching food from the trays of other patients. She would frequently stare at her hands and say, "I'm floating; my body is turning to liquid." She would frequently become very restless, then be found lying on the floor mute and uncommunicative and remain this way for periods ranging for from 30 minutes to 10 hours. She was usually very slow about getting dressed and would stand before her open closet for a half hour or longer before actually getting started. She tended to wear the same outfit of clothing day after day and her hair was usually hanging uncombed about her shoulders. At times she would let the nurse do things for her and at other times she

would insist on doing them by herself. When around other patients she
would usually be found in the corner, or, if the corners were occupied,
she would be in the center of the room staring off into space.

Questions Relating to the Patient Study

1. The nurse can best elicit Miss Lillianthal's participation in activities
   by
   a._____encouraging her to associate with patients with hypomanic behavior.
   b._____encouraging her to read in the day room.
   c._____participating in a quiet simple game alone with the nurse.
   d._____placing her in the center of activities and insisting that she
   participate.

2. In childhood, of the following phases, Miss Lillianthal probably had
   the most difficulty in the

   a._____anal.
   b._____oedipal.
   c._____oral.
   d._____phallic.

3. The primary obstacle in Miss Lillianthal's psychotherapy probably
   would be her

   a._____auditory hallucinations.
   b._____inability to relate to others.
   c._____lack of emotional expression.
   d._____refusal to tell her thoughts.

4. When Miss Lillianthal is staring into space and has not yet dressed
   for the day, the nurse should secure her participation in dressing by
   commenting

   a._____get your clothes out and dress carefully today.
   b._____here are your clothes, now put them on.
   c._____hurry up or you'll be late for breakfast.
   d._____raise up your right foot; now put on your stocking.

5. The goals which would be helpful for Miss Lillianthal in occupational
   therapy activities are to

   a._____develop interest and confidence.
   b._____help externalize emotional reactions.
   c._____offer opportunity for introspection.
   d._____promote contact with reality.

6. Miss Lillianthal's staring into space is an example of

   a._____artistic temperament.
   b._____autistic behavior.

c._____depressive traits.

d._____suspicious tendencies.

7. Miss Lillianthal's comment, "I'm floating, my body is turning to a liquid," is an example of

a._____depersonalization.   c._____rationalization.

b._____projection.   d._____repression.

8. The activities which would be most likely to direct Miss Lillianthal toward reality are

a._____listening to Brahms' Lullaby.

b._____playing a game of checkers.

c._____reading *Paradise Lost.*

d._____walking with the group.

9. The type of relationship which the nurse should promote in her contacts with Miss Lillianthal is

a._____parasitic.   c._____supportive.

b._____submissive.   d._____symbiotic.

10. The measure which the nurse should employ when Miss Lillianthal refuses to eat is to

a._____attempt to discover her reasons for not eating.

b._____discontinue all nourishment between meals.

c._____discontinue all privileges until eating is established.

d._____tell her that if she does not eat she will be tube fed.

11. The objectives which the nurse should make for her first contact with Miss Lillianthal at the time of admission are

a._____to assure Miss Lillianthal of her respect for the patient's individuality.

b._____to facilitate her adjustment by explaining all possible treatment in detail.

c._____to inspire confidence by personal interest.

d._____to seek all the available information from her regarding the past.

12. Actions which would hinder the establishment of rapport with Miss Lillianthal are

a._____attacking an incorrect point of view.

b._____establishing intimate friendship.

c._____orienting the new patient thoroughly to electrotherapy.

d._____stimulating ideas of reference.

13. Miss Lillianthal's illness is most typical of

a._____catatonic schizophrenia.

b._____conversion hysteria.

c._____manic-depressive, depressed phase.

d._____simple schizophrenia.

Questions for Discussion and Student Projects

1. What might the school nurse have done to assist Miss Lillianthal's teacher and mother in regard to Miss Lillianthal's tendency to spend too much time on her books?
2. Why do you think Miss Lillianthal moved to a rooming house on the other side of town when she could have probably saved money by living at home?
3. How do you think Miss Lillianthal's mother should have treated her when she returned from running away from home during childhood?
4. Outline the situations in Miss Lillianthal's childhood that were early symptoms of her illness.
5. Assume that Miss Lillianthal is from your own community. If her symptoms had been noted during her childhood, what agencies would be available to assist with her problems?
6. Why might Miss Lillianthal have been hunting for her father when she ran away from home in her childhood?
7. What could the nurse do to assist Miss Lillianthal in a plan for improving her personal appearance?
8. What might the nurse do when Miss Lillianthal insists on lying on the floor? How might the nurse get Miss Lillianthal to become more communicative?
9. Why is it important that the nurse be very careful about what she says while caring for Miss Lillianthal when she is staring into space and is very uncommunicative?

Questions Relating to the Section in General

1. The spontaneous recovery rate for individuals with schizophrenic reactions is

   a.＿＿＿11 per cent. b.＿＿＿22 per cent. c.＿＿＿33 per cent. d.＿＿＿44 per cent.

2. The diagnosis of schizophrenia is most common in the age group of

   a.＿＿＿10 to 25 years.   c.＿＿＿20 to 35 years.
   b.＿＿＿15 to 30 years.   d.＿＿＿25 to 40 years.

3. The symptoms which characterize a schizophrenic reaction are

   a.＿＿＿bizarre thinking.   c.＿＿＿repressed emotion.
   b.＿＿＿rejection of reality.   d.＿＿＿rigid behavior.

4. Muscular tension is the most obvious characteristic in which type of schizophrenic reaction?

   a.＿＿＿catatonic. b.＿＿＿hebephrenic. c.＿＿＿paranoid. d.＿＿＿simple.

5. The characteristics which portray the schizoid personality are

   a.＿＿＿abstract thinking.   c.＿＿＿psychosexual maturity.
   b.＿＿＿emotional restraint.   d.＿＿＿weak conscience.

6. The symptoms which characterize paranoia in its classical form are

a._____bizarre hallucinations.   c._____persecutory ideas.
b._____inappropriate affect.   d._____systematized delusions.

7. The one type of schizophrenia in which the nurse would most likely encounter the symptom of suspicion is

   a._____catatonic. b._____hebephrenic. c._____paranoid. d._____simple.

8. The individual who would be most apt to reveal a predominantly hostile attitude toward the social community is the one with

   a._____involutional melancholia.   c._____schizophrenia, catatonic.
   b._____manic-depressive, manic.   d._____schizophrenia, paranoid.

9. The factors which are thought to be significant in the etiology of schizophrenic reactions are

   a._____constitutional.   c._____hereditary.
   b._____economic.   d._____racial.

10. When we speak of aggression from the psychiatric viewpoint, we refer to

    a._____controlling other persons.   c._____hostility aimed at injury.
    b._____gaining possession of ob-   d._____initiative in leadership.
    jects.

11. Paranoia usually does not become apparent before the age of

    a._____20 years. b._____30 years. c._____40 years. d._____50 years.

12. The most significant symptom(s) of secondary shock in insulin therapy is (are)

    a._____anorexia.   c._____diaphoresis.
    b._____apprehensiveness.   d._____edema.

13. Emergency ampules which should be immediately available during insulin shock therapy are those containing

    a._____adrenalin.   d._____digitalis.
    b._____Coramine.   e._____glucose.
    c._____dichloramine.   f._____saline.

14. A common complication of insulin shock therapy is

    a._____cardiac failure.   c._____fracture of long bones.
    b._____essential hypertension.   d._____dislocation of vertebrae.

15. In order to give U50 of insulin from a bottle labeled U80, the nurse should withdraw

    a._____8 minims.   c._____12 minims.
    b._____10 minims.   d._____14 minims.

16. During insulin therapy symptoms which would indicate that the patient may be approaching a peripheral vascular collapse are

    a._____cessation of perspiration.   c._____increased pulse rate.
    b._____decreased pulse volume.   d._____a steady drop in blood
    pressure.

17. The behavior disorder which usually responds best to deep insulin coma is

    a._____involutional melancholia.
    b._____manic-depressive, depressed.
    c._____manic-depressive, manic.
    d._____paranoid schizophrenia.

18. The symptom which produces the most immediate reason for action by the nurse during insulin shock therapy is

    a._____absence of the Babinski reflex.
    b._____diminished corneal reflex.
    c._____inability to respond to name.
    d._____the presence of dry hot skin.   •

19. In order to prevent the complication of pneumonia during insulin shock therapy, the nurse should

    a._____avoid changing the patient's position during coma.
    b._____change the patient's position every 10 minutes during coma.
    c._____keep the patient on his back with his face turned toward the nurse.
    d._____turn the patient on his side with his head turned to one side.

20. The first man to use insulin shock therapy in the treatment of psychiatric disorders was

    a._____Freud.   b._____Meduna.   c._____Rush.   d._____Sakel.

21. The reactions which would be evident in an "ideal" sub-coma state during insulin therapy are

    a._____chorea-athetoid movements.   c._____fine tremor.
    b._____drowsiness.   d._____increased sensitivity.

22. Occupational therapy is an important measure in the treatment of the psychiatric patient because it

    a._____offers the "poor" patient an opportunity to pay for part of his care.
    b._____provides a modified normal atmosphere in which the patient may spend part of his time.
    c._____offers a means wherein the individual may achieve a feeling of self-accomplishment.
    d._____facilitates the individual in developing insight of his intrapersonal problems.

23. The activity which is most suitable for the destructive patient is

    a._____crocheting rugs from strips of cloth.
    b._____hammering copper ash trays.
    c._____tearing carpet rags into strips.
    d._____weaving rugs on a hand loom.

24. The factors which the nurse should consider in planning occupational therapy activities for an individual are the

    a._____economic value to the hospital.
    b._____material available for use.
    c._____predominant behavior of the patient.
    d._____ultimate goal to be achieved.

25. A nurse should take precautions when supervising an **extremely** paranoid patient during occupational therapy by

    a._____minimizing the amount of equipment that may be used as weapons by the patient.
    b._____making it clear to the patient that his threats will forfeit his privileges.
    c._____permitting the patient to browse about the room until he chooses a project.
    d._____securing the patient's promise that he will control his aggression toward others.

26. Supplies which are necessary for tooling in leather craft are

    a._____a plate glass surface.   d._____a soft wood surface.
    b._____tap water.   e._____blunt scissors.
    c._____a small chisel.

Questions for Discussion and Student Projects—*(Continued)*

1. Differentiate between the overt symptoms of a patient with paranoia and one with paranoid schizophrenia.
2. Give a brief description of the following types of therapy:

    a. bibliotherapy.   e. deep sleep therapy.
    b. industrial therapy.   f. psychoanalysis.
    c. hypnotherapy.   g. group therapy.
    d. music therapy.

3. Differentiate between the purposes of recreational and of occupational therapy.
4. In what conditions other than schizophrenia might the nurse anticipate finding the overt symptoms of the autistic and suspicious patients?
5. Describe the type of environment the nurse should maintain in a room where patients are receiving insulin therapy.
6. What observations are important for the nurse to make on patients receiving insulin therapy? Why?
7. List 3 measures that the nurse should follow when using hazardous articles in any activity.
8. List 5 factors that the nurse should consider in regard to the patient when encouraging him to select activities.

Section 4. Nursing Care of Depressed and Elated People

"IT'S ALL MY FAULT"—PATIENT STUDY

Mrs. Appel, a 27-year-old Jewish woman, was admitted to the psychiatric unit of the hospital last night as an emergency, after a suicidal attempt. Her husband, the informant, stated that when he returned early from a banquet (the sixth he had attended in 2 weeks), he found Mrs. Appel with her wrists slashed, lying on the floor in the bathroom. He was unable to arouse her.

Mr. Appel is a business executive for a manufacturing concern in a large metropolitan area. They have 2 children, a boy 5 years of age and a girl 3 years of age, and they live in an attractive ranch house in the suburbs. Mrs. Appel, a high school graduate, frequently has thought of continuing her study of music, which she gave up at the insistence of her father when her older brother entered law school. Mrs. Appel's associates all say that she has a good voice and friends request that she sing for them on various occasions. Her father believed that education was strictly for men and that the place for women was in the home.

The husband states that the patient has not been her "usual self" for the past 3 months. She first seemed to lose interest in her home, which has always been a great source of satisfaction to her, with her hobbies of interior decorating and gardening. She has gradually become more impatient with the children and lately has given little attention to her own personal appearance. In response to her husband's inquiries Mrs. Appel would say that she was just a little tired but would refuse to go to the doctor.

The afternoon before Mrs. Appel was hospitalized, the children with several of their friends were playing in and around the patio and at times evidently became quite noisy. In the midst of the furor Mrs. Appel had screamed at them to stop making so much noise. A 3-year-old neighbor boy started running toward home, tripped and fell on the cement, cutting a large gash in his forehead. When Mrs. Appel had run out of the house toward the boy he began screaming, "No, no, go away."

At present this patient is confined to bed. She was seen by the surgeons who sutured her wrists and gave her a blood transfusion. She responds in monosyllables when addressed, except to mention several times that she is responsible for injuring her neighbor's child. She takes fluids when they are offered, but has refused any solid food. This is Mrs. Appel's first hospitalization and the psychiatrist has diagnosed her illness as manic-depressive psychosis, depressed phase.

References

Ingram, Madelene: Principles of Psychiatric Nursing, pp. 187–213, Philadelphia, Saunders, 1949.

Kalkman, Marion E.: Introduction to Psychiatric Nursing, pp. 195–205, 207–220, 263–278, New York, McGraw-Hill, 1950.

Muller, Theresa: The Nature and Direction of Psychiatric Nursing, pp. 157–187, Philadelphia, Lippincott Company, 1950.

Orgel, Samuel Z.: Psychiatry Today and Tomorrow, pp. 249–277, New York, International Universities Press, 1946.

Render, Helena Willis: Nurse-Patient Relationships in Psychiatry, pp. 88–227, New York, McGraw-Hill, 1947.

Thorner, Melvin W.: Psychiatry in General Practice, pp. 148–178, Philadelphia, Saunders, 1949.

Questions Relating to the Patient Study

1. The approach which the nurse should make when taking Mrs. Appel's dinner tray to her is to say

   a._____"It is important that you eat—if you don't we'll have to tube feed you."
   b._____"Don't you want to eat your dinner?"
   c._____"Here is your tray, let me help you butter your bread."
   d._____"We will have to move you to another ward, if you don't eat your dinner."

2. Mrs. Appel should be observed carefully primarily because she may

   a._____develop a secondary infection.
   b._____attempt suicide again.
   c._____develop a reaction to the blood transfusion.
   d._____all of the above.

3. The response which the student nurse should make when Mrs. Appel mentions that she was responsible for the child's injury is to

   a._____listen but say and do nothing.
   b._____ask her, "Why do you think you are responsible?"
   c._____tell Mrs. Appel that she should try to develop more patience with children.
   d._____reflect the patient's feelings.

4. The doctor probably would regard Mrs. Appel's prognosis for the present attack of her illness as

   a._____good.   c._____fair.
   b._____poor.   d._____guarded.

5. The nurse should anticipate that Mrs. Appel's behavior in the future will be that she

   a._____will not have a recurrence of her illness.
   b._____may become elated at a later time.
   c._____will never have another depression once she gets over this one.
   d._____attacks will be more severe each time.

6. The characteristic which should not typify the therapeutic environment established for Mrs. Appel is

a._____democratic.   c._____inflexible.
b._____permissive.   d._____protective.

7. The nurse's therapeutic approach to Mrs. Appel should be based upon

a._____acceptive atmosphere.   c._____individual needs.
b._____genuine interest.   d._____a noncritical attitude.

8. In approaching Mrs. Appel, the best measures to follow in gaining her co-operation are to

a._____establish a close friendship.
b._____reveal your disapproval of her suicidal attempt.
c._____maintain a neutral attitude.
d._____avoid making promises to her.

9. The description which would not characterize an effective plan for Mrs. Appel's re-education is

a._____consistent.   c._____inflexible.
b._____individualized.   d._____practical.

10. Acceptance of Mrs. Appel as a person implies that we

a._____accept her expression of feeling.
b._____refrain from criticizing her action.
c._____respect her ideas and opinions.
d._____show approval of her total behavior.

11. The characteristic which would not be typical of an effective nurse-patient relationship established with Mrs. Appel are

a._____advice given unselfishly.
b._____controlled bond of affection.
c._____definite limits to her action.
d._____freedom from coercion.

12. In an attempt to change Mrs. Appel's concept of herself, the nurse can

a._____avoid showing disapproval of her behavior at any time.
b._____create situations in which she can gain some measure of success.
c._____show disapproval of her behavior when she doesn't eat.
d._____show respect for her as an individual at all times.

13. The motive which would be most helpful to the nurse in establishing an effective relationship with Mrs. Appel is a

a._____desire to follow the doctor's orders.
b._____need to have others dependent upon her.
c._____need to reassure herself of her own integrity.
d._____sincere interest in the individual.

14. Which of the following would not be a therapeutic advantage of hospitalization:

    a.＿＿＿providing an emotionally neutral environment.
    b.＿＿＿removing the patient from the stresses of home life.
    c.＿＿＿relieving the patient of responsibility.
    d.＿＿＿providing rigid schedules.

Questions for Discussion and Student Projects

1. What situational factors probably were significant in precipitating Mrs. Appel's illness?
2. What behavior patterns of Mrs. Appel are typically characteristic of the manic-depressive, depressed reactions?
3. How would you describe Mrs. Appel's usual pattern of relating to others?
4. What do you think are Mrs. Appel's true feelings about her husband? About her children?
5. Outline and describe a plan for Mrs. Appel's nursing care in accord with the following orders written by her physician:

    a. special observation.
    b. intake and output.
    c. high-caloric soft diet.
    d. force fluids.
    e. be acceptive and permissive.
    f. minimize activity.
    g. encourage verbal expression.
    h. offer a minimum of reassurance.

6. How would the nurse respond when Mrs. Appel insisted on doing everything for herself?
7. How would the nurse cope with Mrs. Appel's expression that she is responsible for injuring her neighbor's child?
8. What measures would the nurse find most helpful in encouraging a more adequate nutritional intake?
9. What cues in Mrs. Appel's behavior would alert the nurse that supportive reassurance was needed?

"LET US BE GAY!"—PATIENT STUDY

Mrs. Richard, a 24-year-old housewife, was admitted to an acute psychiatric unit 10 days ago. She flits and dances about the dayroom and jokingly states that she is a "ballerina." She occasionally takes off her dress and uses it for a scarf for her dancing. Mrs. Richard wears heavy make-up and adorns her hair with artificial flowers. At times she becomes irritable when other patients tire of her. She calls them "sourpusses" and occasionally swears at them if they do not agree with her that she is gorgeous. The other day she impulsively kissed the porter as he was cleaning the floor in her room. She later accused him of making sexual advances toward her.

Mrs. Richard's history states that she has been married for 4 months.

Although she was slightly hyperactive before her marriage, she did not become overly so until after her husband, a member of the armed services, was sent to Korea.

Little information has yet been secured in regard to Mrs. Richard's childhood. According to her medical history she is the oldest child and has one sister 2 years younger. Her parents are in their early fifties and seem somewhat baffled by Mrs. Richard's sudden illness. She had the usual childhood illnesses but has not been seriously ill.

She is a high school graduate and attended the Junior College in her home town, an Eastern city with a population of 60,000. In school she made above-average grades with little effort and was very active in extra-curricular activities. After she was graduated she was employed as a secretary in the personnel office of a large business concern. She continued her employment after her marriage. Her work record had been excellent but the company became concerned when she promised several applicants for employment large bonuses and salaries. She was discharged when, without permission, she gave 20 dollars from the company's petty cash fund to a male applicant to buy a new tie.

Questions Relating to the Patient Study

1. The nurse should anticipate that, as she becomes more elated, Mrs. Richard will most likely have

   a._____cerea flexibilities.
   b._____decreased motor activity.
   c._____incoherent speech.
   d._____visual hallucinations.

2. The characteristics which the nurse might anticipate in regard to Mrs. Richard's speech are

   a._____leaving out words when conversing.
   b._____rhyming of words when conversing.
   c._____talking slowly when emphasizing a point.
   d._____talking softly when requested.

3. In carrying out a plan to assist Mrs. Richard in becoming more attractive to others, the nurse should

   a._____insist that she wear the clothing provided by the hospital so she will not tear hers.
   b._____limit the available lipstick and rouge to the more subdued shades.
   c._____offer a variety of lipstick and rouge and suggest that she choose the light shades.
   d._____secure an order to take her shopping for more suitable clothing.

4. In dealing with the problem of Mrs. Richard's obscene, profane language, the nurse should

   a._____avoid criticizing this behavior.
   b._____deduce that the patient is an immoral woman.
   c._____register disapproval by refusing to talk to the patient.
   d._____remind the patient that ladies do not "talk that way."

5. The characteristic typical of manic symptoms shown by Mrs. Richard is

 a._____concentration on details.
 b._____increased motor activity.
 c._____poverty of ideas.
 d._____tolerance of other patient's behavior.

6. In making a nursing care plan for Mrs. Richard, as a general aim for her care the nurse should

 a._____encourage a more optimistic outlook.
 b._____encourage her ability to entertain other patients.
 c._____increase her feelings of security.
 d._____increase her decorative tendencies.

7. At this stage of Mrs. Richard's illness, in regard to eating habits the nurse should appreciate that the patient should

 a._____be served food that she can eat while "flitting" about her room.
 b._____be served large quantities at mealtime so that she will develop regular habits.
 c._____be served a limited amount of fluids because she sprinkles them about her room.
 d._____go to the dining room with others so that she can learn to socialize with them.

8. When patients with Mrs. Richard's diagnosis have delusions with paranoid tendencies, the delusional content which is most characteristic is that

 a._____God is controlling their body with electricity.
 b._____others are having sexual designs in regard to them.
 c._____someone has destroyed a part of their body.
 d._____someone is trying to kill them.

9. In Mrs. Richard's present state, her super ego can best be described as

 a._____intense.
 b._____flexible.
 c._____rigid.
 d._____weak.

10. Mrs. Richard is probably attempting to solve her problems by

 a._____depersonalizing.
 b._____dissociating.
 c._____identifying.
 d._____incorporating.

11. Points for the nurse to remember when caring for Mrs. Richard are to

 a._____adapt the nutritional intake to the activity level.
 b._____redirect energy into constructive channels.
 c._____reduce stimuli in the external environment.
 d._____require a strict adherence to ward routine.

12. The physician wrote an order for Mrs. Richard to have a catheterized urine specimen. When carrying out the procedure the nurse should

    a._____give Mrs. Richard a detailed explanation of the procedure.
    b._____minimize the amount of breakable equipment.
    c._____restrain Mrs. Richard before bringing the equipment to the room.
    d._____secure Mrs. Richard's promise to lie still during the treatment.

13. The nurse should appreciate that, before Mrs. Richard became ill, she was probably described by others as being

    a._____benevolent.
    b._____decisive.
    c._____mystical.
    d._____witty.

Questions for Discussion and Student Projects

1. What types of psychiatric therapies are commonly employed in the total plan of treatment for patients like Mrs. Richard?
2. Why did Mrs. Richard's illness probably become so acute before it was recognized by herself or her associates?
3. What instructions should be given to Mrs. Richard's family in regard to a recurrence of her present illness?
4. What are some of the reasons why Mrs. Richard's parents were so "baffled" by her illness?
5. If the company for which Mrs. Richard was employed would consent to re-employ her after she is well, would you encourage her to pursue this type of work? Why?
6. What information in the Patient Study would be helpful in planning diversional activities for Mrs. Richard? In the light of this information, what activities would be most suitable for Mrs. Richard? How would you approach her in order to secure her interest?
7. Why are the oldest and youngest children in a family more likely to develop psychiatric disorders?
8. What additional data might be helpful to the nurse in planning the care for Mrs. Richard?

Questions Relating to the Section in General

1. The term manic-depressive psychosis is synonymous with

    a._____acute mania.
    b._____involutional melancholia.
    c._____reactive depression.
    d._____none of the above.

2. The incidence of manic-depressive psychosis in women is highest among the

    a._____American Indian.
    b._____Chinese.

    c._____German.
    d._____Jewish.

3. The first attack of manic-depressive psychosis usually occurs at approximately

    a._____15–20 years.
    b._____20–30 years.
    c._____30–40 years.
    d._____40–50 years.

4. The physicochemical treatment which is most commonly used in treating depressed patients is

    a._____electrotherapy.
    b._____hydrotherapy.
    c._____insulin therapy.
    d._____narcotherapy.

5. The characteristic of speech which is typical of the patient in the depressed phase of manic-depressive psychosis is

    a._____accelerated rate.
    b._____increased duration.
    c._____retarded rate.
    d._____none of the above.

6. The depressed patient is suffering primarily from a (an)

    a._____loss, either real or imagined.
    b._____sense of well being.
    c._____increase in home responsibilities.
    d._____increase in occupational responsibilities.

7. When administering oral sedation to a very wealthy and severely depressed patient, the action most acceptable is to

    a._____set the tray of medications on the patient's bedside table while filling the pitcher from the adjoining bathroom.
    b._____offer him water from a paper cup taken from the medication tray.
    c._____give the patient the medicine and then wait in his room until he goes into his adjoining bathroom for water.
    d._____take the medication tray to the kitchen and secure a glass tumbler of water before going to the patient's room.

8. The observation which is the most significant expression of a patient's intent to commit suicide is

    a._____complaining of the high cost of hospitalization.
    b._____mentioning his strong desire to leave the hospital.
    c._____refusing his tray on 3 successive occasions.
    d._____warning others that he intends to commit suicide.

9. In manic-depressive psychosis, the statement most typical in regard to the duration of the illness is that periods

    a._____of depression are usually longer than those of elation.
    b._____of elation are usually longer than those of depression.
    c._____of elation and depression are usually about equal in length.
    d._____between attacks usually become longer as the patient becomes older.

10. In manic-depressive psychosis—depressed phase, the statement most characteristic of the patient's thoughts is that his thoughts

    a._____are appropriate to his moods.
    b._____do not reflect his moods.
    c._____are much faster than his actions.
    d._____are not appropriate to his actions.

11. The most correct statement in regard to a depression is that it is

    a._____a specific psychiatric disorder.
    b._____seldom noted in the average individual.
    c._____a symptom common to several psychiatric disorders.
    d._____found only in those who have a reactive depression.

Questions Relating to the Situation Study

Mrs. Grandy, a housewife aged 47 years, was admitted in a state of intense agitation. She was crying, wringing her hands and imploring everyone to send for the priest so she could confess her many sins before she was "put under the ground." Although her husband and daughter accompanied her to the institution, she stated they were dead and that she too would soon be dead, because she is a "bad woman." She has refused all food for several days, is constipated, and insists that her "bowels are all gone" and her heart "petrified." She responds momentarily to the nurse's reassurance that she will be safe from harm, but continues to repeat that she is a "bad woman" and will soon be "put under ground."

[Items 12 to 18, inclusive, refer to this situation.]

12. Considering the behavior shown by Mrs. Grandy, the nurse would anticipate the probable diagnosis to be

    a._____involutional melancholia.   c._____manic-depressive, depressed.
    b._____involutional, paranoid trend.   d._____schizophrenia, paranoid.

13. The delusional patterns shown by Mrs. Grandy are

    a._____guilt.   c._____nihilism.
    b._____grandiosity.   d._____persecution.

14. To increase Mrs. Grandy's fluid and food intake, the nurse should

    a._____approach her with the idea that she will eat and drink.
    b._____carefully consider the delusional content.

c.____give oral hygiene before meals.

d.____serve small amounts at frequent intervals.

15. In dealing with the problem of constipation the nurse should

    a.____ask the physician to prescribe a daily laxative.

    b.____give at least 4000 cc. of water daily unless contraindicated.

    c.____report constipation to the head nurse.

    d.____take Mrs. Grandy for short walks about the ward.

16. To lessen Mrs. Grandy's agitation the nurse should

    a.____avoid placing her in the center of activities.

    b.____explain any change in activities well in advance.

    c.____give her some gauze and let her help fold dressings.

    d.____spend as much time as possible with the patient.

17. In response to Mrs. Grandy's insistence that her "bowels are gone" and her heart "petrified," the nurse should

    a.____attempt to direct her attention and energy into other channels.

    b.____tell Mrs. Grandy that she is too concerned about herself.

    c.____tell Mrs. Grandy that those feelings will disappear as she improves.

    d.____try to convince her that those ideas are silly.

18. In regard to Mrs. Grandy's hopeless outlook on life, the nurse should

    a.____avoid being overly cheerful herself.

    b.____give constant unobtrusive supervision.

    c.____try to interest her in crocheting a scarf for her daughter.

    d.____tell Mrs. Grandy it would be a sin to take her own life.

19. Electrotherapy was first used in the treatment of psychiatric disorders in

    a.____1917.   b.____1927.   c.____1937.   d.____1947.

20. Complications of electroshock therapy are

    a.____aspiration of fluid.   c.____fractures of the long bones.

    b.____dislocation of the jaw.   d.____laceration of the tongue.

21. The most dramatic response to electroshock therapy is seen in individuals with

    a.____involutional melancholia.

    b.____manic-depressive, depressed phase.

    c.____manic-depressive, manic phase.

    d.____schizophrenia, catatonic type.

22. To prevent aspiration following electroshock therapy the position of the patient should be

    a.____in semi-Fowler's with the head turned toward the nurse.

    b.____flat on the back with the head turned to one side.

c._____flat on the abdomen with the head turned away from the light.

d._____in low Fowler's with the head turned to one side.

23. The preparation of a patient for electroshock therapy is most similar to the preparation of a patient for

a._____deep heat therapy.   c._____electroencephalogram.

b._____electrocardiogram.   d._____general anesthesia.

24. Symptoms which would indicate that the nurse should remove a patient in the neutral stage from a cold wet sheet pack are

a._____chilliness. b._____drowsiness. c._____noisiness. d._____weakness.

25. Mrs. Blythe, a mildly hyperactive patient who is receiving a continuous tub bath, asks that the nurse turn on the light and give her a magazine so that she may read during the treatment. The nurse should

a._____convince the patient that her request cannot be fulfilled under the circumstances.

b._____fulfill the patient's request by supplying her with suitable reading material.

c._____summon another patient to submit Mrs. Blythe's request to the head nurse.

d._____summon an attendant to submit Mrs. Blythe's request to the head nurse.

26. The man who did most toward establishing hydrotherapy on a physiologic basis was

a._____Currie. b._____Fleury. c._____Preissnitz. d._____Winternitz.

27. Under normal conditions hydrotherapy treatment(s) which produce(s) a sedative effect is (are)

a._____cold wet sheet pack, neutral stage.

b._____continuous tub bath 94°–97°F.

c._____continuous tub bath 99°–104°F.

d._____Scotch douche.

28. The precautions the nurse should take when administering a cold wet sheet pack are to

a._____arrange air pockets in the blankets.

b._____avoid the contact of 2 skin surfaces.

c._____maintain the room temperature at 65°F.

d._____observe the condition of the skin.

29. The measure(s) important in the nursing care of an individual receiving a cold wet sheet pack is (are) to

a._____apply a neutral compress to the eyes.

b._____apply a cold compress to the forehead.

c.____place a hot-water bottle to the feet.
d.____place an ice bag to the feet.

30. In general, patients who would respond favorably to stimulative hydrotherapy treatment are those with

a.____combative behavior.   c.____retarded behavior.
b.____depressed behavior.   d.____stuporous behavior.

31. The physiologic effect obtained when giving a hydrotherapy treatment using alternate hot and cold is chiefly

a.____analgesic. b.____circulatory. c.____sedative. d.____antipyretic.

Questions for Discussion and Student Projects

1. In what other psychiatric disorders will the nurse see the symptoms of elation and depression?
2. Differentiate between the underlying psychodynamics of a patient with involutional melancholia and manic-depressive psychosis, depressed phase.
3. Differentiate between the underlying psychodynamics of a patient with elation and one with depression.
4. Compare the rate of first admission to state hospitals of schizophrenic patients and those with manic-depressive psychosis.

Section 5. Nursing Care of Antisocial People

SINFUL OR SICK?—PATIENT STUDY

Mr. Roberts, a 24-year-old service station attendant in a large metropolitan area, was admitted to the hospital 1 week ago. At that time, 8 marijuana cigarettes and a small envelope of tiny white tablets were found concealed in the lining of his shaving kit. During this first week, he was friendly, congenial and frequently offered to assist the nurses with other patients and routine hospital activities. Some of the patients commented that Mr. Roberts had been sent to the ward to watch them because "he isn't crazy."

The social worker's history revealed the following: The father is a soft-spoken, kindly person who talks freely about himself but refers all questions about the home to his wife. The mother organizes information well and seems to have every detail at her fingertips. The patient has 2 older sisters who are apparently happily married and who have no history of "nervous disorders." As a child, Mr. Roberts was frequently sick with "colds" and "stomach upsets." His sisters thought he was frail and often came to his rescue in any difficulty that arose in grade school. During high school, Mr. Roberts was still "frail" but his sisters had tired of making excuses for him and teased him about being a "'sissy."

Mr. Roberts' teacher often asked him what he would like to do when he finished high school. Mr. Roberts hadn't thought about this but his mother had always wanted him to go to college and be a music teacher like her brother. The father thought that since Mr. Roberts was frail he should work on a farm so he could be outdoors more. Bitter family arguments over this conflict started before the patient began kindergarten.

When Mr. Roberts was in the second year of high school, his complaints of being "sick" ceased. The high school principal, however, reported to the family that Mr. Roberts missed 2 or 3 days of school each week. Several petty thefts occurred at school and although circumstances seemed to implicate the patient no definite proof was ever established. The sisters had also missed money from their purses and had accused their brother of taking it. This the mother refused to believe. She frequently referred to the fact that her family had always been "well to do" and that her son could never do such a thing.

When Mr. Roberts finished high school, he secured a position in a loan company but was discharged after a few weeks because he forged a check for 20 dollars. The company did not press charges because the mother repaid the money. The mother blamed this incident on the fact that she had married a "working man with little get up" and that these characteristics in the boy must have come from his father's family.

When a circus came to town, Mr. Roberts secured a job collecting tickets. Without saying anything to his family, he left town with the circus group. After he had been gone for 3 weeks, the police contacted the family to say that Mr. Roberts had been jailed on a charge of driving while intoxicated and being involved in a traffic accident. The mother's attorney was able to get Mr. Roberts released because "he was so young." Mr. Roberts promised he would "be good" and found a job in a service station. In 2 weeks he again disappeared and was heard from when he was jailed on a disorderly conduct charge. The court sent him to the hospital for observation and diagnosis. After a Rorschach and various other psychological tests had been administered, Mr. Roberts was diagnosed as sociopathic personality with drug addiction and alcoholism.

References

Burton, Arthur, and Harris, Robert E., Editors: Case Histories in Clinical and Abnormal Psychology, pp. 338–345, 431–487, 505–516, New York, Harpers, 1947.

Cleckley, Hervey M.: The Mask of Sanity, St. Louis, Mosby, 1941.

Hirsh, Joseph: The Problem Drinker, New York, Duell, Sloan and Pearce, 1949.

Ingram, Madelene: Principles of Psychiatric Nursing, pp. 365–368, 434–439, Philadelphia, Saunders, 1949.

Johnson, Wendell: People in Quandaries, pp. 401–402, New York, Harpers, 1946.

Orgel, Samuel: Psychiatry Today and Tomorrow, pp. 205–215, New York, International Universities Press, 1946.

Steele, Katharine, and Manfreda, Marguerite: Psychiatric Nursing, pp. 296–301, 329–338, Philadelphia, Davis, 1950.

Thorner, Melvin W.: Psychiatry in General Practice, pp. 58–122, 364–389, Philadelphia, Saunders, 1948.

Questions Relating to the Patient Study

1. When Mr. Roberts was 8 years old, the approval of the group most important to him probably was that of his

    a._____parents.
    b._____playmates.
    c._____sisters.
    d._____teachers.

2. The pattern most typical of Mr. Roberts' basic personality is that of

    a._____dependency.
    b._____depression.
    c._____repressed guilt.
    d._____independence.

3. The nurse should anticipate that developing rapport with Mr. Roberts will be established

    a._____without difficulty but within a few days.
    b._____with difficulty over a long period of time.
    c._____with difficulty within a few days.
    d._____without difficulty over a period of weeks.

4. The nursing team should be firm but kind and consistent in their nursing of Mr. Roberts because he

   a.＿＿＿＿does not have a knowledge of the law.
   b.＿＿＿＿has an inflated concept of himself.
   c.＿＿＿＿has never developed a realistic concept of the self.
   d.＿＿＿＿has a strong, rigid super ego.

5. The underlying reason for Mr. Roberts' not assuming social responsibility for his actions was that he

   a.＿＿＿＿did not attend school regularly.
   b.＿＿＿＿drank too much alcohol.
   c.＿＿＿＿lacked a knowledge of the law.
   d.＿＿＿＿none of the above.

6. One of the underlying etiologic factors in Mr. Roberts' illness was

   a.＿＿＿＿alcohol addiction.　　　c.＿＿＿＿marijuana addiction.
   b.＿＿＿＿childhood experiences.　d.＿＿＿＿organic lesions in the brain.

7. The dominant factor in Mr. Roberts' basic personality structure is characterized by a "weak"

   a.＿＿＿＿id.　　　　c.＿＿＿＿super ego.
   b.＿＿＿＿libido.　　d.＿＿＿＿none of the above.

8. The main reason for the Rorschach test was to determine

   a.＿＿＿＿intelligence.　　　　　c.＿＿＿＿vocabulary.
   b.＿＿＿＿reading comprehension.　d.＿＿＿＿none of these.

9. The statement which should be made in regard to Mr. Roberts' behavior is that it

   a.＿＿＿＿was purposeful.　　　c.＿＿＿＿is not motivated.
   b.＿＿＿＿was not purposeful.　d.＿＿＿＿does not have a cause.

10. Mr. Roberts' antisocial traits were probably

   a.＿＿＿＿inherited from his mother's family.
   b.＿＿＿＿inherited from his father's family.
   c.＿＿＿＿inherited from both his mother's and his father's families.
   d.＿＿＿＿not inherited.

Questions for Discussion and Student Projects

1. What etioligic factors in Mr. Roberts' childhood may have contributed to the development of his present behavior patterns?
2. How do you think Mr. Roberts feels about his father?—his mother?—his sisters?
3. Which of Mr. Roberts' behavior manifestations are characteristic of an individual with sociopathic personality?
4. How far should the nurse go in permitting Mr. Roberts to assist her in the routine activities of the ward?

5. Outline and describe a plan for Mr. Roberts' nursing care:

a. What specific occupational and recreational activities would be suitable for Mr. Roberts on the ward? What value would he gain from each activity?

b. The physician has indicated that the nurse should be firm, accepting, objective and astute in her relationships with Mr. Roberts. How would the nurse maintain these attitudes in the following situations?

(1) Mr. Roberts asks the nurse for her home address.

(2) Mr. Roberts is in a 4-bed ward with 3 older men. It has been observed that he is usually very kind to and protective of these men. An attendant, however, overheard Mr. Roberts insisting that one of these elderly men had better hurry and clean his shoes.

(3) Mr. Roberts calls the nurse by her first name and tells her how cute she is.

(4) Mr. Roberts repeatedly asks to stop in the corner drug store while out walking with the group.

(5) Mr. Roberts asks the nurse to play a game of pingpong.

(6) Mr. Roberts is extremely restless after a weekend at home. Monday night he requests that the male attendant remain at his bedside.

(7) Mr. Roberts tells the nurse how sorry he is for all that he has done and states that he is turning over a new leaf. He also comments that Dr. X has been so mean to him that he doesn't want him for his doctor any more because "Dr. X just doesn't understand me."

6. What local and national social agencies are available that might assist in Mr. Roberts' rehabilitation?

7. Would Mr. Roberts be held legally responsible for his conduct? Support your decision.

8. How can the social worker's history be helpful to the nurse in planning Mr. Roberts' nursing care?

9. Mr. Roberts was of draft age. One of his friends commented that "serving in the army would be good for him." How should the nurse respond in this situation?

10. How can the nurse utilize the psychologist's report in planning suitable occupational and recreational activities for Mr. Roberts?

11. What are the similarities and differences between the adult criminal, the juvenile delinquent and the individual with sociopathic personality?

12. What are the legal complications involved in the treatment of individuals with drug addiction, with alcohol addiction and with sociopathic personality?

13. Why are the sociopathic and alcohol individuals sometimes referred to as being antisocial? Differentiate between the terms antisocial and asocial.

Questions Relating to the Section in General

1. A student nurse is accompanying 3 young patients with the diagnosis of alcoholism on a walk. One patient breaks away from the group and disappears over the hill. The closest available telephone is in a tavern across the street. The nurse should

    a._____instruct the 2 remaining patients to return to the hospital while she follows the departed patient.
    b._____accompany the 2 remaining patients to the hospital to insure their safety.
    c._____stop at the tavern with the 2 remaining patients to telephone the hospital.
    d._____take the 2 remaining patients with her to search for the departed patient.

2. The effects of alcohol when taken internally by man are shown first in the area of

    a._____judgment.   c._____specialized skills.
    b._____motor co-ordination.   d._____visual acuity.

3. According to Alcoholic Anonymous, characteristics of the alcoholic individual are

    a._____constitutional predisposition.   c._____inflated ego.
    b._____inferiority complex.   d._____strong super ego.

4. In alcoholic delirium tremens, nursing care measures indicated are to

    a._____give plenty of fluids.
    b._____reduce external stimuli to a minimum.
    c._____supervise constantly during delirium.
    d._____tell the patient it is "foolish" to be afraid.

5. In caring for the patient with alcoholic Korsakoff's syndrome, acute stage, the nurse should

    a._____give daily exercises to the patient's ankles.
    b._____provide a cradle to relieve pressure.
    c._____reduce the patient's body movement to a minimum.
    d._____support his feet to prevent footdrop.

6. Alcohol is a primary etiologic factor in

    a._____Alzheimer's disease.   c._____Korsakoff's syndrome.
    b._____delirium tremens.   d._____Wernicke's syndrome.

7. Tests used to evaluate the individual's intelligence are the

    a._____Army Alpha.   d._____Wechsler-Bellevue.
    b._____Otis.   e._____all of the above.
    c._____Stanford-Binet.

8. The projective test known as the "ink blot test" is the

    a._____Rorschach.   c._____Szondi.
    b._____thematic apperception.   d._____none of the above.

Part Four

Nursing Care of Mothers and the Newborn

Section 1. Nursing Care of the Normal Mother and the Newborn*

STUDY SUGGESTIONS: Before beginning the study of this Section, the student will find it helpful to

A. Review

1. In anatomy and physiology texts: anatomy of the female reproductive tract, reproduction.
2. In nutrition texts: diet in pregnancy.
3. In pharmacology texts: Pitocin, vitamin K.

B. Study: In obstetric texts: Prenatal care, phenomena of labor, nursing care during the puerperium, care of the newborn.

C. Read the additional References listed before attempting to answer the questions relating to each patient study.

THE EXPECTANT FAMILY
Background Review Question

1. Complete the following questions by placing the letter preceding the term in the left-hand column next to the proper descriptive phrase in the right-hand column on this page and on the following page.

a. Goodell's sign.
b. amenorrhea.
c. quickening.
d. Chadwick's sign.
e. decidua.
f. endometrium.
g. tubercles of Montgomery.
h. Hegar's sign.
i. Braxton Hicks sign.
j. nidation.
k. chloasma.
l. pseudocyesis.
m. gravid.
n. parous.
o. striae gravidarum.
p. linea nigra.
q. ptyalism.
r. lightening.

___*k*___mask of pregnancy.
___*j*___implantation.
_____endometrium of pregnancy.
_____sebaceous glands in the areola surrounding the nipples.
_____absence of menstrual flow.
_____softening of lower uterine segment.
_____false pregnancy.
_____mother's first perception of baby's movements.
_____softening of the cervix.
_____lining of the nonpregnant uterus.
_____having borne one or more viable babies.
_____bluish appearance of the vulva and the vagina.
_____pregnant.
_____painless uterine contractions occurring during pregnancy.

* For care of the newborn in the home, see the Pediatric section, pp. 341–345.

_____pertaining to a gonad.

_____increased salivation.

_____dark line on the abdomen extending from the pubis toward the umbilicus.

_____shining purplish lines on the abdomen caused by stretching.

_____the settling of the presenting part into the pelves near or at term.

_____chafed patch of skin accompanied by moisture, usually in the axillae and about the anus and the vulva.

THE EXPECTANT FAMILY—PATIENT STUDY

Mr. and Mrs. Kurz, now in their early forties, had married in 1940. Jackie was born the following year. During the Second World War Mr. Kurz served as an officer in the Field Artillery, seeing action in North Africa and in Italy. While he was away, Mrs. Kurz lived with her mother-in-law, who took care of the baby while she worked in an aircraft factory. After the war Mr. Kurz returned to his former position as assistant manager of a woolen mill in a large New England town, and the family moved into their own home, about a mile outside of town. Both the girls were born at home—Joanne in 1947 and Betty in 1949.

When she realized she was again pregnant, in the summer of 1952, Mrs. Kurz visited her family physician. At this time she learned that he no longer delivered mothers at home, so she was registered at the hospital. Arrangements were made with the woman who had helped them after the girls were born to come to the Kurzes after mother and baby returned from the hospital. The children knew of the expected baby, and were looking forward to their stay with Grandmother and Grandfather Kurz, in town, while their mother was in the hospital. Mr. Kurz also planned to stay there, to be nearer his family.

Joanne and Betty helped their mother to get the baby's layette together. There was little to be purchased—the baby clothes which had been used for Jackie and his sisters would do for the new baby. Jackie and his Dad decorated the small guest room as a nursery, painting the nursery furniture blue in anticipation of another boy.

Early in her pregnancy, Mrs. Kurz had experienced frequency and morning sickness, and had been very tired, but these symptoms had disappeared after the third month. As pregnancy progressed, she noticed swelling of her feet and ankles toward afternoon. Before pregnancy she weighed 135 pounds; at term, her weight was 155 pounds. She planned to nurse this baby, as she had her others. Her past pregnancies and labors had been normal. Jackie had been born in the hospital after a 20-hour labor. Mrs. Kurz remembered little of the experience. Her two daughters had been born at home, after labors of 5 and 6 hours, respectively.

References

Bearg, Philip A., and Wood, Eleanor L.: Community planning for parent education, Publ. Health Nursing 39:256, 1947.

De Lee, Sol T.: Safeguarding Motherhood, Philadelphia, Lippincott, 1950.

Donnelly, Veronica: Protecting the prospective mother in industry, Publ. Health Nursing 44:134, 1952.

Eastman, Nicholson J.: Expectant Motherhood, Boston, Little, Brown, 1947.

Hymes, James L.: How to Tell Your Child about Sex, Public Affairs Pamphlets, #149.

McKinnon, Ann S.: Body mechanics in pregnancy: nursing responsibilities, Publ. Health Nursing 42:595, 1950.

Neisser, Edith G.: How to be a Good Mother-in-Law and Grandmother, Public Affairs Pamphlets, 22 E. 38th Street, New York City 16. (#174, $.20)

———, and Neisser, Walter: Making the Grade as a Dad, Public Affairs Pamphlets, 22 E. 38th Street, New York City 16. (#157, $.20)

Peck, Elizabeth: Mothers' classes answer a community need, Publ. Health Nursing 43:658, 1951.

Public Health Nursing in Obstetrics: Part IV, Maternity Center Association, New York, 1945.

Thoms, Herbert J.: Training for Childbirth, New York, McGraw-Hill, 1950.

Wiedenbach, Ernestine: Safeguarding the mother's breasts, Am. J. Nursing 51:544, 1951.

Questions Relating to the Patient Study

1. During this pregnancy Mrs. Kurz is

   a.———gravida IV, para IV.
   b.———gravida III, para IV.
   c.———gravida III, para III.
   d.———gravida IV, para III.

2. Symptoms one might expect Mrs. Kurz to notice during the first trimester are

   a.———amenorrhea, frequency, quickening.
   b.———frequency, morning sickness, amenorrhea.
   c.———weight gain, lightening, amenorrhea.
   d.———swelling of the ankles, amenorrhea, frequency.

3. Mrs. Kurz experienced frequency in early pregnancy as a result of

   a.———pressure of the enlarging uterus on the bladder.
   b.———urinary infection.
   c.———increased fluid intake.
   d.———desire to experience symptoms of pregnancy.

4. Her morning sickness might be explained by lowered blood sugar due to

   a.———inadequate diet.
   b.———rapid growth of the baby.
   c.———hyperinsulinism.
   d.———hypothyroidism.

5. The tired feeling experienced during the first trimester probably was due to

   a._____inadequate diet.
   b._____low blood sugar.
   c._____hypothyroidism.
   d._____anemia.

6. During pregnancy, Mrs. Kurz would probably note the following with regard to her breasts:

   a._____darkening of the areola, tingling sensation, hardness.
   b._____lightening of the areola, tingling sensation, increased size.
   c._____colostrum, tingling sensation, darkening of the areola.
   d._____increased size, tenderness, flattening of the nipples.

7. Compared to the desired weight gain during pregnancy, Mrs. Kurz' total was

   a._____high.
   b._____low.
   c._____within the expected range.

8. Mrs. Kurz should be instructed to go to the hospital

   a._____as soon as contractions start.
   b._____when contractions become regular.
   c._____when contractions recur every 5 minutes.
   d._____when contractions recur every 2 to 3 minutes.

Questions Relating to the Section in General

1. Assume that you are a public health nurse, visiting the home of Mrs. Kurz. What points should you consider in discussing her personal hygiene during pregnancy?
2. Knowing that Mrs. Kurz planned to nurse her baby, what help should you give her? How should your approach and advice to her differ if she were not planning to nurse her baby?
3. Assume that Mrs. Kurz' physician had been willing to conduct a home delivery. How should the public health nurse help Mrs. Kurz prepare for the event? Take into consideration choice of room, arrangement of furniture, preparation of supplies, preparation of family.
4. Using the Birth Atlas (Maternity Center Association), show how you would explain to Mr. and Mrs. Kurz the physiology of conception and pregnancy, the development of the baby, and the process of labor.
5. Joanne and Betty are of an age where they might be expected to regard a baby as an intruder. How could the rest of the family help them avoid this attitude?
6. What type of information do you believe Jackie should have regarding his mother's pregnancy? If Mr. Kurz asked you about reading material suitable for Jackie, what might you suggest?

Questions Relating to the Section in General

1. Occasionally a laboratory examination is done to confirm the presence of pregnancy. Some of the pregnancy tests are

   a.＿＿＿Aschheim-Zondek, Xenopus, Friedman.
   b.＿＿＿V.D.R.L., Prostigmin, Xenopus.
   c.＿＿＿Friedman, Rubin, Aschheim-Zondek.
   d.＿＿＿Prostigmin, Schick, Mazzini.

2. A positive reaction to these pregnancy tests depends on the presence of

   a.＿＿＿pregnanediol in the blood.
   b.＿＿＿chorionic gonadotropin in the blood.
   c.＿＿＿chorionic gonadotropin in the urine.
   d.＿＿＿pregnanediol in the urine.

3. The woman who is to have such a pregnancy test done should be instructed to

   a.＿＿＿report to the laboratory for a fasting blood specimen.
   b.＿＿＿obtain a clean early-morning urine specimen.
   c.＿＿＿obtain a urine specimen at any time during the day.
   d.＿＿＿report to the laboratory for a catheterized urine specimen.

4. The signs that constitute positive evidence of pregnancy are

   a.＿＿＿enlarging uterus, Braxton Hicks contractions, x-ray visualization of the baby's skeleton.
   b.＿＿＿fetal movements felt by the examiner, Hegar's sign, positive Aschheim-Zondek test.
   c.＿＿＿x-ray visualization of the baby's skeleton, outlining the baby by abdominal palpation, auscultation of the baby's heart sounds.
   d.＿＿＿auscultation of the baby's heart sounds, fetal movements felt by the examiner, x-ray visualization of the baby's skeleton.

5. Many physiologic changes take place in the mother's body during pregnancy, affecting every system.

   a. The average weight of the nonpregnant uterus is 50 Gm., the capacity 2 cc. At term the weight is

      (1)＿＿＿100 Gm., the capacity 4,500 cc.
      (2)＿＿＿1,000 Gm., the capacity 450 cc.
      (3)＿＿＿10 Gm., the capacity 450 cc.
      (4)＿＿＿1,000 Gm., the capacity 4,500 cc.

   b. The total blood volume increases about 20 per cent, resulting in

      (1)＿＿＿pseudo-anemia.
      (2)＿＿＿true anemia.
      (3)＿＿＿nutritional anemia.
      (4)＿＿＿pernicious anemia.

c. The purplish streaks appearing on the breasts and the abdomen are called

(1)＿＿chloasma.
(2)＿＿striae.
(3)＿＿areola.
(4)＿＿alveoli.

6. During pregnancy stasis of the urine and pyelitis usually result from

a.＿＿toxemia.
b.＿＿increase in waste products in the circulation.
c.＿＿impaired kidney function.
d.＿＿pressure of the uterus on the ureters at the pelvic brim.

7. According to the Caldwell-Moloy classification, the normal female pelvis is known as

a.＿＿gynecoid.
b.＿＿anthropoid.
c.＿＿android.
d.＿＿platypelloid.

8. The average external measurements of this type of pelvis are

a.＿＿intercristal 26 cm., interspinous 28 cm., external conjugate 18 cm., bituberous 11 cm.
b.＿＿intercristal 24 cm., interspinous 22 cm., external conjugate 12.5 cm., bituberous 8 cm.
c.＿＿intercristal 32 cm., interspinous 26 cm., external conjugate 21 cm., bituberous 8 cm.
d.＿＿intercristal 28 cm., interspinous 26 cm., external conjugate 20 cm., bituberous 11 cm.

9. The physician doing an internal examination to determine the capacity of a woman's pelvis would expect, in a gynecoid pelvis, to find

a.＿＿sacrum well hollowed, coccyx movable, spines not prominent, pubic arch wide.
b.＿＿sacrum flat, coccyx movable, spines prominent, pubic arch wide.
c.＿＿sacrum deeply hollowed, coccyx immovable, spines not prominent, pubic arch narrow.
d.＿＿sacrum flat, coccyx immovable, spines prominent, pubic arch narrow.

10. X-ray pelvimetry is being done in many places to determine the relationship between the baby's head and the mother's pelvis. To obtain a true relationship, the following conditions must be met:

a.＿＿pregnancy in the last trimester, presenting part engaged.
b.＿＿pregnancy in the second trimester, presenting part breech.

c.____pregnancy close to term, presenting part vertex.
d.____pregnancy close to term, presenting part not engaged.

11. The time between fertilization of an ovum in an oviduct and its implantation in the uterine lining is approximately

a.____9 weeks.
b.____9 days.
c.____9 hours.
d.____9 minutes.

12. The placenta is the organ of exchange between mother and baby. The baby receives food and oxygen and gets rid of waste products by

a.____direct exchange of blood through the placenta.
b.____filtration.
c.____osmosis.
d.____suction.

13. In addition to this function, the placenta produces

a.____chorionic gonadotropin, pregnanediol, estrogen.
b.____chorionic gonadotropin, estrogen, progesterone.
c.____progesterone, lactogen, estrogen.
d.____pituitrin, progesterone, estrogen.

14. In most primigravidae, lightening occurs about 2 weeks before the onset of labor. At this time the mother notices

a.____leg pains, frequency, easier breathing.
b.____constipation, dysuria, abdominal pains.
c.____dyspnea, dysuria, constipation.
d.____frequency, dyspnea, leg pains.

15. The contractions of false labor typically occur at

a.____regular intervals, gradually increase in intensity, discomfort intensified by walking, discomfort located chiefly in the lower back.
b.____irregular intervals, intensity remains the same, discomfort often relieved by walking, discomfort located chiefly in the abdomen.
c.____irregular intervals, intensity remains the same, intervals gradually shortened, discomfort intensified by walking.
d.____regular intervals, intensity increases, intervals remain long, discomfort relieved by walking.

16. The ductus arteriosus and foramen ovale, structures essential to fetal circulation, serve as a means of

a.____by-passing the lungs.
b.____directing arterial blood from the placenta to the baby.
c.____directing venous blood from the baby to the placenta.
d.____by-passing the portal system.

17. In many instances it is to the mother's advantage to continue her employment for a time during pregnancy. Those occupations an expectant mother might ordinarily engage in with safety are

    a._____x-ray technician, dress designing, painting.
    b._____secretarial work, sewing-machine operator, photography.
    c._____sales clerk, receptionist, night nurse.
    d._____dress designing, secretarial work, photography.

Questions for Discussion and Student Projects—(*Continued*)

1. What are the components of a complete history and physical examination of a pregnant woman? What is the significance of each component?
2. Some of the minor complications of pregnancy are morning sickness, heartburn, constipation, dyspnea, varicose veins, cramps in the lower extremities and dependent edema of the feet and the ankles. In discussing these with expectant mothers, how should you explain the cause of each? What measures should you advise for the relief or prevention of these discomforts?
3. Every expectant mother should be familiar with the danger signals associated with pregnancy. With one of your classmates as the mother, show how you would bring these to her attention without unduly alarming her.
4. What facilities are available in your community for education for parenthood? Set up a brief course outline for use in teaching parents. Indicate which topics should be discussed before and which ones after the birth of the baby.
5. In order to teach parents effectively the nurse must be able to interpret medical terms to them. How should you describe each of the following terms to parents:

Membranes.	Fundus.
Os.	Vertex.
Cervix.	Fetal heart.
Uterus.	Symphysis.
Perineum.	Spines (ischial).
Areola.	Secundines.

6. There is a wealth of literature available for parents, with new articles appearing monthly in lay magazines. Evaluate some of the current articles from the standpoints of appeal, readability, validity, and probable effect.
7. What are the predominant cultural groups in your community? On the basis of their eating habits plan for each group a day's menu containing the essential elements in adequate amounts for a woman in the last trimester of pregnancy.
8. What is your interpretation of "natural childbirth"? What points are stressed in preparing parents for this experience? Are there facilities in your community at present for carrying out such a program?

9. Suggested activity for one student: Estimate the cost of having a baby. Include such things as prenatal and hospital care, medications (e.g. iron, calcium), layette, diaper service, nursery furniture and cost of food and medical supervision of the baby during the first year of life.
10. Suggested activity for one student: Investigate the availability of housekeeping services in your community. Are the women willing to remain with families day and night? What is the cost of such service?

THE BIRTH OF A BABY

Background Review Question

1. Complete the following questions by placing the letter preceding the term in the left-hand column next to the correct descriptive phrase in the right-hand column.

a. effacement.	(1)_____parallelism between planes of the fetal head and the mother's pelvis.
b. dilatation.	
c. presentation.	(2)_____enlargement of the external os.
d. viability.	(3)_____entrance into the pelvic inlet of the largest diameter of the presenting part.
e. engagement.	
f. attitude.	(4)_____posture of the baby.
g. position.	(5)_____ability to live.
h. secundines.	(6)_____pertaining to the head.
i. souffle.	(7)_____relation of a fixed point of the presenting part to the mother's pelvis.
j. show.	
	(8)_____that part of the baby nearest the internal os.
	(9)_____blood-tinged mucous discharge from the cervix during labor.
	(10)_____obliteration of the cervical canal.
	(11)_____afterbirth.
	(12)_____soft blowing sound caused by blood current.

THE BIRTH OF A BABY—PATIENT STUDY

As she was sitting down to Saturday lunch, Mrs. Kurz felt the first twinge suggestive of a labor contraction. She noted that the time was 1:10 P.M. At 1:25 there was another mild contraction. By the time she had finished cleaning up after the mid-day meal, contractions were coming every 10 minutes and had become somewhat stronger. She and her husband, with the help of Jackie, got the girls dressed, added the finishing touches to the suitcases that had been packed in advance, and the family was ready for a trip to Grandma's. Joanne and Betty each chose a toy to take along; Jack took his library book. Mr. Kurz called his mother to tell her they were on their way and Mrs. Kurz notified Dr. Miller that she was about to leave for the hospital.

After leaving the children with their grandmother, the Kurzes continued by car to the hospital. Mrs. Kurz had brought with her a completed hospital admission form which she turned over to the clerk, and she was ushered to her room. Her husband was requested to wait in the reception room for word from the doctor. A half hour later, Dr. Miller told him that he had examined Mrs. Kurz and thought she was either in very early labor or in false labor, since the baby had not dropped and the cervix was open only 2 cm. Contractions were now coming at irregular intervals. The doctor showed Mr. Kurz to his wife's room and left to go to his office, across the street.

By 8 P.M., after 5 hours in the hospital, Mrs. Kurz' contractions had ceased. Examination by the obstetrician showed no other change in her condition, and she was discharged. Rather than disturb the youngsters, they went straight home, calling Mr. Kurz' mother from there. They watched television through the 11 o'clock news report, then retired.

At 2 A.M. Sunday Mrs. Kurz was awakened by strong contractions which were coming at 5-minute intervals. Again she and her husband dressed and started for the hospital immediately after calling Dr. Miller. By the time they reached the hospital at 3 o'clock her contractions were only 3 minutes apart. She was taken directly to the delivery room. Ten minutes later the membranes ruptured spontaneously and the baby was born. Dr. Miller attended the spontaneous vertex delivery. The perineum remained intact. The placenta was delivered by Schultz mechanism, 5 minutes after the birth of the baby. Mrs. Kurz was given Pitocin 1 cc. (h) following the third stage.

The couple were delighted with their son, and ready to name him— Thomas, after Mr. Kurz, Sr. Baby Thomas cried lustily while the nurse was caring for him. He was cleansed, had silver nitrate instilled in each eye, received an injection of vitamin K, and the cord was checked for bleeding. Identical name bracelets were put on mother and baby, and he was taken to the nursery after being shown once again to his mother and then to his father.

References

Bookmiller, Mae M., and Bowen, George Loveridge: Textbook of Obstetrics and Obstetric Nursing, pp. 363–379, Philadelphia, Saunders, 1949.

Javert, Carl T.: The immediate postpartum period as a fourth stage of labor, Am. J. Obstet. and Gynec. 54:1028, 1947.

Owen, Ruth E., and Denman, Lucille G.: Experiences in childbirth, Am. J. Nursing 51:26, 1951.

Read, Grantly Dick: An outline of physiological labor, Am. J. Obstet. and Gynec. 54:702, 1947.

Questions Relating to the Patient Study

1. Mrs. Kurz' labor probably would be classified as

   a._____rapid.
   b._____inertial.
   c._____prolonged.
   d._____operative.

2. Following this type of labor the nurse should be particularly alert for signs of

   a._____aspiration.
   b._____inverted uterus.
   c._____hematoma.
   d._____hemorrhage.

3. Immediately following the third stage, the nurse caring for Mrs. Kurz would hope to find the fundus

   a._____contracted, at the xiphoid.
   b._____relaxed, at the symphysis.
   c._____contracted, at the umbilicus.
   d._____relaxed, at the xiphoid.

4. If the fundus were not as desired the nurse should inform the physician and

   a._____massage the fundus.
   b._____take Mrs. Kurz' blood pressure.
   c._____compress the fundus to expel clots.
   d._____apply a sandbag to the patient's abdomen.

5. Mrs. Kurz was given Pitocin to

   a._____help her relax.
   b._____stimulate circulation to the uterus.
   c._____stimulate contraction of the uterus.
   d._____relieve pain.

6. Silver nitrate was used in Baby Thomas's eyes to prevent

   a._____syphilitic infection.
   b._____gonorrheal infection.
   c._____*Monilia* infection.
   d._____*Trichomonas* infection.

7. Vitamin K was given to him to reduce the possibility of

   a._____infection.
   b._____dehydration.
   c._____malnutrition.
   d._____bleeding.

8. As the nurse working with Mrs. Kurz as she was delivering her baby, you should have instructed her to

   a._____pant during contractions.
   b._____bear down during contractions.
   c._____hold her breath during contractions.
   d._____do abdominal breathing.

Questions for Discussion and Student Projects

A. Relating to the Patient Study

1. Using a baby doll, demonstrate how you should care for Baby Thomas immediately after his birth. In your hospital who is responsible for the care of the eyes and of the cord, and for the identification of the newborn? How are babies resuscitated if necessary? Who is responsible?

2. Mr. and Mrs. Kurz are accustomed to home confinements. What reactions should you anticipate to a hospital confinement? How could you help them to feel comfortable in this situation?

3. As the nurse caring for Mrs. Kurz during her intrapartal period, what care should you give her? What is the extent of the charting that would be expected of you (in your hospital) with regards to such a situation?

B. Relating to the Section in General

1. Suggested activity for one student: Follow a couple through the mother's admission to the hospital. In what ways have the hospital personnel (including clerks, cashiers, elevator operators, aides, secretaries, nurses and doctors) helped to make the couple feel comfortable?

2. In many hospitals preadmission forms are given to expectant mothers (as well as other patients) whenever possible. What is the value of this policy?

3. What facilities are available at your hospital for the men whose wives are in labor? Plan a waiting room for expectant fathers, considering location, communications, interior decorations, available food service, books, etc.

4. What are the principles upon which you should base your care of a mother in labor? In your hospital what is expected of the nurse caring for a mother in the first stage of labor? Second stage? Third stage? Fourth stage?

5. Be prepared to discuss the significance of each of the following points to be observed in timing contractions during labor:

   Interval between contractions.
   Duration of contractions.
   Strength of contractions.
   Degree of uterine relaxation between contractions.
   Reaction of the mother to contractions.

   In your hospital how often is a nurse expected to time contractions? How should they be recorded?

6. What facts must the nurse know about a mother in labor in order effectively to report her condition to the supervising nurse?

7. Enumerate the responsibilities of the nurse and the doctor to the mother in labor who has been prepared for physiologic labor

(natural childbirth). How should the nurse assist the mother at the points of emotional menace? What is the ideal rôle of the husband of such a woman, during her labor?

8. Using a fetal doll and a bony pelvis, demonstrate the mechanism of labor and management of the second stage, the head having engaged as right occiput anterior.
9. Describe how you should manage a situation in which a mother delivers her baby before the physician arrives at her bedside.
10. Describe your approach to a mother having her first baby, as you carry out the admission procedures required in your hospital.
11. Describe the nurse's responsibilities in preparing a mother for a rectal examination during labor.

Questions Relating to the Section in General

1. The second stage of labor begins with

   a._____true labor contractions.
   b._____full dilatation and effacement of the cervix.
   c._____rupture of the membranes.
   d._____birth of the baby.

2. The second stage of labor ends with

   a._____birth of the baby.
   b._____delivery of the placenta.
   c._____delivery of the placenta and membranes.
   d._____repair of the laceration or episiotomy.

3. Signs which may announce the approaching second stage are

   a._____inability to bear down, frequency, perspiration on the upper lip and the bridge of the nose.
   b._____bulging perineum, desire to bear down, rupture of the membranes.
   c._____desire to bear down, increase in show, tremors of the lower extremities.
   d._____bulging perineum, hiccoughs, tremors of the lower extremities.

4. When alone with a mother who is delivering her baby the nurse should

   a._____deliver the presenting part between contractions.
   b._____have the mother bear down to deliver the baby during a contraction.
   c._____hold the mother's legs together until help arrives.
   d._____go after assistance.

5. Abdominal palpation is done to determine

   a._____presentation, engagement, dilatation.
   b._____effacement, engagement, dilatation.
   c._____position, presentation, engagement.
   d._____viability, descent, position.

6. If the physician learns from abdominal palpation that the baby's back is toward the mother's left and slightly anterior, the head is well flexed and cannot be dislodged from the pelvic inlet, he would chart his observations as

    a._____LOA, floating.
    b._____LOP, floating.
    c._____LOP, engaged.
    d._____LOA, engaged.

7. With descent constant, the proper order of mechanisms of labor with the baby in ROA position are

    a._____flexion, rotation, extension, restitution.
    b._____flexion, restitution, rotation, extension.
    c._____rotation, flexion, restitution, extension.
    d._____extension, rotation, flexion, restitution.

8. The mechanism by which a baby's head is delivered in the occiput anterior position is

    a._____flexion.
    b._____rotation.
    c._____extension.
    d._____restitution.

9. When the placenta is expelled with the fetal side outermost, the mechanism is known as

    a._____Duncan.
    b._____Credé.
    c._____Schultz-Ahlfeld.
    d._____Schultz.

10. When the placenta is expressed by compression of the fundus, the method is called

    a._____Duncan.
    b._____Credé.
    c._____Schultz-Ahlfeld.
    d._____Schultz.

11. In the immediate care of an infant after birth, usually the first step is

    a._____removal of mucus from the nose and the mouth.
    b._____administration of vitamin K.
    c._____administration of oxygen.
    d._____stimulation of crying.

12. Many obstetricians and pediatricians recommend that the cord not be clamped and cut until pulsation has ceased. They believe that in this way

    a._____hemorrhage may be prevented.
    b._____breathing may be stimulated.

   c._____the infant's blood volume may be increased.

   d._____the placenta will be separated more easily.

13. The normal range of fetal heart rate usually is considered to be

   a._____100–140 beats per minute.

   b._____60–100 beats per minute.

   c._____120–160 beats per minute.

   d._____140–180 beats per minute.

14. Dr. Grantly Dick Read has noted 4 points during labor at which a mother is most likely to require reassurance and medication. These "points of emotional menace" are

   a._____2 cm. dilatation, 6 cm. dilatation, 8 cm. dilatation, birth of the head.

   b._____6 cm. dilatation, 8 cm. dilatation, head on the pelvic floor, early crowning.

   c._____2 cm. dilatation, 4 cm. dilatation, 8 cm. dilatation, 10 cm. dilatation.

   d._____6 cm. dilatation, 8 cm. dilatation, head on the pelvic floor, birth of the shoulders.

15. Pitocin is used in obstetrics in preference to pituitrin because Pitocin has

   a._____stronger oxytocic action.

   b._____vasodilator action.

   c._____no vasopressor action.

   d._____less oxytocic action.

MOTHER AND BABY GET ACQUAINTED
Background Review Question

1. Complete the following questions by placing the letter preceding the term in the left-hand column next to the proper descriptive phrase in the right-hand column.

a. lanugo.	(1)_____product of the sebaceous glands around the penis and the prepuce, and in the region of the clitoris and the labia minora.
b. vernix caseosa.	
c. meconium.	
d. Moro reflex.	
e. asphyxia.	(2)_____uterine discharge following delivery.
f. melena neonatorum.	
g. miliaria.	(3)_____excessive amount of urine.
h. icterus neonatorum.	(4)_____jaundice of the newborn.
i. smegma.	(5)_____blood in the stools of newborn infants.
j. lochia.	
k. engorgement.	(6)_____congestion of the breasts.
l. lactation.	(7)_____fine hair covering the body of the fetus.
m. involution.	

n. polyuria.
o. dysuria.
p. colostrum.
q. puerperium.
r. postpartum.

(8)_____secretion of milk.
(9)_____failure of the infant to breathe immediately after birth.
(10)_____creamy substance covering the baby at birth.
(11)_____period from the end of labor until the time the genital organs and tract have returned to approximately their prepregnant state.
(12)_____infection of the mouth of the newborn.
(13)_____sudden movement of the baby when startled, consisting of drawing up the legs, opening the arms widely then closing the arms.
(14)_____black tarry stools seen in the first few days of life.
(15)_____abatement or diminution of symptoms.
(16)_____breast secretion during pregnancy and the first few days after delivery.
(17)_____irritation of the skin due to excessive clothing or heat.
(18)_____after childbirth.
(19)_____painful micturition.
(20)_____process by which the uterus returns to normal size and condition after childbirth.

MOTHER AND BABY GET ACQUAINTED—PATIENT STUDY

Mrs. Marsh, the nurse from the nursery, brought Baby Thomas to Mrs. Kurz for his first feeding period. The baby did not seem to be hungry so Mrs. Marsh suggested that they take this opportunity to inspect him. As they looked over the baby, the nurse pointed out the characteristics of a normal newborn infant, brought out some of the points in his care and answered the mother's questions.

As they finished inspecting the baby, he made it known that he was ready to be fed. Mrs. Marsh put the baby to breast, explaining to Mrs. Kurz the procedure used in that hospital, and left the two alone. The baby sucked vigorously for a few minutes, then went back to sleep. When Mrs. Marsh returned later to check on the progress of the feeding, she found Mrs. Kurz gently caressing the sleeping infant.

References

Burke, Bertha S., and Stuart, Harold C.: Nutritional requirements during lactation and pregnancy, J.A.M.A. 137:119, 1948.
Fries, Margaret E.: The Importance of Mother and Baby Rooming Together,

in Problems of Early Infancy, New York, Josiah Macy, Jr., Foundation, 1947.

Jeans, Philip, Rand, Winifred, and Blake, Florence: Essentials of Pediatrics, pp. 146–154, Philadelphia, Lippincott, 1946.

Peto, Marjorie: The normal newborn infant, Am. J. Nursing 52:1353, 1952.

Ribble, Margaret: The Rights of Infants, New York, Columbia, 1943.

Richmond, Julius B.: Health supervision of infants and young children, Am. J. Nursing 52:1460, 1952.

Sellew, Gladys: Nursing of Children, pp. 52–55, 270–282, Philadelphia, Saunders, 1948.

Simmons, Leo W.: The manipulations of human resources in nursing care, Am. J. Nursing 51:452, 1951.

Spock, Benjamin: Baby and Child Care, New York, Pocket Books, 1946.

State of California, Department of Public Health, Bureau of Maternal and Child Health, *Straight from the Start*, 1944.

Thoms, Herbert: Training for Childbirth, pp. 63–72, New York, McGraw-Hill, 1950.

Questions Relating to the Patient Study

1. One of the questions which Mrs. Kurz asked the nurse was "whether the baby should wear a 'belly band.' " The nurse should explain that a band is not recommended because

   a._____it makes additional work.

   b._____bands are usually not kept in the proper position.

   c._____cord stumps heal more satisfactorily when uncovered.

   d._____babies show fewer symptoms of colic when bands are not used.

2. Mrs. Kurz noticed that the baby's eyes were swollen and red. Mrs. Marsh should explain that this is

   a._____due to the silver nitrate used in the eyes.

   b._____normal for newborn infants.

   c._____the result of a rapid delivery.

   d._____a reaction to the vitamin K.

3. The mother asked Mrs. Marsh why the baby's hands and feet were cold and blue. The nurse should have told her this was because the

   a._____baby was exposed while they were inspecting him.

   b._____circulation of the blood to the extremities is not yet well established.

   c._____oxygen in the room is inadequate.

   d._____baby's respirations are shallow and irregular.

4. Mrs. Kurz commented that her other babies had lost weight during the first few days of life. The nurse should assure her that this is normal, and because of

   a._____inadequate food intake.

   b._____inability to use fluids properly.

   c._____passage of urine and feces.

   d._____an unknown cause.

5. Mrs. Marsh should tell the mother that weight lost during the first few days of life should be regained by the

    a._____sixth to tenth day.
    b._____fourteenth to sixteenth day.
    c._____sixteenth to twentieth day.
    d._____tenth to fourteenth day.

6. In answer to Mrs. Kurz' question about whether or not the baby can see, the nurse should tell her that he can

    a._____see only moving figures.
    b._____distinguish light from dark.
    c._____distinguish colors but not shapes.
    d._____not see at all.

7. Mrs. Kurz expressed concern one day when she noticed that the baby's eyes were crossed. The nurse should tell the mother that

    a._____this is common during the first year of life.
    b._____the condition will be reported to an eye specialist.
    c._____the eye muscles of co-ordination are undeveloped in a newborn infant.
    d._____it is nothing to cause her worry.

8. If Mrs. Kurz' breasts become so full that Baby Thomas has difficulty grasping the nipple and areola, the nurse should

    a._____discontinue breast feeding.
    b._____express some milk manually.
    c._____give the mother a nipple shield.
    d._____notify the physician.

9. During visiting hours one evening Mr. Kurz told the nurse on the postpartum floor that he was afraid Joanne and Betty would be jealous of the new baby. The nurse should suggest that the parents

    a._____ignore the girls; they'll outgrow their jealousy.
    b._____tell them they are supposed to love their baby brother.
    c._____leave them with their grandmother until the new baby is settled at home.
    d._____take each of them a baby doll at the time Baby Thomas is taken home.

Questions for Discussion and Student Projects

A. Related to the Patient Study

    1. Describe how Mrs. Kurz should be taught to care for Baby Thomas at home. Include bathing, diapering, feeding, clothing, addition of orange juice, arrangements for sleeping and any other points she might need to have reviewed.

2. Suppose Mrs. Kurz asks you how to prevent irritated or excoriated buttocks. List 4 or 5 causes of sore buttocks and describe a method recommended for the prevention of each.
3. Describe how you should instruct Mrs. Kurz in a safe, easy way to care for diapers.
4. As you are taking Baby Thomas to breast one day, the mother asks you what is meant by self-demand feeding. Explain in your own words to your classmates how best to describe this kind of management to Mrs. Kurz.
5. List the ways in which Baby Thomas may indicate his hunger.
6. How should you answer Mrs. Kurz when she asks you the value of having the baby circumcised before taking him home from the hospital? In your hospital, what is the care of a baby following circumcision? What should you do if you find such a baby bleeding?
7. Assume that Mrs. Kurz had been delivered at home. Show how you, a public health nurse, should instruct the family in the care of the mother and the new baby.

B. Related to the Section in General

1. Using a doll in the classroom, demonstrate how you determine accurately the length of a newborn infant.
2. Suggested project for one student: Investigate the weekly cost of diaper service in your community. How many diapers are needed weekly or daily for one infant? What provisions are made by the diaper service to assure absolute safety for babies?
3. Using an infant doll, demonstrate the procedure followed in your hospital in giving daily care to a newborn infant. What observations should you make at this time? What is the extent of the charting that is expected of the nurse?
4. Individual technic is recommended in the hospital care of newborn infants. What does this term mean to you? Describe how individual technic can be achieved in a centralized nursery.
5. Centralized nurseries (nurseries housing a large number of babies) were instituted as a result of the increase in the number of hospital confinements. Discuss the advantages and disadvantages of this plan. How can the advantages be maintained, at the same time reducing the disadvantages?
6. In your hospital what care is given the cord stump? Upon what principles is this care based?
7. Compare the various methods of preparing infant formulae. Be prepared to discuss the advantages and disadvantages of each method. Explain how you would use materials and equipment usually found in the home in preparing formulae by each of these methods.
8. Describe how you should teach a new mother and baby the technic of breast feeding. What are the points that should be emphasized? (As a basis for this, consider the anatomy and physiology of the breast.)

9. Compare the technics used in the care of the breasts of a nursing mother. Take into consideration comfort of the mother, simplicity, adequacy, adaptability and cost.

10. How should the diet of a lactating mother differ from that of a pregnant woman? In what ways can the differences in needs be met?

11. In many places the procedures for giving perineal care are undergoing critical evaluation. Two of the main issues are whether to use cotton balls or tissue, and whether to use tap water or sterile water. Be prepared to present the pros and cons of each of these.

12. In giving care to a mother on the morning following her delivery, what teaching points should you include?

13. Some obstetricians advocate that exercises be done in the postpartum period. Be prepared to discuss the kinds of exercises most frequently used, and the rationale behind their use.

14. With one of your classmates as the mother, show how you would stress to her the importance of the follow-up examination by her physician. How would you impress upon her the importance of health supervision of her baby?

15. What are the recommended policies with regard to visitors on a postpartum floor? What are the reasons for these recommendations?

16. What is the policy in your hospital with regard to showing babies?

17. Early ambulation is an established practice in many obstetric units. In your hospital, what changes in policies and procedures have been made or would have to be made to meet the demands of this practice? Take into consideration perineal care, breast and formula feeding, bathing and change of linen.

18. What is meant by rooming-in? What are the stated advantages of this plan for the care of mothers and babies?

19. Assume that you have been delegated the responsibility of organizing a teaching program for mothers in your postpartum unit. Construct a course outline, indicating what you would teach, the number and length of classes, who should teach and the equipment and teaching aids you consider necessary for such a project.

20. Are there facilities available in your community for health supervision in the home by public health nurses of mothers and babies? What method of referral is used between the hospital and public health nursing agency?

21. Assume that one of the mothers to whom you are assigned is depressed and weeping, on her third postpartum day. Insofar as you know, there is nothing wrong with either her, her baby or her family. What are the possible causes of her depression? What should be your course of action?

22. A mother under your care, who is due to go home the following day, tells you that her 5-year-old daughter has just come down with the measles. What suggestions would you have to offer her regarding plans for leaving the hospital?

Questions Relating to the Section in General

1. The average weight and length of term infants at birth is

   a._____8–9 pounds, 19–20 inches.
   b._____7–7½ pounds, 19–20 inches.
   c._____6½–7 pounds, 20–21 inches.
   d._____8½–9 pounds, 21–22 inches.

2. The circumference of the average infant's head at birth is

   a._____35 cm.
   b._____30 cm.
   c._____25 cm.
   d._____38 cm.

3. The anterior fontanel is an opening in the skull formed by the

   a._____parietal and occipital bones.
   b._____frontal and occipital bones.
   c._____temporal and frontal bones.
   d._____parietal and frontal bones.

4. Respirations in early infancy are described as

   a._____irregular, abdominal, 35–45 per minute.
   b._____regular, abdominal, 25–35 per minute.
   c._____regular, noisy, 35–45 per minute.
   d._____irregular, quiet, 45–55 per minute.

5. The average pulse rate of newborn infants is

   a._____100–120.
   b._____150–160.
   c._____120–150.
   d._____110–130.

6. If undisturbed, in 24 hours the newborn infant will sleep

   a._____18–20 hours.
   b._____20–22 hours.
   c._____16–18 hours.
   d._____14–16 hours.

7. Measures which have been found useful in the reduction of crying in nurseries are

   a._____self-demand feeding, picking up crying infants.
   b._____self-demand feeding, ignoring crying infants.
   c._____rigid feeding schedule, talking to babies in a soothing voice.
   d._____rigid feeding schedule, picking up crying infants.

8. Icterus neonatorum, or physiologic jaundice, frequently is seen in newborn infants. The basis for this phenomenon is

a.____rapid increase in red blood cells, blocked bile duct.

b.____rapid destruction of red blood cells, immature function of the liver.

c.____contamination of the cord, rapid destruction of white blood cells.

d.____blocked bile duct, immature function of the liver.

9. Fetal circulatory structures not needed for extrauterine life are

a.____ductus arteriosus, foramen ovale, pulmonary artery, hypogastric arteries.

b.____ductus venosus, foramen ovale, portal vein, ductus arteriosus.

c.____foramen ovale, pulmonary artery, ductus venosus, umbilical vein.

d.____umbilical vein, foramen ovale, ductus venosus, ductus arteriosus.

10. Of the 5 special senses, those having the highest development at birth are

a.____touch and taste.

b.____touch and hearing.

c.____hearing and smell.

d.____vision and taste.

11. The lochial discharge in the early postpartum period consists of blood, mucus and particles of decidua from the placental site. The nurse should expect, under normal conditions, to note this type of lochia for approximately

a.____1 day.

b.____3 days.

c.____5 days.

d.____7 days.

12. The names given to the types of lochia, in order of their appearance, are

a.____rubra, alba, serosa.

b.____serosa, alba, rubra.

c.____rubra, serosa, alba.

d.____alba, serosa, rubra.

13. The menstrual flow of a woman who does not nurse her baby is likely to return

a.____within 6 weeks after labor.

b.____within 8 weeks after labor.

c.____as soon as her breasts dry up.

14. After-pains result from the contractile efforts of the uterus to

a.____return to its normal size.

b.____expel blood clots.

c.____return to its normal position.

15. After-pains are experienced most frequently by

    a._____multiparae before nursing.
    b._____multiparae after nursing.
    c._____primiparae before nursing.
    d._____primiparae after nursing.

16. A mother who is receiving ergotrate following delivery should be warned that

    a._____it probably will make her dizzy.
    b._____she may become nauseated.
    c._____it will make her breasts dry up.
    d._____she may experience after-pains.

17. The nurse may consider as normal the immediate reactions to delivery of

    a._____chill, exhaustion, tremors.
    b._____chill, exhaustion, slightly elevated temperature.
    c._____exhaustion, slightly elevated temperature, elevated pulse rate.
    d._____sharp rise in temperature, tremors.

18. A chill following delivery is usually the result of

    a._____nervous reaction and exhaustion, exposure during delivery.
    b._____exposure during delivery, sudden reduction of intra-abdominal pressure.
    c._____sudden reduction of intra-abdominal pressure, nervous reaction and exhaustion.
    d._____concealed hemorrhage, exposure during delivery.

19. After the birth of the baby, lactation is stimulated by

    a._____estrogen.
    b._____progesterone.
    c._____androgen.
    d._____lactogen.

20. Prior to delivery the action of this hormone was inhibited by the secretion of

    a._____estrogen by the placenta.
    b._____progesterone by the ovaries.
    c._____androgen by the ovaries.
    d._____lactogen by the pituitary.

21. Colostrum, the forerunner of milk, usually is secreted

    a._____during pregnancy, for 2 weeks following delivery.
    b._____during pregnancy, for 3 days following delivery.
    c._____for 3 days following delivery.
    d._____for 2 weeks following delivery.

Section 2. Nursing Care in Problems of Sterility

STUDY SUGGESTIONS: Before beginning the study of this Section, the student will find it helpful to

A. Review

1. In physiology texts: reproduction.

B. Study

1. In obstetric nursing, gynecologic and genitourinary texts: sterility.

C. Read the additional References listed before attempting to answer questions relating to each patient study.

THE CHILDLESS HOME—PATIENT STUDY

Mr. and Mrs. Calvin had been classmates at the State Teachers College. Soon after graduation they had married and both started to teach in the high school of a large Southern town. Their home was an old structure, which Mrs. Calvin had furnished tastefully with antiques. In anticipation of having a family, one room had been set aside to be used as a nursery. Among its contents were an old wooden cradle, a low armless rocking chair and a music box that played "Rock-a-Bye Baby."

After 5 years of marriage, Mrs. Calvin had not yet become pregnant, though she and her husband were very anxious to have children. She consulted her family physician, Dr. Fletcher, about her problem, explaining tearfully that her husband was blaming her for the lack, and she was afraid their marriage was being threatened as a result of the situation. After talking to her for a while, the doctor suggested that she visit the local Planned Parenthood Clinic, where she would have available to her the services of a marriage counselor as well as that of personnel who were specially trained in problems of sterility. Mrs. Calvin accepted the doctor's suggestion and made an appointment to go to the clinic the following week.

On her first visit to the clinic, Mrs. Calvin's social and medical history was taken by a nurse. Appointments were made for the following week for Mrs. Calvin to see the gynecologist, and Mr. Calvin the urologist.

References

Beck, Sr. M. Berenice: The Nurse, Handmaid of the Divine Physician, Philadelphia, Lippincott, 1945.

Boyle, Frances, Cohen, Hedwig, Hernandez, Marion, and Stahle, Pauline: The Nurse and Planned Parenthood, New York, Planned Parenthood Corporation of America, Inc.

Jeffers, Frances C.: Preparation for marriage, Am. J. Nursing 51:514, 1951.

Levy, John, and Monroe, Ruth: The Happy Family, New York, Knopf, 1938.

Marsh, Helen Rome: Psychologist can help in planning for Baby's adoption, The Child 14:68, 1949.

Stone, Abraham: Marriage counseling and the nursing profession, Am. J. Nursing 51:658, 1951.

————: Infertility, Am. J. Nursing 47:606, 1947; or Planned Parenthood, New York, Federation of America, (1952). (Booklet.)

————, and Stone, Hannah: Marriage Manual, New York, Simon and Schuster, 1952.

Walsh, Jane A: Twelfth grade girls study the problems of marriage and family living, *Publ. Health Nursing* 44:181, 1952.

Questions Relating to the Patient Study

1. Mrs. Calvin's social and medical history was taken by the nurse. Mrs. Calvin was told that one of the methods they would use in trying to help the couple to become pregnant was a review of her basal temperature record. This would be done in order to

   a.————determine the day during the menstrual cycle that ovulation usually occurs.

   b.————determine the probable date of onset of the next menstrual period.

   c.————discover the presence of existing infection.

   d.————determine her normal temperature range.

2. In keeping a basal temperature chart Mrs. Calvin will be instructed to take her temperature

   a.————rectally, at mid-day.

   b.————rectally, before retiring.

   c.————by mouth, before rising.

   d.————rectally, before rising.

3. Mrs. Calvin's temperature chart followed the typical pattern————as shown in the chart on p. 502.

4. After reviewing Mrs. Calvin's history, and making physical and pelvic examinations, the gynecologist did a test to determine the patency of the oviducts. This is called the

   a.————Hubner test.

   b.————Rubin test.

   c.————Kohlmer test.

   d.————Coombs test.

5. In doing a Rubin test, patent tubes are indicated by

   a.————shoulder pain.

   b.————abdominal cramps.

   c.————uterine cramps.

   d.————chest pain.

6. The urologist examined Mr. Calvin, and asked that he bring in a specimen of semen so that the activity and the number of normal spermatozoa could be determined. Some of the factors which may affect the production or activity of spermatozoa adversely are

a._____excessive physical activity, sexual excess, constitutional diseases.
b._____sexual abstinence, acid environment of spermatozoa, nutritional disorders.
c._____endocrine disorders, sexual excess, acid environment of spermatozoa.
d._____sexual abstinence, endocrine disturbances, developmental anomalies.

Questions Relating to the Situation Study

1. Had Mrs. Calvin come to you, as a friend, rather than to her physician, what should have been your course of action?
2. Suggested activity for one student: With one of your classmates as Mrs. Calvin, explain the purpose and the method of keeping a basal temperature record.

Questions Relating to the Section in General

1. Preparation for family living usually begins

   a._____in infancy.
   b._____in the pre-school period.
   c._____during adolescence.
   d._____during the engagement period.

2. The average life span of an ovum, under favorable conditions, is about

   a._____72 hours.
   b._____48 hours.
   c._____24 hours.
   d._____6 hours.

3. Under favorable conditions, the average life span of a spermatozoon is about

   a._____72 to 96 hours.
   b._____48 to 72 hours.
   c._____24 to 48 hours.
   d._____12 to 24 hours.

4. Obstruction of the oviducts is among the chief cause of sterility in women. Some other causes are

   a._____rachitic pelvis, congenital anomalies of the uterus, nutritional anemia.
   b._____fixed retroversion of the uterus, infantile uterus, nutritional anemia.
   c._____congenital anomalies of the uterus, hormonal imbalance, infantile uterus.
   d._____hormonal imbalance, rachitic pelvis, nutritional anemia.

5. It has been found that the woman is responsible for infertility in approximately

   a._____60% of the instances.
   b._____100% of the instances.

c._____20% of the instances.
d._____80% of the instances.

6. The childhood disease which frequently leads to inflammation of the testes and subsequent sterility is

a._____mumps.
b._____scarlet fever.
c._____diphtheria.
d._____measles.

7. Suppose a married woman asks your advice concerning the adoption of a baby. You should tell her

a._____to consult her family physician.
b._____to seek legal counsel.
c._____that most adoptions have proved unsatisfactory.
d._____to visit an authorized adoption agency.

8. In adopting a child, prospective parents usually are

a._____investigated by a social worker, given the child for a temporary trial period.
b._____discouraged in adopting a very young infant, urged to accept a child of either sex.
c._____encouraged to delay adoption for at least 5 years after marriage, investigated by a social worker.
d._____charged a fee by the social agency, given the child for a temporary period.

9. An adopted child should be told that he is adopted

a._____at the time he starts to school.
b._____before playmates have an opportunity to tease him.
c._____gradually, from the time he can understand.
d._____at the beginning of adolescence.

Questions for Discussion and Student Projects

1. Suggested activity for one student: Write to the Planned Parenthood Clinic nearest you for information regarding its program. What services does the clinic offer the community?
2. What is your understanding of the term "premarital counseling"? "Marriage counseling"? What qualifications is it desirable for a marriage counselor to have? How would you go about locating a marriage counselor in your community?
3. Who do you believe should assume the responsibility for the preparation of a child for family living? When should this preparation begin? What are the major areas you feel should be covered in preparing a child for family life?
4. Briefly describe the development and the transportation of a spermatozoon and an ovum. At what points may there be interferences which may result in sterility? What are some of the causes of sterility?

5. What do you consider to be the nurse's function in advising a person who consults her about contraceptive methods?
6. Explain the physiologic basis for the rhythm method of contraception.
7. On the Federal, state and local levels, what legislation has been passed to control the sale and distribution of contraceptive materials?
8. Project for one student: Consult with a priest to obtain the Roman Catholic view regarding contraception and artificial insemination.
9. What is artificial insemination? Under what circumstances may this procedure be done? What precautions are observed by the physician?
10. Suggested activity for one student: Contact a social worker regarding adoption. In what ways can the adopting parents foster in the child a feeling of belonging? If, after the legal phase of the adoption had been completed, a child was found to be mentally defective, what course of action would be open to the parents? How is a child's behavior and development evaluated before he is placed for adoption?

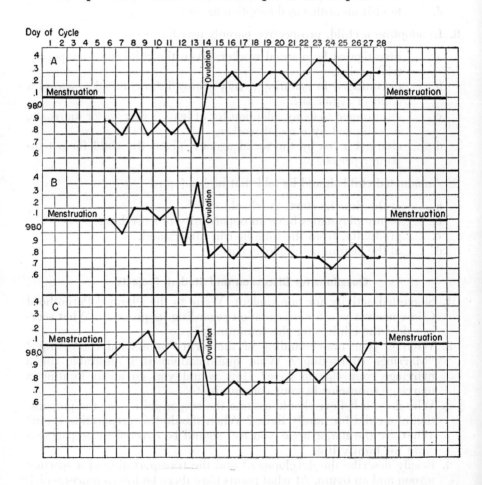

Section 3. Nursing Care of Mothers with Complications*

STUDY SUGGESTIONS: Before beginning the study of this Section, the student
will find it helpful to

A. Review
   1. In medical nursing texts: cardiac diseases, diabetes, syphilis, tuberculosis.
   2. In pharmacology texts: picrotoxin, vitamin K.
   3. In physiology texts: blood typing, Rh factor.

B. Study
   1. In nutrition texts: nutrition in pregnancy, diet in pre-eclampsia.
   2. In obstetric nursing texts: each of the conditions considered, cesarean
      section and forceps delivery, postpartum complications.

C. Read the additional References listed before attempting to answer questions
   relating to each patient study.

THE UNMARRIED MOTHER—PATIENT STUDY

Anita Jackson came to the admission ward of the hospital near her home
during the third month of pregnancy. She told the doctor she had been
spotting for 3 days, and now had moderate cramps. Until this time she
had had no difficulty with the pregnancy, and had not seen a doctor.
Speculum examination showed the cervix to be closed. The vulva and the
vagina were of a bluish color. The physician told her she would have to
be admitted to the hospital immediately, and left orders for morphine
sulfate 0.011 Gm. every 4 hours as necessary, and complete bed rest.

The bleeding and cramps gradually subsided by the fourth hospital day.
Anita was permitted out of bed on her sixth day, and was discharged from
the hospital 2 days later.

Anita was a thin, attractive, single girl of 24. She lived in a 3-room
apartment with her parents and 4 younger brothers and sisters, and contributed generously to the family upkeep from her salary as a sewing-
machine operator in a shirt factory. A nurse about her own age had been
assigned to care for Anita, and the two girls became quite friendly. Anita
confided in the nurse that she and her boy friend had been going together
for 3 years but that they couldn't marry since both were depended upon
by their families for support. She had told him about the pregnancy, and
both were looking forward to having a baby. Neither foresaw any difficulties with their families.

References

Burke, Bertha S.: Diet and nutrition during pregnancy, Am. J. Nursing 52:
1378, 1952.

* Cardiac diseases, diabetes, syphilis and tuberculosis are also considered in Part
One of this Study Guide. For disorders of the genitourinary system in pregnancy, see
pp. 131–136. Abortions are considered in the Medical-Surgical Nursing section, pp. 281–
282.

Confidential Nature of Birth Certificates, Children's Bureau Publication No. 332, Federal Security Agency, January 1949. (10¢)

Services for Unmarried Mothers and Their Children, Children's Bureau, Federal Security Agency, 1945. (10¢)

Questions for Discussion and Student Projects

1. Assume that you are the nurse in the situation. What should you have done when Anita told you her story?
2. Draw up a nursing care plan to be used for Anita during her early hospitalization. What kinds of information should be recorded by the nurse about Anita? What points should be stressed in teaching her? In your hospital, what is meant by complete bed rest?
3. In your community, what provisions could be made for the continued supervision of Anita's health following her discharge from the hospital?
4. On the basis of your knowledge of weight gain with relation to pregnancy and childbearing, should Anita be encouraged to gain more than the usual 15 to 20 pounds during pregnancy, so that she will not be underweight after she has had her baby?
5. With one of your classmates as Anita, plan with her a 3-day menu, taking into consideration her likes and dislikes and her limited budget, as well as the fact that the other family members will be eating with her.
6. In the event Anita did not marry before the birth of her baby, to what agency in your community might she be referred for assistance in planning for hospitalization and later care of the baby?

Questions Relating to the Patient Study

1. Anita's symptoms and the doctor's findings were suggestive of

   a._____inevitable abortion.
   b._____threatened abortion.
   c._____septic abortion.
   d._____therapeutic abortion.

2. Bluish discoloration of the vulva and the vagina is referred to as

   a._____Hegar's sign.
   b._____Goodell's sign.
   c._____Braxton Hicks's sign.
   d._____Chadwick's sign.

3. Morphine was ordered for her in order to

   a._____induce sleep.
   b._____stop uterine contractions.
   c._____reduce restlessness.
   d._____reduce bleeding.

4. She was placed on complete bed rest in an attempt to

   a._____induce sleep.
   b._____stop uterine contractions.

    c._____reduce restlessness.

    d._____reduce bleeding.

5. To keep Anita on complete bed rest, the nurse should see that she is

    a._____occupied, understands the reason for the order, understands what activities she may engage in.

    b._____unoccupied, understands the reason for the order, understands what activities she may engage in.

    c._____occupied, not told the reason for the order, understands what activities she may engage in.

Questions Relating to the Section in General

1. To give morphine sulfate 0.011 Gm. (gr. ⅙) from morphine sulfate 0.016 Gm. (gr. ¼) tablets, dissolve

    a._____one 0.016-Gm. tablet in minims xv of sterile water, discard minims v and administer minims x of the solution.

    b._____two 0.016-Gm. tablet in minims xx of sterile water, discard minims v and administer minims xv of the solution.

    c._____one 0.016-Gm. tablet in minims xx of sterile water, discard minims v and administer minims xv of the solution.

    d._____two 0.016-Gm. tablets in minims xv of sterile water, discard minims v and administer minims x of the solution.

2. Some of the other causes of bleeding in early pregnancy are hydatidiform mole, erosion of the cervix, ectopic pregnancy and carcinoma of the cervix. Hydatidiform mole describes the condition in which there is a

    a._____cystic degeneration of the chorion.

    b._____nodular cervix.

    c._____patulous cervix.

    d._____hypertrophy of the decidua.

3. Hydatidiform mole is characterized by

    a._____continuous bleeding, rapid decrease in the size of the uterus, destruction of the fetus.

    b._____destruction of the fetus, slow increase in the size of the uterus, intermittent bleeding.

    c._____rapid growth of the uterus, destruction of the fetus, intermittent bleeding.

4. Ectopic pregnancy usually results from the

    a._____rupture of a uterine pregnancy.

    b._____failure of a sperm to fertilize an ovum.

    c._____implantation of a fertilized ovum outside the uterine cavity.

    d._____failure of a fertilized ovum to implant.

5. The most common type of ectopic pregnancy is tubal. Within a few weeks after conception the tube may rupture, causing

    a._____sudden excruciating lower abdominal pain.

    b._____continuous dull lower abdominal pain.

   c.____painless vaginal bleeding.
   d.____intermittent uterine contractions.

6. Carcinoma of the cervix is rarely seen during pregnancy. When such a diagnosis is made, the course of action is to

   a.____allow the baby to go to term, then do a Porro-cesarean section.
   b.____allow the baby to go to viability, then do a Porro-cesarean section.
   c.____amputate the cervix, and allow the baby to go to term.
   d.____do an immediate radical hysterectomy.

Questions for Discussion and Student Projects—(*Continued*)

1. What should be your approach to the couple who has lost a baby in early pregnancy?
2. Why are pregnancy tests done at intervals following the expulsion of a hydatidiform mole? Is it possible for a woman who has had a hydatidiform mole to have a normal pregnancy in the future?
3. What are the laws in your state regulating the registration of births? Does the birth certificate indicate whether or not the child's parents were married at the time of his birth? Enumerate some of the instances in which a person might be called upon to show his birth certificate.
4. Occasionally mothers who are bleeding in early pregnancy are given stilbestrol from the onset of bleeding to the termination of pregnancy. Estimate the total cost of this drug to the mother who starts in the sixteenth week of her pregnancy to take 15 mg. of stilbestrol daily, increasing the dosage by 5 mg. a week until her fortieth week.
5. Explain the physiologic basis of the use of stilbestrol in threatened abortion.

THE COMMON LAW WIFE—PATIENT STUDY

Mrs. Thompson was relieved when at last the nurse beckoned her to the examining room. She had arrived for her first antepartum clinic visit promptly at 8:30 A.M. Half an hour later she was directed to a dressing room, given a cotton gown and told to remove all clothing but her shoes, to put on the gown and to sit on the bench until called. The 15-minute wait had seemed an eternity.

During his examination of Mrs. Thompson, the resident learned that this was her fourth pregnancy. The first 3 had terminated in spontaneous abortions at 3, 5 and 6 months, respectively. She had not been under a doctor's care during any of these pregnancies. The present pregnancy had been uneventful to date. Her last menstrual period began February 14— 5 months ago; she had felt life for the first time 2 weeks ago.

Following her dismissal from the examining room the social service worker talked with Mrs. Thompson. An excerpt from her record follows:

Common law marriage of 10 years, duration. Patient 35, husband 47. Both had grade school education. Living in basement of apartment building in which he is janitor. Patient works by day as domestic. No hospitalization, will try to pay part of hospital bill.

Reluctant to discuss pregnancy. Doesn't know how they'll manage financially after the baby is born.

A blood sample taken at the time of her first clinic visit demonstrated a strongly positive reaction indicating syphilis. The public health nurse contacted Mrs. Thompson in her home and arrangements were made for her hospitalization for penicillin therapy.

Reference

Huse, Betty, and Aufranc, W. H.: A proposal for joint action against congenital syphilis, The Child 14:182, 1950.

Stone, Emerson: Newborn Infant, pp. 196–204, 257–260, Philadelphia, Lea and Febiger, 1946.

Wegman, Myron E.: Congenital syphilis, Pediatrics vol. 7, 1950.

Questions Relating to the Patient Study

1. The dose of penicillin indicated for Mrs. Thompson is

    a.____4,000,000 units in 12 days.
    b.____40,000 units daily for 10 days.
    c.____450,000 units daily for 12 days.
    d.____4,000,000 units in 3 days.

2. With immediate antiluetic therapy Mrs. Thompson's pregnancy will probably terminate

    a.____prematurely, the infant having congenital syphilis.
    b.____before the baby is viable.
    c.____at term, the infant free from syphilis.
    d.____at term, the infant having congenital syphilis.

3. Mrs. Thompson's history of pregnancies

    a.____has no particular significance.
    b.____follows a pattern seen frequently in syphilitic women.
    c.____is indicative of endocrine dysfunction.
    d.____is typical of a habitual aborter.

4. The sign of pregnancy reported by Mrs. Thompson was

    a.____Braxton Hicks's.
    b.____lightening.
    c.____Goodell's.
    d.____quickening.

5. Mrs. Thompson's expected date of confinement is

    a.____November 7.
    b.____December 7.
    c.____December 21.
    d.____November 21.

6. Mrs. Thompson was considered to be a gravida

    a.____IV, para I.
    b.____IV, para O.

c.——I, para IV.
d.——IV, para II.

7. The tests which are done to determine the presence of syphilis **are**

   a.——Mazzini, Friedman, Wassermann.
   b.——Kline, Kahn, Kolmer.
   c.——Kolmer, Kline, Aschheim-Zondek.
   d.——Wassermann, Xenopus, Mazzini.

8. Syphilis usually is not infectious in the

   a.——primary stage, secondary stage.
   b.——secondary stage, latent stages.
   c.——latent stages, congenital.

Questions for Discussion and Student Projects

1. Assume that you are the public health nurse mentioned in the patient study. Plan your preparation for the visit and your approach to Mrs. Thompson.
2. Estimate the cost of penicillin used in treating Mrs. Thompson. What provisions might be made if she were unable to pay for the treatment?
3. In your locality, what resources would be available to the social worker in planning aid for Mrs. Thompson? What is the law regarding the man's legal responsibilities in common law marriages in your state?

Questions Relating to the Section in General

1. The causative agent in syphilis is

   a.——*Monilia albicans.*
   b.——Welsh bacillus.
   c.——*Treponema pallidum.*
   d.——*Trichomonas vaginalis.*

2. The manifestation most frequently associated with the first stage of syphilis is

   a.——general skin eruption.
   b.——condylomata lata.
   c.——chancroid.
   d.——chancre.

3. The action of penicillin is

   a.——bacteriostatic.
   b.——bacteriocytic.
   c.——antiseptic.
   d.——antibiotic.

4. The syphilitic placenta is

   a.——large, pale, edematous.
   b.——large, dark, thin.

c._____of average diameter, pale, edematous.
d._____of small diameter, pale, edematous.

5. Timely treatment of the syphilitic woman will benefit

a._____only the mother.
b._____the mother and the baby.
c._____only the baby.

6. Some of the common sites of gonorrheal infection in the female are the

a._____urethra, oviducts, Bartholin's glands.
b._____eyes, mouth, Skene's glands.
c._____mouth, urethra, Skene's glands.
d._____Skene's glands, oviducts, mouth.

7. If infection occurs at birth, symptoms of ophthalmia neonatorum usually appear within

a._____5 or 6 days.
b._____2 to 3 days.
c._____24 hours.
d._____10 days.

Questions for Discussion and Student Projects—(*Continued*)

1. What are the laws in your community regarding premarital and prenatal serologic examinations?
2. Discuss the possible educational, medical and legal measures which can help in the prevention of venereal diseases.
3. Describe the procedure followed by a physician in your community in reporting venereal diseases. What attempt is made to seek out contacts?
4. Describe the policy in your hospital regarding (a) care of the mother with active syphilis before, during and after labor, and (b) care of the baby.
5. What are the characteristics of an infant with congenital syphilis? Approximately when does each of these characteristics appear?
6. Describe the symptoms and course of a gonorrheal infection in a woman. If an existing gonorrheal infection is not cured during pregnancy, what precautions should be observed by the nurse for her own protection?
7. Describe the course of gonorrheal ophthalmia neonatorum. What law in your state is designed to prevent this disease?
8. Consider the antepartum unit of the out-patient department of your hospital or community. What suggestions have you for improving it from the standpoint of the comfort of the expectant mother? How could their waiting time be used for teaching?

MATERNAL TRAGEDY—PATIENT STUDY

When admitted to the hospital at 3:00 P.M., Mrs. Stewart seemed alert and calm but could not recall anything that had happened since noon. Mr. Stewart told the physician that his wife had been complaining of severe pain in the upper abdomen all morning, had had a convulsion at about noon and another while they were on their way to the hospital. For about a week she had been bothered by headaches and "blind spots." He had noticed that her face had become quite full.

The Stewarts, both in their early thirties, had been married for 8 years. They owned a new ranch-type house in the suburbs of a large city, where he is employed as a radio engineer. Mrs. Stewart, a former model, has not been employed since their marriage. Aside from managing their home, she devotes a great deal of time to working with charitable organizations, remaining active throughout her pregnancy.

Mrs. Stewart is a primigravida. She has been under the care of an obstetrician; her pregnancy had been normal until the thirty-eighth week, when the symptoms described began to appear. Admission examinations showed

Blood pressure 190/112.
Albuminuria 4+.
Fetal heart rate 140.
Uterus irritable.
Cervix effaced, dilated 2 cm.
Presenting part at the spines.
Membranes intact.

A diagnosis of eclampsia was established. Membranes were ruptured artificially and fractional doses of pitocin given. During her labor Mrs. Stewart was given morphine 0.016 Gm. every 2 hours, and 50 per cent magnesium sulfate 2 cc. on the alternate hours. An indwelling catheter was inserted; her average output was 30 cc. every 4 hours. She was placed in an oxygen tent shortly after admission. After an inertial labor of 27 hours, during which time she had 6 convulsions, a mid-forceps extraction was done to deliver a 6-pound stillborn infant. Mrs. Stewart died a few minutes after the delivery of her baby.

References

Eastman, Nicholson J., et al.: Definition and classification of toxemias brought up-to-date, *The Mother* pp. 10–11, Summer, 1952.

————: Williams' Obstetrics, New York, pp. 778–785, Appleton-Century-Crofts, 1950.

Scharr, Henry A., Nagle, Richard A., and Priest, Benjamin: The patient's spiritual needs, Am. J. Nursing 50:75, 1950.

Zabriskie, Louise, and Eastman, Nicholson J.: Nurses' Handbook of Obstetrics, pp. 224–236, Philadelphia, Lippincott, 1952.

Questions Relating to the Patient Study

1. The symptom experienced by Mrs. Stewart, which often warns of impending convulsions in the toxic mother, was

    a._____headaches.
    b._____severe epigastric pain.
    c._____scotoma.
    d._____all of the above.

2. 50 per cent magnesium sulfate was given to Mrs. Stewart to

   a.____reduce her blood pressure.
   b.____stimulate labor contractions.
   c.____reduce edema of the brain.
   d.____increase peristalsis.

3. Mrs. Stewart's loss of memory following her first convulsion was

   a.____a danger signal.
   b.____to be expected.
   c.____of no significance.

4. The severe epigastric pain experienced by Mrs. Stewart probably was

   a.____a warning of impending convulsions.
   b.____a warning of impending labor.
   c.____the result of a bad digestive upset.
   d.____of no significance.

5. Fractional doses of pitocin were given to

   a.____stimulate uterine contractions.
   b.____reduce the blood pressure.
   c.____provide sedation.
   d.____increase urinary output.

6. Low urinary output was an indication of

   a.____low fluid intake.
   b.____excessive perspiration.
   c.____high sodium intake.
   d.____kidney impairment.

7. Death of the baby probably was caused by

   a.____injury during a convulsion.
   b.____birth injury.
   c.____insufficient tissue oxidation.
   d.____imperfect expansion of the lungs.

8. The cause of Mrs. Stewart's convulsions probably was

   a.____hypertension, edema of the brain.
   b.____arteriolar spasm, scotoma.
   c.____hypertension, arteriolar spasm.
   d.____edema of the brain, scotoma.

Questions for Discussion and Student Projects

1. An important point in the care of Mrs. Stewart was the reduction of external stimuli. What is the reason for this? Describe measures which should be taken to provide a quiet environment, including instruction of hospital personnel and visitors, placement of the patient within the unit and organization of nursing activities.

2. Set up a unit in the classroom as you would for Mrs. Stewart. With one of your classmates as the patient, demonstrate what you should do during one of her convulsive seizures.

3. With one of your classmates as Mr. Stewart, explain the reasons for such orders as "no visitors" and "use oxygen tent." How would you respond to his questions: "Just what is wrong with my wife? Will she be all right? Will the baby be all right?"

Questions Relating to the Section in General

1. Three warning signs of pre-eclampsia are

    a._____sudden weight gain, hypertension, albuminuria.
    b._____nausea and vomiting, hypertension, albuminuria.
    c._____sudden weight gain, diplopia, albuminuria.
    d._____diplopia, nausea and vomiting, hypertension.

2. The diet often prescribed for the pre-eclamptic mother is

    a._____low sodium, low protein, high carbohydrate.
    b._____low sodium, low protein, low carbohydrate.
    c._____high sodium, high protein, high carbohydrate.
    d._____low sodium, high protein, low carbohydrate.

3. The sodium intake is reduced in toxemias of pregnancy in an effort to reduce

    a._____hypertension.
    b._____edema.
    c._____scotoma.
    d._____albuminuria.

4. Among the foods the pre-eclamptic mother may eat are

    a._____canned soups, carbonated beverages, frozen vegetables.
    b._____carbonated beverages, frozen vegetables, fresh fruits.
    c._____fresh fruits, fresh vegetables, shellfish.
    d._____fresh fruits, fresh vegetables, red meats.

5. In talking with an expectant mother, you would advise her to keep her appointments with her doctor so that he would be able to

    a._____check her for signs of abnormalities.
    b._____check on the growth of the baby.
    c._____help her to maintain a state of good health.
    d._____teach her the danger signs.

6. On admission to the hospital, the mother with severe pre-eclampsia would be placed in a

    a._____semi-private room with plenty of sunlight, have unlimited visitors.
    b._____semi-private darkened room, have unlimited visitors.
    c._____single darkened room, have no visitors.
    d._____single room with plenty of sunlight, have no visitors.

7. Pre-eclampsia and eclampsia are disorders which are

    a._____peculiar to the first trimester.
    b._____peculiar to the second trimester.
    c._____peculiar to the third trimester.
    d._____apt to occur at any time during pregnancy.

8. The patient with the diagnosis of chronic hypertensive disease has an elevated blood pressure

    a._____only on exertion.
    b._____before she becomes pregnant.
    c._____only in the second and third trimesters.
    d._____none of the above.

9. The purpose of bed rest in pre-eclampsia is to

    a._____reduce blood pressure by lowering body metabolism.
    b._____conserve energy in view of the impending labor.
    c._____reduce the incidence of headaches.
    d._____reduce contact with other patients.

10. After delivery of the pre-eclamptic mother

    a._____danger of convulsions has passed.
    b._____symptoms disappear immediately.
    c._____chronic hypertensive disease develops.
    d._____symptoms disappear gradually.

11. In the treatment of eclampsia, magnesium sulfate should be administered

    a._____rectally.
    b._____intramuscularly.
    c._____orally.
    d._____intravenously.

Questions for Discussion and Student Projects— (*Continued*)

1. What are the methods of choice in the treatment of pre-eclamptic and eclamptic toxemias in your hospital? Be prepared to explain the rationale behind these treatments.
2. What measures can be taken to reduce the incidence of pre-eclampsia? Consider the doctor and the nurse, as well as the patient and her family?
3. Consider the various laboratory tests that might be done for the pre-eclamptic mother in your hospital. What is the significance of each of these tests?
4. What instructions would you give to a pre-eclamptic mother who had been advised to go on a low-sodium diet, with regard to foods which may be eaten, foods to be avoided, preparation of meals and planning family menus around her diet?
5. Investigate the procedure followed by your hospital when a patient is placed on the serious list. How is the immediate family notified? What

is the policy, generally, regarding visitors? List your responsibilities in preparing the patient and the room for a visit by a clergyman.

6. Suggested activity for one student: consult with the clergymen of the various religious groups to determine under what conditions an infant is baptized by hospital personnel. How should you baptize an infant? How is the baptism registered in the parish?

7. From your knowledge of the uses, action and administration of pitocin, how should you care for a mother receiving the drug during labor? How does Pitocin differ from pituitrin?

8. Review the topic of forceps operations. How are they classified? What are the indications? Compare the mortality rates of forceps extractions with those of cesarean sections and of vaginal deliveries.

BILLY HAS A LITTLE SISTER—PATIENT STUDY

The Morrisons live in a furnished 3-room apartment on the third floor of a tenement. Mr. Morrison works as a night watchman in a nearby factory; Mrs. Morrison supplements their income by crocheting doilies, potholders, etc., to order. Their first child, Billy, was 18 months old when Mrs. Morrison again became pregnant. Billy is a lively youngster who requires considerable supervision, since his greatest joys are climbing and turning on gas jets.

Mrs. Morrison's second pregnancy was uneventful until the thirty-fourth week, at which time she started to bleed vaginally. The clinic doctor ordered her to remain in bed at home. Intermittent bleeding continued; there was no associated pain. Her blood pressure and pulse and the fetal heart rate remained within normal limits. The following week the bleeding became more profuse and Mrs. Morrison was admitted to the hospital. At this time the doctor estimated the baby's weight to be about 5 pounds. Some of the orders left for her were:

> Blood typing; Rh factor and crossmatch 500 cc. of whole blood.
> Report unusual bleeding.
> Mol iron tab. II t.i.d. p.c.

Four days after admission to the hospital she passed several small clots and the bleeding increased, becoming continuous. She was prepared and taken to the operating room, where a low cervical cesarean section was done and a 6-pound baby girl delivered. The diagnosis of central placenta previa was confirmed.

Reference

Lam, Conrad R.: What is "shock"? Am. J. of Nursing 51:116, 1951.

Questions Relating to the Patient Study

1. Mol iron was given for the purpose of

    a._____replacing hemoglobin lost in bleeding.
    b._____providing iron for the baby.
    *c._____increasing the number of red blood cells.
    d._____building up resistance to infection.

2. It was given after meals to

    a._____reduce achlorhydria.
    b._____reduce loss of appetite.
    c._____reduce gastric irritation.
    d._____secure maximum solution in the gastric juice.

3. Mrs. Morrison's history was

    a._____typical of placenta previa.
    b._____suggestive of premature separation of the placenta.
    c._____typical of both placenta previa and premature separation of the placenta.
    d._____atypical of placenta previa.

4. Mrs. Morrison's doctor estimated the weight of her baby by

    a._____funduscopic examinations.   c._____palpation.
    b._____auscultation.   d._____vaginal examination.

5. Cesarean section was postponed as long as possible because

    a._____the later it is done, the safer it is for the mother.
    b._____the longer the baby remains in utero, until term, the better chance it has to survive.
    c._____it is done only as a last resort.
    d._____it is not a safe procedure while a mother is bleeding.

6. The doctor performed a cesarean section to

    a._____provide the safest method of delivery for the mother.
    b._____provide the safest method of delivery for the baby.
    c._____provide the safest method of delivery for both the mother and the baby.
    d._____avoid having Mrs. Morrison exert herself during labor.

7. Compared to lochia following a vaginal delivery, Mrs. Morrison's lochia would be expected to be

    a._____the same in amount and odor.
    b._____of the same odor, less in amount.
    c._____less in amount, with a foul odor.
    d._____of the same odor, greater in amount.

8. Mrs. Morrison was told that nursing

    a._____the baby would help the healing of the abdominal wound.
    b._____is not permitted following a cesarean section.
    c._____is not possible following a cesarean section.
    d._____would aid involution.

9. The doctor refrained from doing a vaginal examination to

    a._____reduce the possibility of infection.
    b._____avoid aggravation of bleeding.
    c._____avoid discomfort to Mrs. Morrison.
    d._____avoid injury to the baby.

Questions for Discussion and Student Projects

1. Assume that you have been assigned to care for Mrs. Morrison on her admission to the hospital. Outline a plan for her nursing care. Be prepared to discuss the reason for each point you have included. Discuss in detail the emotional aspects of her care. What do you think might be Mr. Morrison's feelings regarding his wife's condition? What are your responsibilities toward him?

2. What would be the responsibilities of the public health nurse visiting Mrs. Morrison while she was confined to bed at home, before her admission to the hospital? What instructions should she give to the patient? To her family? What suggestions should she make regarding the care of Billy? Regarding provision for adequate rest for Mr. Morrison?

3. In the event a vaginal examination had been indicated, what preparation would have been required? What would be your duties before, during and after the examination?

4. What points would you cover in preparing Mrs. Morrison for surgery? What preparation should be made for the reception of the baby?

5. Should Mrs. Morrison be permitted to nurse her baby if she so desires? Why?

6. What are the salient points in the postoperative care of Mrs. Morrison? Do you think she should be placed on a postpartum or postoperative floor? Why?

Questions Relating to the Patient Study—(*Continued*)

1. A second major cause of bleeding in the last trimester of pregnancy is premature separation of the placenta. Of these signs and symptoms, a patient with this complication might present

   a.＿＿decrease in size of the uterus, cessation of contractions, visible or concealed hemorrhage.
   b.＿＿tense and tender uterus, concealed or visible hemorrhage, shock.
   c.＿＿increase in size of the uterus, visible bleeding, no associated pain.
   d.＿＿shock, decrease in size of the uterus, absence of external bleeding.

2. Premature separation of the placenta is also known as

   a.＿＿abruptio placenta.
   b.＿＿placenta previa.
   c.＿＿placenta acreta.
   d.＿＿placenta increta.

3. In premature separation of the placenta, shock is

   a.＿＿seldom seen.
   b.＿＿often greater than bleeding would seem to indicate.
   c.＿＿often less than bleeding would seem to indicate.
   d.＿＿always seen.

4. Premature separation of the placenta frequently is associated with

    a._____syphilis.
    b._____tuberculosis.
    c._____toxemia of pregnancy.
    d._____multiple pregnancy.

Questions for Discussion and Student Projects—*(Continued)*

1. Why is postpartum hemorrhage frequently associated with placenta previa? What are the nurse's responsibilities in the prevention and control of postpartum hemorrhage? List as many other causes of postpartum hemorrhage as you can. Why might each of these predispose a mother to hemorrhage?
2. Review the signs of shock. What measure would you take if you found an undelivered mother in shock? A postpartum mother? Consider the effect of your activities on the mother; on her visitors; on other patients; on their visitors.
3. What are the ways in which premature separation of the placenta and placenta previa endanger the life of the infant? What are the signs of fetal distress?
4. Compare the types of cesarean sections as to safety to the mother and the baby, site of incision and ease of operation. Under what conditions might each be chosen? List as many indications as you can for a cesarean section. Why might each of these conditions require a section?
5. Suggested activity for one student: find out from a pharmacist the retail price of several widely used iron preparations. Compare the costs to the mother who has been instructed to take the average dose of iron during the last trimester of pregnancy and during lactation.

THE SOLDIER'S BRIDE—PATIENT STUDY

Robert Gilbreth was inducted into the Army upon being graduated from high school. Within a few months he married his high-school sweetheart, Virginia, and they rented a furnished 1-room apartment near the post to which he was assigned. A year later Pfc. Gilbreth was sent to Korea and Mrs. Gilbreth returned to her parents' home.

Mrs. Gilbreth had been diabetic since the age of 13, and had been under the supervision of an internist. Upon returning to her parents' home, she visited her physician who confirmed her suspicion of an existing pregnancy and referred her to an obstetrician for care. Throughout her pregnancy she was followed closely by both specialists. During this time she kept herself busy helping with the housework and preparing for the baby. She wrote her husband daily and received frequent letters from him.

Approximately 2 months before term, she was admitted to the hospital; she weighed 140 pounds, having gained 15 pounds in 2 weeks, had moderate hydramnios and edema of the legs and hands. At the time of admission her blood pressure was 120/70, blood sugar 128 mg., N.P.N 30.8, urine sugar negative. The baby's heart rate could not be heard and fetal movement could not be palpated, although Mrs. Gilbreth insisted she could feel the baby moving. The report of the flat plate of the abdomen stated that the baby was of approximately 8 months' gestation, breech presentation. A low cervical cesarean section was performed and a living baby boy delivered, birth weight 9 pounds 1 ounce, birth length 21 inches.

At birth the baby was very edematous. By the time he was 4 days old he had lost 1 pound 4 ounces. Regular feedings had been established and the baby seemed to be doing very well.

Following the operation, Mrs. Gilbreth received an infusion of 1,000 cc. of 5 percent glucose in water, to which regular insulin, 20 units, had been added. Her postoperative course was uneventful. Through the efforts of the American Red Cross her husband was returned home after 6 months in Japan, in time to take his wife and son, Bobby, home from the hospital.

References

Betzold, Virginia: How safe is your mask? Am. J. Nursing 43:59, 1943.
Eastman, Nicholson J.: Williams' Obstetrics, pp. 633–640, New York, Appleton-Century-Crofts, 1950.
Frobischer, Martin, Jr.: Practical disinfection in hospitals, Am. J. Nursing 45: 610, 1945.
Petkauskos, Mary, and White, Pricilla: Pregnancy complicating diabetes mellitus, Am. J. Nursing, 48:300, 1948.
Redmond, Grace C.: Tuberculosis nursing technics, Am. J. Nursing 51:399, 1951.

Questions Relating to the Patient Study

1. In all probability, the fetal heart could not be heard because of

    a._____hydramnios.
    b._____a thick abdominal wall.
    c._____the breech presentation.
    d._____the short period of gestation.

2. Mrs. Gilbreth's blood sugar was

    a._____slightly elevated.
    b._____greatly elevated.
    c._____within normal range.
    d._____lower than normal.

3. Usually, the baby born of a diabetic mother is

    a._____of average length, underweight.
    b._____of average length, heavier than normal.
    c._____longer and heavier than normal.
    d._____about the same in weight and length as other babies.

4. The baby whose mother is diabetic, but whose father is neither diabetic nor a carrier, will be

    a._____nondiabetic, a carrier.
    b._____diabetic, a carrier.

    c._____diabetic, a noncarrier.
    d._____nondiabetic, a noncarrier.

5. In a low cervical cesarean section, the uterine incision is made in the

    a._____lower portion of the cervix.
    b._____upper portion of the cervix.
    c._____lower uterine segment.
    d._____upper uterine segment.

Questions for Discussion and Student Projects

1. Outline a plan for the nursing care of Mrs. Gilbreth before and after her operation. Review the signs and symptoms of hypoglycemic shock and of diabetic coma. What emergency measures would you take if you found Mrs. Gilbreth in coma? In shock?
2. What are some of the maternal and infant complications which are frequently associated with diabetes? Why are they so often seen in this condition? What measures can be taken to prevent their development?
3. What are the important points in the nursing care of Bobby? How would you determine the presence of hypoglycemic shock in a newborn infant?
4. Would you have been able to be of any help to Mrs. Gilbreth had you found her, during her pregnancy, to be despondent over the absence of her husband? If so, how?

Questions Relating to the Section in General

1. In addition to diabetes, tuberculosis and heart disease frequently are seen in women of childbearing age. A woman with active tuberculosis often

    a._____improves during pregnancy, suffers a relapse after delivery.
    b._____remains the same during pregnancy, suffers a relapse after delivery.
    c._____remains the same during pregnancy, improves following delivery.
    d._____does poorly during pregnancy, improves following delivery.

2. A mother with active tuberculosis should

    a._____nurse her baby if she so desires, not otherwise care for it.
    b._____not nurse her baby, otherwise care for it.
    c._____not nurse her baby, not care for it.
    d._____nurse her baby, otherwise care for it.

3. A cardiac mother in labor usually is

    a._____permitted to have a normal second stage.
    b._____delivered by cesarean section at term.
    c._____delivered by forceps as soon as she reaches the second stage.
    d._____delivered by cesarean section as soon as the baby is viable.

4. Typical symptoms of pyelitis are pain over the

    a._____sacral region, low-grade fever, night sweats.
    b._____lumbar region, high fever, chills.
    c._____sacral region, high fever, night sweats.
    d._____lumbar region, low-grade fever, chills.

5. German measles is of importance during pregnancy because of the

    a._____tendency of the mother to abort.
    b._____interference with oxygenation of the blood.
    c._____increased incidence of congenital defects.
    d._____danger of sepsis.

6. The vaginal discharge typical of *Trichomonas vaginalis* is

    a._____scant, thin, watery, nonirritating.
    b._____moderate, blood-tinged mucus, nonirritating.
    c._____profuse, white, irritating.
    d._____profuse, yellow, irritating.

7. A baby born of a mother who has *Monilia* vaginitis may develop

    a._____thrush.
    b._____gonorrhea.
    c._____impetigo.
    d._____diarrhea.

8. *Monilia* vaginitis responds readily to treatment with

    a._____silver nitrate.
    b._____penicillin.
    c._____gentian violet.
    d._____boric acid.

Questions for Discussion and Student Projects—(*Continued*)

1. What are some of the discomforts often experienced by the expectant mother? How would you explain the causes of these to a mother? What points might be included in teaching the expectant mother to help prevent these from occurring? What advice could you give with regard to overcoming these conditions?
2. Theoretically, hyperemesis gravidarum is caused by one or more of the following factors: neurosis, toxicity, alteration of hormonal production, alteration of gastric motility. On what basis may each be thought to cause excessive vomiting?
3. Discuss in detail the nursing care you think should be given a cardiac woman in labor.
4. What are the policies in your hospital regarding the care of a mother with active tuberculosis? Where is she placed during labor? Where is she delivered? What is the aftercare of these rooms? Where is she placed after delivery? Is her baby sent to the newborn nursery?
5. What instructions would you give to the mother who had been told in antepartum clinic to take a vinegar douche?

A COMPLICATED LABOR

Background Review Question

1. Complete the following questions by placing the letter preceding the term in the left-hand column next to the proper descriptive phrase in the right-hand column.

a. version.	(1)____a drug agent used to obliterate memory.
b. rotation.	
c. frank breech.	(2)____one or both feet presenting.
d. footling breech.	(3)____painful, slow or difficult labor.
e. complete breech.	(4)____turning a baby in utero to change the presenting part.
f. dystocia.	
g. amnesic.	(5)____both legs extended so that the feet are near the face.
h. analgesic.	
i. anesthesia.	(6)____turning a baby in utero to change the position.
	(7)____a drug agent used to relieve discomfort.
	(8)____a drug agent used to hasten labor.
	(9)____a subdivision of the uterine surface of the placenta.
	(10)____a drug agent used to produce loss of feeling.
	(11)____feet and legs flexed on the thighs, thighs flexed on the abdomen, so that feet and buttocks present.

A COMPLICATED LABOR—PATIENT STUDY

Miss Watkins, a student nurse, reported on duty at 11 P.M. and was assigned to care for Mrs. Shaw, who was in the labor room. Some of the information she obtained about the patient from her record is as follows:

Admission not—6 P.M. 3/12/53
    Age: 20.
    Race: Negro.
    Religion: Baptist.
    Gravida IV, para III.
    Usual childhood diseases.
    Past pregnancies uneventful:
        1949—living male, at term, birth weight 7 pounds.
        1950—living male, at term, birth weight 6½ pounds.
        1952—living male, at term, birth weight 7½ pounds. Died of pneumonia at 3½ months.
    Present pregnancy at term. No medical care. No signs and symptoms of toxemia.
    Abdominal examination: ROP engaged. Estimated weight of baby 7½–8 pounds.
    Rectal examination: Cervix effaced, dilated 4 cm. Sagittal suture in the right oblique. Presenting part 1 cm. above spines.

Contractions started at 5 P.M., 3/12, now every 4 minutes. Membranes ruptured spontaneously at 10 A.M., 3/12. Slight show.
10 P.M.
Cervix dilated 6–7 cm., presenting part at spines.
Demerol 100 mg., scopolamine 0.00043 Gm. (gr. 1/150) stat.
Penicillin 300,000 units every 12 hours.
Nurses' notes—10:45 P.M.
Contractions every 3–4 minutes lasting 40–45 seconds, moderate to strong. Sleeps between contractions, wakens and cries out with contractions. Voided 200 cc., perineal care given. Moderate show. Temperature 98.2°, pulse 88, respirations 20. Blood pressure 124/80. Fetal heart rate 140, right lower flank.

By 2 A.M. contractions were weaker, coming at 5-minute intervals, and Mrs. Shaw was becoming restless between contractions. The fetal heart rate was 144, blood pressure 124/76, temperature 98°, pulse 110, respirations 22. In response to Miss Watkins' call the obstetric resident examined Mrs. Shaw again and found no change. He ordered morphine sulfate 0.016 Gm. (gr. ¼) to be given immediately, and started an infusion of 500 cc. of 10 per cent glucose in distilled water.

Mrs. Shaw slept soundly until 5 A.M., at which time she was awakened by strong contractions coming at 2-minute intervals. Examination showed her to be in second stage, the presenting part just below the spines, position ROP. At 6:50 A.M., after almost 2 hours in the second stage of labor, Mrs. Shaw was prepared for delivery. Under nitrous oxide anesthesia a left mediolateral episiotomy and forceps rotation were done, and a 9-pound baby girl was delivered by low forceps extraction at 7:20 A.M. Pitocin 1 cc. was given hypodermically, and the episiotomy was repaired. During this time the circulating nurse cared for the baby, whose condition appeared to be excellent. At 7:30 Mrs. Shaw began to bleed excessively. The placenta was removed manually, Ergotrate 1 cc. was given intravenously and the bleeding ceased.

Mrs. Shaw had reacted fully from the anesthesia by 7:50 A.M., but was kept in the delivery room to be observed until 9 o'clock. During this time the nurse showed the infant to its mother, and Mrs. Shaw held her baby until it was time for her to be taken to her room and the baby to the nursery.

References

Abraham, Leo M., and Dyer, Isadore: Significance of the fetal heart rate in pregnancy and labor, New Orleans M. and Surg. Jour. 102:245, 1949.
Dieckman, William J., et al.: The placental stage and postpartum hemorrhage, Am. J. Obstet. and Gynec. 54:415, 1947.
Hospital and hospitality, Briefs, p. 13, Winter 1949.
Hurlburt, Maretta, and Oscadal, Julia M.: The obstetric recovery room, Am. J. Nursing 49:136, 1949.

Questions Relating to the Patient Study

1. In reading Mrs. Shaw's record, the initials ROP should indicate to Miss Watkins that the presentation is

   a._____vertex.
   b._____brow.
   c._____breech.
   d._____chin.

2. "ROP" should also tell her that the baby faced the

   a._____left anterior portion of its mother's pelvis.
   b._____right anterior portion of its mother's pelvis.
   c._____left posterior portion of its mother's pelvis.
   d._____right posterior portion of its mother's pelvis.

3. The landmark used to indicate the presenting part was the

   a._____sinciput.
   b._____sacrum.
   c._____occiput.
   d._____mentum.

4. The spines referred to by the doctor are the ischial spines. They are located at

   a._____the inlet.
   b._____the outlet.
   c._____midpelvis.

5. Mrs. Shaw probably received the penicillin because she was

   a._____showing signs of infection.
   b._____predisposed to infection due to early rupture of the membranes.
   c._____predisposed to infection due to the presence of vaginal bleeding.
   d._____showing signs of fatigue.

6. Mrs. Shaw's labor was fairly typical of

   a._____primary uterine inertia.
   b._____secondary inertia.
   c._____cervical dystocia.
   d._____outlet dystocia.

7. At 5 A.M. Mrs. Shaw was found to be in the second stage of labor This means that the cervix was dilated

   a._____4 cm.
   b._____6 cm.
   c._____8 cm.
   d._____10 cm.

8. The physician did an episiotomy to enlarge the introitus and to

   a._____make the delivery easier for the mother.
   b._____prevent a traumatic tear of the perineum.
   c._____shorten the first stage.
   d._____prevent infection.

9. Failure of the presenting part to rotate, necessitating a forceps rotation in Mrs. Shaw's case, is known as

    a._____transverse arrest.
    b._____midpelvic arrest.
    c._____persistent occiput posterior.

10. Following the forceps rotation, the sagittal suture was in the

    a._____right oblique of the mother's pelvis.
    b._____anteroposterior diameter of the mother's pelvis.
    c._____transverse diameter of the mother's pelvis.
    d._____left oblique of the mother's pelvis.

11. The probable cause of Mrs. Shaw's bleeding during the third stage of labor was

    a._____partial separation of the placenta.
    b._____uterine atony.
    c._____retained placental lobe.
    d._____multiparity.

12. The nurse caring for Mrs. Shaw during the fourth stage of labor should be particularly alert for signs of hemorrhage to which she would be predisposed because of

    a._____multiparity, precipitate labor.
    b._____prolonged third stage, multiparity.
    c._____persistent occiput posterior, obstetric operations.
    d._____obstetric operations, large baby.

Questions for Discussion and Student Projects

A. Relating to the Patient Study

1. In addition to your basic points in caring for any woman in the first stage of labor, what *other* points should you have included, had you been responsible for Mrs. Shaw? In the second stage? Third stage? Fourth stage?
2. Describe your preparation of Mrs. Shaw for an operative delivery. In your hospital, what are the responsibilities of the nurse during an operative delivery? What additional supplies would be needed for manual removal of the placenta?
3. What was the rationale behind the administration of morphine and intravenous fluids?
4. Mrs. Shaw had had no prenatal supervision. With one of your classmates as Mrs. Shaw, show how you as a nurse caring for her on the postpartum unit would impress upon her the value of early and continuous care during future pregnancies.

B. Relating to the Section in General

1. Review the kinds of forceps used in your hospital. What characteristics are common to all forceps? How do the forceps differ? What

type forceps would be used for outlet or low forceps extractions? Rotations? Difficult extractions? Aftercoming head in a breech extraction?

2. How does primary uterine inertia differ from secondary uterine inertia in cause, in characteristics and in treatment?

3. At birth what are the physical characteristics of a baby who has presented as a frank breech? Brow? Face? What should be told the parents of such babies with regard to these characteristics?

4. What should be your course of action if you answered a mother's call bell and found her membranes had ruptured and the umbilical cord had prolapsed from the vagina?

5. What action should a nurse take upon finding that a newly delivered mother had an inverted uterus?

6. Artificial rupture of the membranes, frequently done to induce labor, is considered an obstetric operation. Discuss the nurse's responsibilities with regard to such a procedure. Include the preparation of the mother, observation and recording.

7. What are the nurse's duties in preparing a mother for, and administering, Demerol? Scopolamine? Rectal ether? Nembutal? What care should be given the mother following the administration of each of these agents?

8. How should you prepare a mother for a general anesthetic? What are your responsibilities in preparing a mother for spinal anesthesia? Local anesthesia?

9. What is the nursing care of a mother who is receiving continuous caudal anesthesia?

Questions Relating to the Section in General

1. Breech presentation occurs in approximately

   a._____33% of all deliveries.
   b._____23% of all deliveries.
   c._____13% of all deliveries.
   d._____3% of all deliveries.

2. The greatest danger encountered during labor with a breech presentation is

   a._____prolapsed foot.
   b._____prolapsed arm.
   c._____prolapsed cord.
   d._____precipitate delivery.

3. Occasionally a baby lies in the transverse (shoulder presentation). The operation usually done to correct this is

   a._____version.
   b._____rotation.
   c._____perineorrhaphy.
   d._____craniotomy.

4. Cephalopelvic disproportion may be due to
   a.____pelvic tumors, spina bifida, large baby.
   b.____anencephalus, contracted pelvis, hydrocephalus.
   c.____contracted pelvis, hydrocephalus, large baby.
   d.____hydramnios, hydrocephalus, pelvic tumors.

5. Rupture of the uterus occurs in an area of weak musculature such as
   a.____lower uterine segment, cervix.
   b.____lower uterine segment, site of cesarean section scar.
   c.____site of cesarean section scar, cervix.
   d.____cervix, upper uterine segment.

6. The precipitating cause of uterine rupture may be
   a.____cephalopelvic disproportion, obstetric operation.
   b.____injudicious use of Pitocin during labor, precipitate delivery.
   c.____premature separation of the placenta, obstetric operation.
   d.____premature labor, cephalopelvic disproportion.

7. Signs of impending rupture of the uterus are
   a.____continuous severe pain in the lower abdomen, absence of uterine contractions, extreme excitement.
   b.____frequent strong contractions, continuous severe pain in the lower abdomen, extreme excitement.
   c.____frequent strong contractions, loss of discretion, continuous severe pain in the lower abdomen.
   d.____absence of uterine contractions, boardlike abdomen, loss of discretion.

8. Indications of a ruptured uterus are
   a.____cessation of uterine contractions, continuous abdominal pain, signs of shock.
   b.____violent uterine contractions, continuous abdominal pain, signs of shock.
   c.____cessation of uterine contractions, external hemorrhage, cessation of abdominal pain.
   d.____uterine atony, cessation of abdominal pain, sign of shock.

9. A laceration which involves the skin, mucous membrane and muscles of the perineal body is called a
   a.____first-degree laceration.
   b.____second-degree laceration.
   c.____third-degree laceration.

10. Many physicians feel it is necessary to listen to the fetal heart rate immediately after rupture of membranes, to look for indications of
   a.____precipitate delivery.
   b.____premature separation of the placenta.
   c.____prolapsed cord.
   d.____placenta previa.

11. Some of the signs which may indicate fetal distress are

    a._____absence of fetal movements, increase in fetal heart rate during a contraction, presence of true meconium at the introitus.
    b._____increase in fetal activity, decrease in fetal heart rate during a contraction, meconium-stained amniotic fluid.
    c._____presence of true meconium at the introitus, decrease in fetal heart rate between contractions, absence of fetal movements.
    d._____meconium-stained amniotic fluid, increase in fetal heart rate between contractions, increase in fetal activity.

12. The generally accepted definition of postpartum hemorrhage is loss of blood in excess of

    a._____200 cc.
    b._____500 cc.
    c._____50 cc.
    d._____800 cc.

13. A woman in labor who has received an amnesic probably will be

    a._____irrational, groggy, quiet.
    b._____rational, wakeful, quiet.
    c._____irrational, restless, groggy.
    d._____rational, restless, groggy.

14. An example of an amnesic is

    a._____Demerol.
    b._____scopolamine.
    c._____morphine.
    d._____atropine.

15. Used in labor, morphine reduces pain but may also

    a._____interfere with the baby's breathing if given within 4 hours of delivery.
    b._____interfere with the mother's rest.
    c._____prevent relaxation of the uterus between contractions.
    d._____prevent the mother from using her expulsive efforts.

16. The actions of Demerol are

    a._____amnesic, analgesic.
    b._____amnesic, antispasmodic.
    c._____antispasmodic, analgesic.
    d._____analgesic, anesthetic.

17. Scopolamine usually is given in gradually decreasing doses, starting with 0.00043 Gm. (gr. $\frac{1}{150}$), then 0.00032 Gm. (gr. $\frac{1}{200}$), and finally 0.00022 Gm. (gr. $\frac{1}{300}$). To give gr. $\frac{1}{300}$ from gr. $\frac{1}{150}$ tablets, you should dissolve

    a._____2 tablets in minims xv of sterile water and administer.
    b._____1 tablet in minims xxx of sterile water, discard minims xv of the solution and administer the remaining minims xv.

    c.____2 tablets in minims xx of sterile water, discard minims v of the solution and administer the remaining minims xv.

    d.____1 tablet in minims xx of sterile water, discard minims v and administer the remaining minims xv.

18. To give gr. $\frac{1}{200}$ from tablets gr. $\frac{1}{300}$ of scopolamine, you should dissolve

    a.____2 tablets in minims xv of sterile water and administer.

    b.____1 tablet in minims xxx of sterile water, discard minims xv of the solution and administer the remaining minims xv.

    c.____1 tablet in minims xxx of sterile water, discard minims xv of the solution, add 1 tablet to the remaining minims xv and administer.

    d.____1 tablet in minims xx of sterile water, discard minims v and administer the remaining minims xv.

19. Continuous caudal anesthesia may be used

    a.____throughout labor.

    b.____only in the first stage of labor.

    c.____only in the second stage of labor.

    d.____only in the third stage of labor.

20. The route of administration of saddle-block anesthesia is

    a.____local infiltration.

    b.____spinal.

    c.____intravenous.

    d.____inhalation.

RELIEF OF PAINFUL BREAST FEEDING

Background Review Question

1. Complete the following questions by placing the letter preceding the term in the left-hand column next to the proper descriptive phrase in the right-hand column.

a. endometritis.	(1)____inflammation of the cellular tissue surrounding the uterus.
b. phlebothrombosis.	
c. thrombophlebitis.	(2)____localized inflammation of the membrane lining the uterus.
d. engorgement.	
e. agalactia.	(3)____excessive congestion of the breasts due to lymphatic or venous stasis.
f. phlegmasia alba dolens.	
g. galactorrhea.	
h. subinvolution.	(4)____thrombosis of a vein without inflammation of the walls of the vein.
i. parametritis.	
j. mastitis.	
	(5)____thrombosis associated with inflammation of the walls of the vein.

(6)_____absence of milk secretion.

(7)_____inflammation of the breast.

(8)_____whitish discharge from the vagina.

(9)_____failure of a part to return to normal size and condition after enlargement from functional activity.

(10)_____excessive secretion of milk.

(11)_____increasing the secretion of milk.

(12)_____inflammation of a femoral vein following delivery.

RELIEF OF PAINFUL BREAST FEEDING—PATIENT STUDY

Mrs. Ellis had agreed hesitantly to breast-feeding her first baby, Louise, but, when she saw how eagerly the baby nursed, she felt sure she had made the right decision. When the baby was 3 days old, the nurse noticed Mrs. Ellis wincing when the baby was put to her right breast. She said that the right nipple had become quite tender. A small crack could be seen, so the mother was given a nipple shield. The baby adjusted readily to this new method of feeding.

Following the order of Mrs. Ellis' physician, the affected nipple was touched with a silver nitrate stick after each feeding, and the use of the shield was continued. These treatments were discontinued in 2 days and no further difficulty was experienced.

References

Davies, Velma, and Pratt, J. P.: Stimulation and maintenance of lactation, Am. J. Nursing 46:242, 1946.

Kohl, Richard M.: The psychiatric aspects of obstetric nursing, Am. J. Nursing 48:422, 1948.

Thompson, Morton: The Cry and the Covenant, New York, Doubleday, 1949.

Questions Relating to the Patient Study

1. The cause of Mrs. Ellis' cracked nipple may have been due to

   a._____multiparity.
   b._____the baby biting the nipple.
   c._____lack of milk supply.
   d._____putting the baby to breast too soon after birth.

2. In applying the silver nitrate to the nipple, Mrs. Ellis' nurse should take care to

   a._____apply it to both nipples to prevent cracking of the unaffected one.
   b._____touch the entire nipple.
   c._____apply it several times to insure adequate cauterization.
   d._____touch the area, only once.

3. In addition to silver nitrate, some agents which may be used in the treatment of cracked nipples are

   a.____benzoin tincture, Peruvian balsam, heat lamp.
   b.____Merthiolate tincture, Peruvian balsam, argyrol.
   c.____heat lamp, iodine tincture, argyrol.
   d.____Zephiran tincture, benzoin tincture, Merthiolate tincture.

4. Patients most apt to develop cracked nipples are

   a.____Scandinavian women.
   b.____Spanish women.
   c.____Negro women.
   d.____Indian women.

5. In the treatment of cracked nipples, the basic principle is

   a.____antisepsis.
   b.____antibiosis.
   c.____asepsis.
   d.____antigens.

6. When a nurse notices that a mother's breasts are engorged she should

   a.____massage them gently.
   b.____apply external cold.
   c.____remove the supporting brassière.
   d.____discontinue the baby's nursing.

7. Breast abscesses develop readily following

   a.____engorgement.
   b.____agalactia.
   c.____parametritis.
   d.____cracked nipples.

8. Symptoms of mastitis are

   a.____gradual rise in temperature, blanching and swelling of the affected breast.
   b.____sharp rise in temperature, blanching and swelling of the affected breast.
   c.____gradual rise in temperature, swelling and redness of the affected breast.
   d.____sharp rise in temperature, swelling and redness of the affected breast.

Questions for Discussion and Student Projects

A. Relating to the Patient Study

   1. Describe how you should teach Mrs. Ellis and her baby to use a nipple shield.
   2. List 5 methods or measures which have been recommended for the prevention of cracked nipples.

3. Compare manual expression of milk, the electric breast pump and the hand breast pump as to simplicity, adequacy, cost and time required.

B. Relating to the Section in General

1. What is the difference between residual urine and retention of urine? How can you distinguish between the uterus and a distended bladder in the early postpartum period? List the measures you should use to try to get a mother to void.
2. Discuss in detail the nursing care of a mother with puerperal infection. What measures should be taken to maintain lactation during the period of the mother's isolation?
3. Discuss puerperal morbidity under the following headings:

   a. Definition (according to Joint Committee on Maternal Welfare).
   b. Possible causes.
   c. Treatment and nursing care.

4. Discuss puerperal infection under the following headings:

   a. Historical: How and by whom were the cause and the prevention discovered?
   b. Incidence: (1) Factors which have decreased the incidence. (2) Type of delivery with which puerperal infection is most commonly associated.
   c. Treatment and nursing care.

5. What is meant by "postpartum" psychosis? Is this a direct result of childbirth, or precipitated by childbirth? What symptoms characterize the onset of this disorder? How is it treated in your institution?

Section 4. Nursing Care of the
Unusual Newborn*

STUDY SUGGESTIONS: Before beginning the study of this Section, the student
will find it helpful to

A. Review

   1. In pharmacology texts: pitocin, stilbestrol.
   2. In physiology texts: the Rh factor.

B. Study

   1. In obstetric nursing texts: congenital anomalies, premature birth,
      pudendal block.

C. Read the additional References listed before attempting to answer questions
   relating to each patient study.

PREMATURE TWINS

Background Review Question

1. Place the letter preceding the term in the left-hand column in the space
   to the left of the proper descriptive phrase in the right-hand column.

   a. blepharitis.
   b. monozygotic twins.
   c. atelectasis.
   d. superfetation.
   e. nystagmus.
   f. amnion.
   g. chorion.
   h. dizygotic twins.
   i. superfecundation.
   j. anoxemia.
   k. anoxia.

   (1)_____rapid involuntary oscillation of the
        eyeballs.
   (2)_____twins resulting from fertilization of
        2 ova.
   (3)_____conception during a pregnancy.
   (4)_____successive fertilization of 2 or more
        ova from the same ovulation.
   (5)_____imperfect expansion of the lungs at
        birth.
   (6)_____innermost fetal membrane.
   (7)_____insufficiency of tissue oxidation.
   (8)_____outermost fetal membrane.
   (9)_____twins resulting from fertilization of
        1 ovum.

PREMATURE TWINS—PATIENT STUDY

At 6 A.M. on January 6, Mrs. Stankowski was awakened by a sudden
gush of water from the vagina. Contractions were felt for the first time,
and were irregular, but within an hour had become regular, occurring at
10-minute intervals. After the family had their breakfast, Mrs. Stankowski and her husband took the children, Rose and Stanley, to her mother's
home, then drove to the hospital, arriving at 8:40 A.M. Mrs. Stankowski

* Congenital anomalies are also considered in the section on Nursing Care of Children,
pp. 334–340.

was admitted and sent immediately to the labor room; her husband remained in the admitting office to give the necessary information to the clerk.

The notations made by Dr. Grimm, the obstetric resident, after he had examined Mrs. Stankowski, included

Age: 30.
Occupation: housewife.
Religion: Hebrew.
Obstetric history:
  Gravida III, para II.
  Last menstrual period May 21.
  Expected date of confinement February 28.
  1947—term pregnancy; living male, 8½ lbs.; hospital delivery, 15-
    hour labor; no complications.
  1949—term pregnancy; living female, 8 lbs.; hospital delivery, 6-
    hour labor; no complications.
  Present pregnancy normal. No toxic signs or symptoms; no bleeding.
Family history:
  Mother, father and one sister living and well. No history of twins.
Medical history:
  Usual childhood diseases.
  Appendectomy 13 years ago.
Abdominal examination:
  Twins. One vertex deeply engaged; second baby presenting breech.
  Contractions q. 3–4 minutes, strong, lasting 50–60 seconds. Fetal
  heart rates: lower right quadrant 140; upper left quadrant 152.
Rectal examination:
  Cervix completely effaced, dilated 8 cm.
  Vertex below spines.
  Membranes ruptured.

A vitamin-K preparation was administered hypodermically; no other medication was given. Mrs. Stankowski was taken to the delivery room and a pudendal block was done. At 9:15 A.M. a right mediolateral episiotomy was made and a 4-pound baby boy was delivered by low forceps extraction. The second bag of waters was ruptured artificially at 9:40 A.M., followed by the spontaneous breech delivery of a second boy, weight 3 lbs. 6 oz. Both babies breathed spontaneously. After checking the fundus for the possibility of another child, Dr. Grimm ordered pitocin 1 cc. to be given hypodermically.

Both infants were placed in incubators and given continuous oxygen. After 24 hours, gavage feedings were started. Mrs. Stankowski felt she would not have enough milk to feed her 2 babies, and refused the doctor's suggestion that she pump her breasts. She was given stilbestrol to dry up her breasts.

References

Carson, A. L., Jr.: Prematurity in relation to obstetric care, *The Child* 14:155, 1950.

Clarke, Erma E.: The premature infant goes home, Am. J. Nursing 52:882, 1952.

Dunham, Ethel C.: Premature Infants, Washington, D. C., Children's Bureau Publ. #325, 1948.

Greene, Doris M., and Zetzsche, Louise: Premies are human beings too," Publ. Health Nursing 44:253, May, 1952.

Losty, Margaret A., Orlofsky, Irene, and Wallace, Helen M.: A transport service for premature babies, Am. J. Nursing 50:10, 1950.

Wollinger, Elgie M.: Nursing care of the premature infant, Am. J. Nursing 45:898, 1945.

Questions Relating to the Patient Study

1. During her next pregnancy, Mrs. Stankowski would be classified as gravida

   a.____IV, para III.
   b.____III, para IV.
   c.____IV, para IV.
   d.____III, para III.

2. A pudendal block involves injecting an anesthetic agent into the

   a.____spinal column.
   b.____cauda equina.
   c.____perineal area.
   d.____abdominal wall.

3. Mrs. Stankowski was given a pudendal block in preference to a general anesthetic because

   a.____it does not cause respiratory embarrassment in the infant.
   b.____it acts rapidly.
   c.____she wanted to be awake for the birth of her babies.
   d.____it acts as a respiratory stimulant.

4. The delivery of the second twin was not hastened because

   a.____uterine circulation had to be re-established.
   b.____Mrs. Stankowski was tired after having delivered the first baby.
   c.____the instrument table had to be reset.
   d.____it is advisable to allow the uterus to decrease in size gradually.

5. In the nursing care of Mrs. Stankowski immediately postpartum, the nurse would be particularly alert for signs of

   a.____hemorrhage.
   b.____eclampsia.
   c.____sepsis.
   d.____psychosis.

6. Mrs. Stankowski would be predisposed to the above complication because of

   a.____premature labor.
   b.____multiple pregnancy.

    c.____prolonged labor.

    d.____premature rupture of membranes.

7. Pitocin is a

    a.____synthetic preparation similar to progesterone.

    b.____derivative of pituitrin with the vasoconstrictor element removed.

    c.____derivative of pituitrin with the vasoconstrictor element added.

    d.____synthetic preparation resembling ergotrate.

8. Stilbestrol is a synthetic preparation simulating one of the functions of estrogen, which is

    a.____reduction of the amount of mammary gland tissue.

    b.____reduction of secretions by causing diuresis.

    c.____inhibition of lactogenic hormone.

    d.____inhibition of "maternal instinct."

9. The Stankowski twins were placed in incubators because

    a.____it was necessary to limit exposure.

    b.____they needed the added protection from infection.

    c.____they had to be protected from drafts.

    d.____their heat-regulatory mechanisms were not functioning properly.

10. Each twin was given vitamin K to

    a.____decrease the danger of intracranial hemorrhage.

    b.____prevent hemorrhagic disease of the newborn.

    c.____prevent menstruation.

    d.____decrease the number of petechiae.

11. Vitamin K should be administered

    a.____subcutaneously.

    b.____intramuscularly.

    c.____orally.

    d.____rectally.

Questions for Discussion and Student Projects

1. How does premature labor differ from term labor? Describe the nursing care of Mrs. Stankowski during her labor.
2. Had Mrs. Stankowski told you that she wanted to dry up her breasts because she would not have enough milk to feed 2 babies, how should you have responded?
3. Before the twins are discharged from the hospital, what information would be needed about the Stankowski home? How could this information be obtained? How might Mrs. Stankowski be prepared to assume the care of her 2 babies?
4. Suggested project for one student: Discuss with a rabbi the significance of the ritual of circumcision. How should the procedure be modified in the case of the Stankowski twins?

Questions Relating to the Section in General

1. A premature infant may be defined as an infant weighing

    a.____3,500 Gm. or less.
    b.____3,000 Gm. or less.
    c.____2,500 Gm. or less.
    d.____2,000 Gm. or less.

2. The incidence of prematurity in the United States is

    a.____7 to 11% of all births.
    b.____0.7 to 1% of all births.
    c.____15% of all births.
    d.____3% of all births.

3. In the first month of life, prematurity accounts for

    a.____40% of the deaths.
    b.____5% of the deaths.
    c.____0.5% of the deaths.
    d.____25% of the deaths.

4. The 3 leading causes of prematurity are

    a.____multiple births, toxemia of pregnancy, antepartum hemorrhage.
    b.____multiple pregnancy, antepartum hemorrhage, fixed retroversion of the uterus.
    c.____toxemia of pregnancy, antepartum hemorrhage, myomata uteri.
    d.____tuberculosis, toxemia of pregnancy, syphilis.

5. Among the early complications of prematurity are

    a.____atelectasis, anemia, anoxia.
    b.____jaundice, anemia, intracranial hemorrhage.
    c.____dehydration, anemia, anoxia.
    d.____atelectasis, intracranial hemorrhage, dehydration.

6. Some of the later complications associated with prematurity are

    a.____jaundice, retrolental fibroplasia, vitamin deficiency.
    b.____anemia, retrolental fibroplasia, rickets.
    c.____jaundice, anemia, retrolental fibroplasia.
    d.____vitamin deficiency, anemia, jaundice.

7. The increased incidence of retrolental fibroplasia in the United States is due to a (an)

    a.____higher birth rate.
    b.____lower mortality rate in small prematures.
    c.____increase in premature births.
    d.____increase in the number of mothers who work during pregnancy.

8. An infant with retrolental fibroplasia presents the following signs:

 a.____small eyeballs, persistence of gray-blue iris, nystagmus.
 b.____dilated pupils, conjunctivitis, persistence of gray-blue iris.
 c.____conjunctivitis, nystagmus, dilated pupils.
 d.____blepharitis, photophobia, small eyeballs.

9. The underlying cause of intracranial hemorrhage in premature infants is

 a.____an excessive number of erythrocytes.
 b.____anoxia.
 c.____vitamin-A deficiency.
 d.____fragility of blood vessels.

10. Among the immediate causes of intracranial hemorrhage in premature infants are

 a.____precipitate delivery, injudicious use of forceps.
 b.____injudicious use of forceps, prolonged first stage.
 c.____use of morphine during labor, precipitate delivery.
 d.____prolonged first stage, use of morphine during labor.

11. Principles in the nursing care of an infant with intracranial hemorrhage are

 a.____conservation of heat, force fluids.
 b.____conservation of heat, gentle handling.
 c.____gentle handling, elevation of the foot of the crib.
 d.____conservation of heat, elevation of the foot of the crib.

12. The temperature of an incubator should be maintained between

 a.____92°–95°.
 b.____95°–98°.
 c.____88°–92°.
 d.____85°–88°.

13. The humidity of an incubator should remain between

 a.____55 to 65%.
 b.____50 to 55%.
 c.____60 to 65%.
 d.____65 to 70%.

14. Superfetation usually results in

 a.____fraternal twins.
 b.____death of the baby.
 c.____paternal twins.
 d.____quintuplets.

15. The following are characteristic of monozygotic twins:

 a.____2 placentas, 2 amnions, 2 chorions.
 b.____1 placenta, 2 amnions, 2 chorions.
 c.____1 placenta, 1 amnion, 1 chorion.
 d.____1 placenta, 2 amnions, 1 chorion.

1. What measures can be taken to reduce the incidence of prematurity? To lower premature mortality? What is being done in various sections of the country about this problem?

2. Write to your State Department of Health for literature on premature care. What are the existing facilities within your state for the care of premature babies?

3. Describe a plan for caring for a 4-pound baby in the home, including bed, provision of heat, prevention of burns, care of skin, clothing and feeding. Who in the family would you teach to care for the baby?

4. Describe the measures that generally are recommended to be carried out in caring for prematures, in order to prevent infections, such as gastro-intestinal, skin, etc.

5. Suggested activity for one student: Prepare a summary of the condition known as retrolental fibroplasia. A booklet on the subject may be obtained by writing to M & R Laboratories, Columbus 16, Ohio.

6. What are some of the problems you would anticipate a mother having to face who, expecting 1 baby, delivered twins? How should you help her in the solution of the problems?

7. In your hospital, how are premature babies cared for? What kind of incubator do you use? What other kinds are there? In what ways do they differ? What are the advantages and disadvantages of each. (Suggested project for one student.)

THE BABY WITH A DEFORMITY—PATIENT STUDY

Mr. and Mrs. Alder, both in their late twenties, were the parents of 2 girls, Joyce, 3½ years old, and Suzanne, 2 days old. Mrs. Alder had worked as a receptionist after her graduation from a business school, and until her marriage 5 years ago. Mr. Alder was a bookkeeper who had gone to school evenings to complete requirements for a Bachelor of Arts degree. The couple had been careful to see that Joyce was prepared for the arrival of a sister or a brother by giving her simple explanations and frank answers to her questions. The family had spent many happy hours working together to prepare for the expected baby. Two months before the expected arrival of the baby, Joyce had gone with her parents to choose her new bed, which she had been using ever since its purchase.

Mrs. Alder had been well throughout her second pregnancy. Suzanne, 7 pounds 8 ounces, was born after a 20-hour labor. Examination revealed congenital absence of the left hand. No other deformities were noted.

After a brief telephone conversation with Mr. Alder, Mrs. Alder, Senior, the baby's grandmother, came to the hospital and asked the nurse on duty in the nursery about her grandchild. Some of her questions were:

Just what is wrong with the baby?
What caused the deformity?
What does the baby's arm look like?
When may I see the baby?
When will the doctor be able to fix the baby's arm?

References

Battersby, J. S., and Greve, M. L.: Modern treatment of atresia of the esophagus, Am. J. Nursing 50:158, 1950.

Brown, Ivan W., Jr.: Present status of the Rh factor, Am. J. Nursing 48:14, 1948.

Gilbert, Margaret Shea: Biography of the Unborn, Baltimore, Williams and Wilkins, 1948.

Jeans, Philip, Rand, Winifred, and Blake, Florence G.: Essentials of Pediatrics, pp. 286–291, Philadelphia, Lippincott, 1946.

Nelson, Waldo E.: Mitchell-Nelson Textbook of Pediatrics, Philadephia, Saunders, 1951.

Spock, Benjamin: Baby and Child Care, New York, Pocket Books, 1951.

Stone, Emerson L.: The Newborn Infant, Philadelphia, Lea and Febiger, 1945.

Wright, Lucille, and Prince, Charles L.: Hypospadius, Am. J. Nursing 46:686, 1946.

Zabriskie, Louise, and Eastman, Nicholson J.: Nurses' Handbook of Obstetrics, Philadelphia, Lippincott, pp. 248–252, 520–524, 1952.

Questions Relating to the Patient Study

1. Considering her parity, Mrs. Alder's labor was

    a._____unusually long.
    b._____of average duration.
    c._____shorter than average.

2. Congenital amputation usually is associated with

    a._____syphilis.
    b._____hydramnios.
    c._____oligohydramnios.
    d._____German measles.

3. During the period of hospitalization, the baby should

    a._____be fed in the nursery.
    b._____not be shown to Mr. Alder.
    c._____be taken to her mother for feeding.

4. When the baby's grandmother asks to see the baby's hand, she should be

    a._____told that she wouldn't want to see it; it is unpleasant to look at.
    b._____referred to the physician.
    c._____told that she will see the baby when she is taken home.
    d._____shown the baby, including the deformity.

5. In their handling of Suzanne, the Alders should

    a._____give her more attention because of her deformity.
    b._____give her less attention to avoid causing jealousy in Joyce.
    c._____treat her as they would a normal baby.

Questions for Discussion and Student Projects

1. Assume you were the nurse in the situation when Mrs. Alder, Sr., came to the hospital. How should you have responded to her questions? With one of your classmates as the grandmother, act out the scene as you think it might have occurred.
2. From your knowledge of the situation, who do you think should prepare Mrs. Alder to see her baby for the first time? Who should explain the deformity to Mr. Alder? Should the grandparents be permitted to see the baby?
3. When taking the baby to her mother for the first time, what should be your approach? What are some of the questions that might be asked by the Alders? How should you handle these questions?
4. Consider the normal growth and development and play activities of the infant and baby. What adjustments will Suzanne have to make?
5. How do you think the parents might feel when friends stop to see the baby? How do you suppose they will explain the situation to Joyce?
6. What advice should you give Mrs. Alder if she asks what she can do to help Joyce to adjust to having another child in the home?

Questions Relating to the Section in General

1. The alert nurse is often the one who first notices indications of disorders of the newborn infant. Complete the following question by placing the letter preceding the disorder in the left-hand column in the blank to the left at the proper descriptive phrase in the right-hand column.

a. imperforate anus.	(1)＿＿vomiting immediately after feeding.
b. pilonidal cyst.	(2)＿＿edema of the scalp.
c. hypospadius.	(3)＿＿bleeding from body orifices.
d. mongolism.	(4)＿＿absence of stools.
e. atresia of the esophagus.	(5)＿＿white curd-like patches in the mouth.
f. cryptorchidism.	(6)＿＿copious discharge of pus beginning on the second or third day.
g. erythroblastosis fetalis.	
h. cephalohematoma.	
i. hemorrhagic disease.	
j. Erb's palsy.	
k. hydrocele.	(7)＿＿relaxation of ligaments of the joints allows the baby to assume bizarre positions.
l. caput succedaneum.	
m. thrush.	
n. gonorrheal conjunctivitis.	
o. impetigo.	(8)＿＿urethral opening at the base of the penis.
p. fracture of the clavicle.	
q. congenital dislocation of the shoulder.	(9)＿＿depression over the sacrum.
	(10)＿＿testicles not palpated in the scrotum.
	(11)＿＿blisterlike lesion easily broken.

(12)_____jaundice appears within 24 hours after birth.

(13)_____swelling limited to the area of a cranial bone.

(14)_____flaccid paralysis of the arm.

(15)_____collection of fluid around the testicle.

2. Caput succedaneum

   a._____requires surgery to correct.

   b._____clears spontaneously within a week.

   c._____clears spontaneously in about a month.

   d._____remains as a permanent defect.

3. A cephalohematoma will

   a._____be absorbed within a week if properly massaged.

   b._____be absorbed in 5 to 6 weeks; no treatment is indicated.

   c._____heal rapidly following incision and drainage.

   d._____heal rapidly following aspiration.

4. The signs which would indicate the presence of erythroblastosis fetalis in a 2-day-old infant are

   a._____jaundice, edema, bleeding from body orifices.

   b._____diarrhea, convulsions, fever.

   c._____edema, excessive crying, subnormal temperature.

   d._____jaundice, absence of stools, projectile vomiting.

5. The nursing care indicated by the presence of erythroblastosis fetalis consists of

   a._____cool sponges, maintenance of the dorsal position, gavage feedings, oxygen as needed.

   b._____additional warmth, oxygen as needed, frequent change of position, feedings as indicated by the infant's condition.

   c._____medicine-dropper feedings, elevation of the foot of the crib, isolation technics, additional warmth.

   d._____breast feeding, elevation of the foot of the crib, oxygen as needed, cool sponges.

6. The treatment for severe erythroblastosis fetalis is

   a._____replacement transfusion with Rh-negative blood.

   b._____replacement transfusion with Rh-positive blood.

   c._____vitamin-K therapy.

   d._____liver and iron therapy.

7. The incidence of erythroblastosis fetalis is about

   a._____1:1,000.

   b._____1:400.

   c._____1:5,000.

   d._____1:50.

8. The proportion of Rh-positive people according to race is approximately

    a._____93% Negro, 95% white, 1% yellow.
    b._____83% Negro, 85% white, 99% yellow.
    c._____93% Negro, 85% white, 99% yellow.
    d._____85% Negro, 93% white, 10% yellow.

9. Erb's palsy is due to

    a._____heredity.
    b._____birth injury.
    c._____developmental defect.
    d._____nutritional deficiency of the mother.

10. Harelip and cleft palate are repaired, respectively,

    a._____both within a few weeks of birth.
    b._____when the child is 6 months old, at the age of 1 year.
    c._____within a few weeks after birth, at 5 to 6 years of age.
    d._____both at 2 years of age.

11. Engorgement of the breasts occurs relatively frequently in newborn infants. To prevent infection

    a._____massage gently.
    b._____apply local heat.
    c._____refrain from manipulation or treatment.
    d._____apply a tight binder.

12. Occasionally during birth the infant sustains a fracture of one clavicle. Signs of such fracture are

    a._____failure to move the arm on the affected side, absence of the Moro reflex on the affected side.
    b._____excessive crying when picked up, shortening of the arm on the affected side.
    c._____failure to nurse vigorously, drowsiness.
    d._____absence of the Moro reflex on both sides, excessive crying when picked up.

13. Treatment of a fractured clavicle in the newborn is

    a._____watchful waiting.
    b._____a plaster-of-Paris cast to the clavicle involved.
    c._____immobilization of the shoulder and the arm on the affected side.
    d._____taping of the arm to the chest on the affected side.

14. The sign on which a diagnosis of epidemic diarrhea of the newborn can always be made is

    a._____listlessness and fretfulness.
    b._____marked dehydration.
    c._____noisy, rapid expulsion of a large yellow watery stool.
    d._____noisy, rapid expulsion of frequent small watery stools.

Questions for Discussion and Student Projects—(*Continued*)

1. Using a life-size doll, demonstrate how you should inspect a newborn infant for physical deformities.
2. List the important points in the nursing care of newborn infants with the following disorders:

   a. spina bifida and hydrocephalus.
   b. harelip and cleft palate.
   c. thrush.
   d. impetigo.
   e. gonorrheal conjunctivitis.

3. What help could you give to the parents of a child born with a physical deformity? Consider such aspects as explanations to other children, attitude toward the deformed child, future pregnancies, etc.
4. What are the characteristics of a mongoloid infant at birth? How should the parents of such a baby be advised regarding his expected development, the kind of care he will require, and the desirability of placing him in an institution? What advice should be given them concerning future pregnancies?
5. Under usual circumstances the Rh-positive trait is dominant. How is it possible for an Rh-negative mother and an Rh-positive father to produce an Rh-negative child? Explain the physiologic basis for the anemia sometimes seen in the Rh-positive infant of an Rh-negative mother.

Section 5. Planning for the Nursing Care of Mothers and Their Babies in the Hospital

In the previous Sections, several mothers and their babies have been described. In this last Section, you are asked to consider facilities and methods which will provide the best possible emotional and physical care for these mothers and their babies. Attention will be directed toward environment, physical facilities, and effective assignment of personnel.

STUDY SUGGESTIONS: Before beginning the study of this Section, the student will find it helpful to review

1. The nursing care needs of the mothers and the babies listed as hospitalized in this group.
2. The summary Section of Part One, Nursing Care of Adult Patients with Medical and Surgical Disorders.

The references in this Section supplement those listed in the Section cited above and in Section 5 of Part Two, Nursing Care of Children.

Listed are the names and the diagnosis of each of the mothers who, with their babies, are hospitalized in the obstetric unit described in this Section.

Mrs. Kurz—normal pregnancy delivered at term.

Anita Jackson—3 months' gestation; vaginal bleeding.

Mrs. Morrison—34 weeks' gestation; vaginal bleeding; cesarean section.

Virginia Gilbreth—32 weeks' gestation; diabetes mellitus; cesarean section.

Mrs. Stewart—38 weeks' gestation; eclampsia; cesarean section, maternal death.

Mrs. Shaw—operative delivery at term; postpartum hemorrhage.

Mrs. Stankowski—32 weeks' gestation; twins; operative deliveries.

Mrs. Alder—normal pregnancy delivered at term; baby has congenital amputation of left hand.

Mrs. Ellis—normal pregnancy delivered at term.

References

McLendon, P. A., and Parks, John: Nurseries Designed for Modern Maternity, Modern Hosp. 65:46, 1945.

Modern Standards in Adequate Facilities for Obstetric Care, Children's Bureau, Federal Security Agency, Washington 25, D.C. (Reprint from *Hospitals*, February 1946.)

Randall, Margaret: Ward Administration, pp. 156–174, Saunders, Philadelphia, 1949.

Standards and Recommendations for Hospital Care of Maternity Patients, Children's Bureau Publication #314, Federal Security Agency, Washington 25, D.C., 1946. (10¢)

Standards and Recommendations for Hospital Care of Newborn Infants, The American Academy of Pediatrics, Evanston, Ill., 1948.

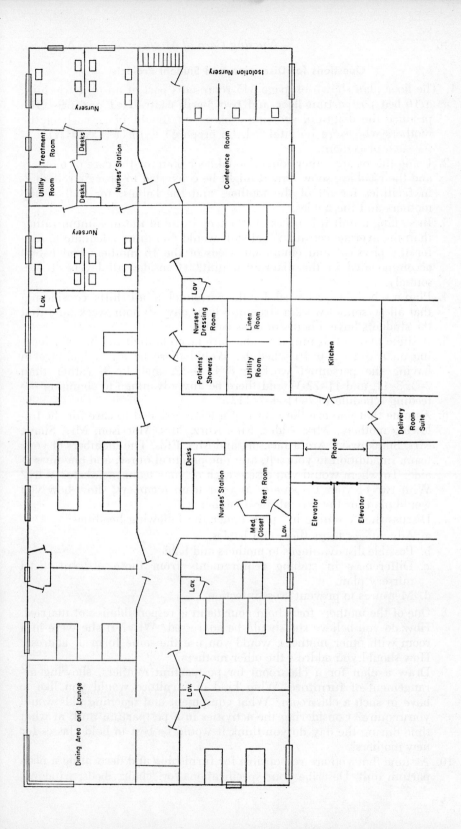

Questions for Discussion and Student Projects

1. The floor plan shown on page 545 represents part of an obstetric unit, a 16-bed postpartum floor and two 8-crib centralized nurseries. Reproduce the diagram, showing where you should place each of the mothers who were hospitalized. Be prepared to discuss your reasons for such placement.

2. Using this or any other conventional floor plan for the care of mothers and their babies, show how it might be converted to provide rooming-in facilities for all of the mothers and the babies; for half of the mothers and the babies.

3. In staffing a unit it is necessary to keep in mind the maximum rather than the average census. What staff would you think adequate to care for the physical and emotional needs of the 16 mothers and babies accommodated in the diagramed unit? (Consider all levels of personnel).

4. Plan a schedule for 1 week for the personnel on all shifts, considering that all personnel work a straight 8-hour day, 40-hour week; and that the students have 5 hours of class weekly.

5. Assume that in this unit the babies are taken to their mothers for feeding on a 6–10–2–6–10 schedule. Would there be any advantage in having the personnel working 8–4, 4–12, and 12–8, rather than 7–3, 3–11, and 11–7? Would there be any advantage to changing the feeding schedule to 7–11–4–7–11?

6. Assume that you are the leader of a team assigned to care for the following mothers: Mrs. Alder, Mrs. Kurz, Mrs. Morrison, Mrs. Shaw, Mrs. Stankowski, Anita Jackson, and Mrs. Ellis. The members of your team, in addition to yourself, are: one practical nurse, and one nurse's aide. To whom would you assign each of your team members? Why? With two of your classmates as your team members, show how you would plan for the care of these mothers.

7. Discuss the "rooming-in" plan under the following headings:
   a. Advantages to mothers and babies.
   b. Possible disadvantages to mothers and babies.
   c. Differences in staffing requirements from those of centralized nursery plan.
   d. Measures to prevent cross-infection.

8. One of the mothers for whom your team is responsible is not married. How do you believe she should be addressed? Why? If she were in a room with other mothers, would you use the same form of address? How should you address the other mothers?

9. Draw a plan for a classroom for postpartum mothers, showing arrangement of furniture. What kind of furniture would you like to have in such a classroom? What equipment and teaching aids would you require? Considering the activities in a postpartum unit, at what time during the day do you think it would be best to hold classes for new mothers?

10. Assume that you are responsible for furnishing and decorating a postpartum unit. Describe your specifications for: chairs, beds, windows,

lighting, bedside stands, floors, walls, ceilings, storage space for the mothers' personal belongings.

11. Should mothers who are ambulatory be permitted to eat in a dining area, rather than at their bedsides or in bed? Be prepared to state your reasons.
12. What activities in the nursery, directly related to baby care, can be safely carried out by practical nurses? Nurse's aides?
13. Describe how individual technic can be carried out in a centralized nursery. What is the value of this technic?
14. What are the advantages of a "self-demand" feeding program? In a centralized nursery, where babies are taken to their mothers for feeding, how may a self-demand feeding program be carried out? How may a strict feeding schedule be modified to incorporate some of the advantages of a self-demand feeding program?

Index

Index

Entries and page references set in **boldface** refer to items of extensive coverage in the text.

A

Abdominal distention, 278
Abdominal paracentesis, of children, 360
Abortion, 281–282
  threatened, 503–506
    morphine sulfate in, 504–505
    stilbestrol in, 281–282, 506
Abscess, general, 54
  of breast, 530
  of lung, 31
Accidents, legal aspects in, 224–225
  prevention of, 200, 225, 265, 294, 364
    in pediatric unit, 361
Acid (*see under* descriptive term)
ACTH, in arthritis, 192–193
  in leukemia, 394–395
  in rheumatic fever, 397–398
Addiction, drug, 410, 468–472
Addison's disease, 184
Adjustment, patterns of, 438, 469
Adolescence, behavior problems in, 419–423
  child development in, 407–409, 422–423
Adoption, 501, 502
Adrenalin, 36, 37
After-pains, 496, 497
Aggressive behavior, 453, 460
Agitated patient, 464–466
Albuminuria, 120
Alcohol sponge, 223
Alcoholism, 468, 472
Allergy, 157, 161
  antihistaminics in, 160
  diet in, 160–161
  in infancy, 324–326
Amebic dysentery, 100–104
  diet in, 101
Aminophylline, in acute glomerulonephritis, 127, 128
  in asthma, 159
Ammonium chloride, 40, 41
Amnesics, in labor, 527

Amputation, congenital, 538–540
  of breast, 150–156
  of legs, 56–61
Anaphylactic shock, 160
Anemia, 65, 66
  pernicious, 65–67, 68–71
    hydrochloric acid in, 70
    liver extract in, 71
  secondary, diet in, 364
Anesthesia, caudal, 525–528
  in eye surgery, 254
  nitrous oxide, 152, 153
  procaine, 82
  pudendal block, 534
Aneurysm, of carotid artery, 216
Angina, Ludwig's, 80, 81
Angiography, 216
Anomalies, cardiac, 365–371
Antihistaminics, in allergies, 160
  in common cold, 8
Antisocial people, 468–472
Antitoxin, tetanus, 292
Anxiety, 435, 436, 437
Appendectomy, 104–105
Argyrol, 253
Arteriosclerosis, 48, 225, 226, **229–233**
  cerebral, 440–445
Artery, carotid, aneurysm of, 216
Arthritis, ACTH in, 192–193
  aspirin in, 190–191
  atrophic, 193
  Cortisone in, 192, 193
  diet in, 191
  gold salts in, 192, 193
  hypertrophic, 193
  rheumatoid, 189–192
  vitamin D in, 191
Artificial respiration, 294–295
Asocial people, 471
Aspirin, in arthritis, 190–191
Assignment of nursing personnel, in medical-surgical unit, 300–303
  in obstetric unit, 544, 546
  in pediatric unit, 426
Asthma, 157–160
  aminophylline in, 159